PRAISE FOR

HOPE FOR CANCER

What Dr. Jimenez consistently gets are *positive results*. One important reason for this is his realization that "one size does *not* fit all." The message consistently relayed: hope should always remain, even in patients with the most advanced cases of cancer—many of whom have been given death sentences by their mainstream medicine oncologists. Nothing is ever promised by Dr. Jimenez, but positive results are nearly always delivered. No one should succumb to cancer without taking a trip to see Dr. Jimenez. It's that simple.

DR. THOMAS E. LEVY, MD, JD
Cardiologist
Author of *Curing the Incurable* and *Hidden Epidemic*
Member, Orthomolecular Medicine Hall of Fame (2016)
PeakEnergy.com

In my nearly three decades as an integrative doctor, I've never come across a book that both inspires and educates cancer patients and their caregivers as much as this brilliant piece of work. The exceptional knowledge and experience in the pages of *Hope for Cancer* truly helps to turn fear to hope. Dr. Jimenez not only wrote a book that could potentially change the lives of my patients, but also one that reminded me of the power of faith that exists in all beliefs and religions.

DR. CHATCHAI SRIBUNDIT, MD
CEO and Founder, Absolute Health Regenerative Clinic, Thailand
www.absolute-health.org

If I didn't know any better, I would say it was a "chance" meeting when I bumped into Dr. Jimenez for the first time at a Cancer Control Society conference in 2014, when he agreed to do an impromptu interview for our docu-series, *The Quest for the Cures Continues*. That meeting sparked a friendship between me, Dr. Jimenez, his wife, Marcy, and my wife, Charlene. It is seldom that you find a physician who is so willing to test the boundaries of what is possible, while staying rooted in the centuries-old, time-tested principles of medicine that we all trust. Dr. Jimenez is full of compassion and represents the best from a bygone era, blended perfectly with our biased vision of the physician-of-the-future.

TY BOLLINGER, DOCUMENTARY FILM PRODUCER
Author of *New York Times* Best Seller *The Truth About Cancer*
Founder, The Truth About Cancer Organization
TheTruthAboutCancer.com

Since I have witnessed the positive outcome of Dr. Jimenez's 7 Key Principles of Cancer Therapy in many patients, I am so excited to share his book with others. It is evidence-based natural medicine at its finest, balanced with faith, hope, love and generosity. This book is a must read for anyone on a cancer healing journey!

 Dr. Veronique Desaulniers, DC
Author of *Do Your Hormones Cause Breast Cancer?*
Founder, Breast Cancer Conqueror™
BreastCancerConqueror.com

Throughout this book, Dr. Jimenez weaves his magic by showing us how a holistic approach using his 7 Key Principles, sprinkled with a good dose of hope, can be a game changer in healing from cancer. I have personally been witness to the wonderful results obtained at Hope4Cancer where patients learn how to heal in body, mind, and spirit.

 Dr. Lucia Guadalupe González Frutis, MD, PHD
Obstetrician/Gynecologist
Professor, Department of Gynecology UAEM, Mexico

It has been said there is no truth. That is not correct. In a world of chaos, there is meant to be order and reason. We are facing a tsunami of cancer and Dr. Jimenez brings order and truth to what is a threatening and confusing circumstance for patients, family and friends. One of my favorite verses is, "Faith is the assurance of what we hope for, the certainty of things we do not see" (Hebrews 11:1). It is my hope these pages hold answers to your questions and bring you faith and hope for your future.

 Dr. Robert Banner, MD, CCFP, FCFP, FRCP, IFMCP, Dip CAPM/AAPM, ABIHM, COT, CPT
President, North American Academy of Neural Therapy, Canada
DrRobertBanner.com

From the very first word of the preface, to the final word of the last chapter, this book will encourage and inspire you. Cancer attacks at all levels: body, mind, and spirit. Dr. Jimenez's holistic approach provides hope and restoration to so many who have failed conventional cancer therapies. He has been a pioneer in seeking out and implementing powerful innovative healing treatments to defeat cancer, and understands that the body was created to heal. Join him and grab a hold of that truth and arise victorious!

 Jenny Hrbacek, RN
Author of Amazon Best Seller *Cancer Free! Are You Sure?*
CancerFreeExperts.com

Dr. Jimenez is a leader in challenging Western medicine's status quo by incorporating a more holistic approach to cancer treatment. His protocols support the body toward wellness by fortifying the immune system to work at an optimum. His rapid adoption of the latest knowledge and technology in integrative cancer therapy, combined with his respect for natural medicine indigenous to different parts of the globe, lay at the very heart of his cancer curative success rate. He represents the future of cancer therapy in a wiser world—available today.

FRAN DRESCHER, ACTRESS, COMEDIAN, AND WRITER
Cancer Survivor, Healthcare Advocate and Educator
Founder, Cancer Schmancer Movement

True spiritual health holds an important place in the comprehensive process of healing. Dr. Jimenez logically gives us an insight to the Spirit-Soul-Body connection. His principles are timeless. A must read for every seeker of wellness.

DR. JEANNE N. STRYKER, MD
Interventional Oncologist
StrykerInterventionalSpecialists.com

This book is brilliant and complete, and Dr. Jimenez is a true doctor—which means "teacher." He shows his patients how integrative medicine, combined with lifestyle changes, can improve their prognosis by changing their body's internal environment. This book brings sanity to the current established barbaric and unscientific medical treatment of cancer. History will show Dr. Jimenez to be a humanitarian and genius. Read and incorporate this book into your lifestyle. Cancer is reversible without toxic therapies. This book is your road map to recovery from cancer.

DR. PATRICK QUILLIN, PHD, RD, CNS
Author of *Beating Cancer With Nutrition*
PatrickQuillin.com

A treasured resource for patients embarking on what has become a treacherous journey in cancer treatment. The juxtaposition of a strong spiritual foundation and an evidence-based integrative approach has been beautifully and succinctly laid out. And for doctors starting out in integrative cancer treatment, this book is at the leading edge of state of the art.

DR. VIJAENDREH SUBRAMANIAN, MBBS, MRCOG
Gynecologist-Oncologist
Founder and Director, Dr. Vijae Integrative Cancer Care Center, Malaysia

Hope for Cancer is a powerful testament to re-introducing the personalized element into cancer treatments, while maintaining the appropriate integrative medical approach. Dr. Jimenez's humanity and his focus on patient wellness comes through. To cancer patients who are frightened into compliance with harsh and painful medical procedures, this book offers a ray of hope and other more encouraging possibilities.

DR. SUNDARDAS D. ANNAMALAY, ND, PHD, MD(MA), DSC
Author of *Vitality and Anti-Aging* and *The Science of Healing Water*
CEO and Clinic Director, Natural Therapies Research Centre, Singapore
Professor of Natural Medicine, Youngson Institute of Natural Science, Australia

Applying the 7 Key Principles and the vital strategies described in this book can lead a patient to a point where they can call their cancer a "disease of the past." I have never heard Dr. Jimenez say, "I treat the patient's cancer." Instead, he treats the patient with cancer, an approach that prevails throughout his book. After thoroughly reading and properly utilizing the methods described here, I believe you will unlock the secrets to health and vitality in the future.

DR. SHINICHIRO AKIYAMA, MD, PHD, FACP
Director, Saisei Mirai Clinic Group, Japan
Visiting Professor, Dept. of Medical Oncology, McGill University, Canada

Dr. Jimenez's lifelong commitment to empower and educate cancer patients is reflected in his 7 Key Principles of Cancer Therapy. With this holistic approach, he helps them remove fear and replace it with faith. Love is the basic ingredient that makes this book a must-read treasure.

DR. CARLOS OROZCO, MD, BSC, MSC, ND, PHD, FPAMS
Author of *Coherence: Integration of Energy and Boosting Your Longevity*
Integrative Physician and Researcher, Australia

From the hand of God, Dr. Jimenez shares with us his experiences in the integrative management of cancer patients. It's a fascinating read that opens a window of hope to those who must face this disease, offering the best integrative treatments available in the world. *Hope for Cancer* is written with passion for life, and teaches us to believe that there is always hope.

DR. JAIME ESCOBAR OROZCO, MD
Medical Surgeon, Chief Medical Officer, Centro Medico Biologico Ser Vital and Hope4Cancer Treatment Centers, Colombia
Specialist, Biological Medicine

It is with the deepest sorrow that I mourn the loss of my dear friend, Dr. Jaime Escobar Orozco, who passed away on May 7, 2020. He left behind a legacy of love, learning and hard work. May he rest in peace in the arms of God!

This ground-breaking book establishes the validity of a new guiding aperture of successful cancer treatment beyond the circular, flat-world approaches of invasive slash and burn, which typically result in harsh and less-than-favorable results. Everyone you know and love should read this remarkable work regardless of their health condition—learn from the best and take to heart the inherent central-core message weaving its way inexorably throughout the pages. Brilliant!

DR. ROBERT CASS, ND
Founder and Master Formulator, Physica Energetics
PhysicaEnergetics.com

As an integrative oncologist my hope is that *Hope for Cancer* will be translated into many different languages so it can benefit cancer sufferers worldwide. Thanks, Dr. Jimenez, for sharing this knowledge with all of us— it brings out hope, faith and encouragement, and a real proof that cancer is no longer a death sentence!

DR. BILLY NJUGUNA, MD
Oncologist
Founder and President of African Genetics Neoplasms Foundation
Medical Director, Kwanc Institute of Integrative Medicine & Research, Kenya

Rarely do you see a book on cancer by an MD who has the audacity to put the "Whole Person" concept in Chapter 1. And rarer still, one who puts his patients front and center, and not his treatments. I couldn't put the book down after starting the first chapter—regretting that I should have finished my dinner first. Dr. Jimenez has made this book a human(e) endeavor, showing that cancer treatments need not be toxic, mutilating or exceedingly expensive. This book really is what the title says: there's always *Hope for Cancer*.

DR. HOMER LIM, MD
Author of the *Cancer Nutrition Course*
Integrative Oncologist, Akesis Holistic Health, Philippines
CancerHealerPh.com

Masterfully written with a profound simplification of the experience acquired over 25 years of caring for oncological patients with an integrative and holistic approach. It makes us reflect on the importance of doctors acting as helpers of nature and as guides for the sick in the healing process, where faith and hope are essential. *Hope for Cancer* is a useful and necessary guide in the prevention and treatment of cancer.

DR. VIVIAN BORROTO RODRÍGUEZ, MD
Professor and Researcher, University of Medical Sciences, Cuba
President, Cuban Society of Ozone Therapy

Hungry for hope? So was I. My cry for hope was answered as I stepped through the doors of Hope4Cancer where the atmosphere radiates the light and love of our Healer, Jesus Christ. When Jesus moves in, fear moves out. Delivered with his signature voice of compassion, Dr. Jimenez pioneers this comprehensive approach to non-toxic, whole-person healing that addresses body, soul, and spirit. Engaging patient stories blended with the 7 Key Principles unlock the shackles of fear slapped on at the time of diagnosis. You aren't alone. There is help. There is hope. Come on in . . . you won't just read these pages, you will experience them.

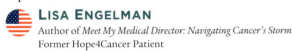
LISA ENGELMAN
Author of *Meet My Medical Director: Navigating Cancer's Storm*
Former Hope4Cancer Patient

In *The Art of War* Sun Tzu says, "Know the enemy and know yourself; in a hundred battles you will never be in peril." Therefore, in order to effectively treat cancer, it is necessary to clearly understand that cancer is a complex disease. Knowing this complexity, Dr. Jimenez has presented 7 Key Principles of Cancer Therapy that vastly improve a cancer patient's chances for a complete recovery.

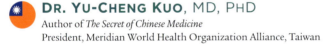
DR. YU-CHENG KUO, MD, PHD
Author of *The Secret of Chinese Medicine*
President, Meridian World Health Organization Alliance, Taiwan

Hope for Cancer transcends teaching—it helps you relinquish fear as it equips you with a battle plan as you fight with hope. With decades of experience, Dr. Jimenez knows what works and what doesn't, and his matchless faith in God offers a contagious confidence to lead the way through frightening and confusing uncertainty.

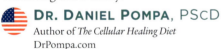
DR. DANIEL POMPA, PSCD
Author of *The Cellular Healing Diet*
DrPompa.com

Dr. Jimenez reveals the scientific truth from the bottom of his heart with conviction. *Hope for Cancer* is an excellent revelation of his practical wisdom, evidenced by long years of enduring research studies, and a positive and holistic approach toward curing and mitigating the pains of ailing patients. Everyone must read this book to know the truth about cancer.

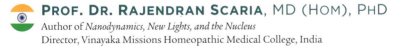
PROF. DR. RAJENDRAN SCARIA, MD (HOM), PHD
Author of *Nanodynamics, New Lights, and the Nucleus*
Director, Vinayaka Missions Homeopathic Medical College, India

When I was diagnosed with bladder cancer in 2011, the urologist immediately recommended the traditional cancer treatment: a lengthy surgery to remove my bladder, followed by chemo and radiation. I did none of this. Instead, while researching alternative possibilities, Hope4Cancer resonated with me. After consulting with Dr. Jimenez, I was on my way to the Hope4Cancer Treatment Centers. I followed the program religiously and remain cancer-free to this day!

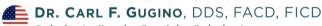
DR. CARL F. GUGINO, DDS, FACD, FICD
Orthodontist; Founder, Great Lakes Orthodontics
Former Hope4Cancer Patient

Dr. Jimenez puts the patient in control in the battle against cancer. Using the 7 Key Principles of Cancer Therapy, the patient has hope and a path to true healing: physically, emotionally, and spiritually.

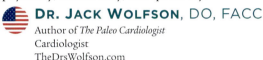
DR. JACK WOLFSON, DO, FACC
Author of *The Paleo Cardiologist*
Cardiologist
TheDrsWolfson.com

Every now and then, an individual stands tall in the crowd, ahead of their time. Dr. Jimenez proves himself as one those unusual thought leaders. "Hope for Cancer" is a brilliant and timely work with a well-thought-out and structured approach to integrative treatment and prevention of cancer from an author who embraces a value-based approach to medicine embedded in the concepts of faith, hope, love, and generosity. This book was long overdue and does not disappoint. Within its pages, you will find an excellent guide to understand a facet of medical knowledge in which even well-trained physicians are deeply misinformed. Read and understood carefully, "Hope for Cancer" will advance the health of all humanity, giving hope to millions who have been, in some way or the other, touched by cancer.

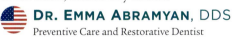
DR. EMMA ABRAMYAN, DDS
Preventive Care and Restorative Dentist

I first met Dr. Jimenez in 2011 after I was "fired" by my doctor for not consenting to radiation treatments following surgery for aggressive prostate cancer. My wife, Sheri, and I knew we were in the right place when, after our consult at Hope4Cancer, Dr. Jimenez held our hands and began to pray for God to lead and direct us, and for God's healing in my body. This book will educate and inspire you, whether you are dealing with cancer or not.

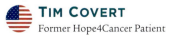
TIM COVERT
Former Hope4Cancer Patient

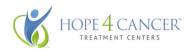

HOPE
for
CANCER

**7 PRINCIPLES TO REMOVE FEAR
AND EMPOWER YOUR HEALING JOURNEY**

Antonio Jimenez
MD, ND

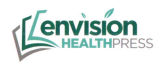

Envision Health Press
10900 Research Blvd., Ste 160C, Unit #2010
Austin, TX 98759

©2019 by Antonio Jimenez

All rights reserved. No part of this book may be reprinted, reproduced, transmitted, or utilized in any form by any mechanical, photographic, electronic, or other means, now known or hereafter invented, including photocopying, microfilming, and recording, or in any information storage or retrieval system—other than for "fair use" as brief quotations embodied in articles and reviews—without written permission from the publisher.

This book describes medical information that is entirely based on the training, research, and clinical experience of the author. The information in this book and its resources is not intended to be used in any way to diagnose, treat, cure, or prevent any disease. There is no explicit or implicit attempt by the author to render professional advice or services to the reader. The information is not presented here to take the place of advice you would receive from your physician or health care provider, or to advocate for any treatment. Given that there is always some risk involved, the reader accepts complete responsibility for any adverse effects or consequences arising from following any suggestions, treatments, procedures, preparations, or supplements described in this book. The author believes it to be a sign of wisdom, not cowardice, to seek further professional medical opinions, and encourages the reader to do so.

Library of Congress Control Number: 2020901338

Jacket and Interior Design: Rob Williams, InsideOutCreativeArts.com
Copy Editor: Kyle Duncan
Content Editor: Subrata Chakravarty
Illustrators: Subrata Chakravarty, Mike Paschal

> Jimenez, Antonio
> *Hope for Cancer: 7 Principles to Remove Fear and Empower Your Healing Journey*
> Antonio Jimenez
> Hardcover ISBN: 978-1-7329033-0-2
> MEDICAL/ALTERNATIVE AND COMPLEMENTARY

Unless otherwise noted, all Scripture quotations are from the New International Version®. NIV®. Copyright © 1973, 1978, 1984, 2011 by Biblica, Inc.TM Used by permission of Zondervan. All rights reserved worldwide. www.zondervan.com

Scripture quotations identified HCSB are from the Holman Christian Study Bible®, Copyright © 1999, 2000, 2002, 2003, 2009 by Holman Bible Publishers. Used by permission. hcsb ® is a federally registered trademark of Holman Bible Publishers.

Scripture quotations identified NLT are from the Holy Bible, New Living Translation®. Copyright © 1996, 2004, 2015 by Tyndale House Foundation. Used by permission of Tyndale House Publishers, Inc., Carol Stream, Illinois, 60188. All rights reserved.

REVISED   21 22 23 24 25 | 7 6 5 4 3 2

CONTENTS

Foreword by Dr. Gustavo Vilela, MD 13
Acknowledgments 17
Preface 19

The Fundamentals of Cancer and Healing

1. **HEALING THE WHOLE PERSON:** Spirit, Soul and Body 27
   Testimonial: *Adriana's Story (Pancreatic Cancer)*

2. **ABOUT CANCER AND ITS CAUSES** 53

3. **NOVEL AND SAFE METHODS TO SCREEN, DIAGNOSE AND TRACK CANCER** 71
   Testimonial: *Rivi's Story (Bile Duct/Pancreatic Cancer)*

The 7 Key Principles of Cancer Therapy

4. **EFFECTIVE INTEGRATIVE CANCER THERAPIES** 101
   ⚛ Key Principle #1: *Non-Toxic Cancer Therapies*

5. **TOOLS THAT EMPOWER YOUR IMMUNE SYSTEM** 137
   〰 Key Principle #2: *Immunomodulation*
   Testimonial: *Charles' Story (Bladder Cancer)*

6. **NUTRITION BASED ON THE GARDEN OF EDEN** 165
   🌿 Key Principle #3, Part 1: *Full Spectrum Nutrition*

7. **SUPPLEMENTS THAT REPAIR AND RESTORE YOUR BODY** 199
   🌿 Key Principle #3, Part 2: *Full Spectrum Nutrition*
   Testimonial: *Juan's Story (Kidney Cancer)*

8. **DETOXIFY TO HEAL AND LIVE LONG** 225
    💧 **Key Principle #4:** *Detoxification*

9. **OXYGEN:** The Foundation for a Vibrant Life 251
    O₂ **Key Principle #5:** *Oxygenation*
    Testimonial: *Isabel's Story (Ovarian Cancer)*

10. **PARASITES, VIRUSES, FUNGI AND BACTERIA:** Their Role in Cancer and How to Treat Them 271
    ☀ **Key Principle #6:** *Restore the Microbiome*

11. **LIFESTYLE TOOLS FOR HEALING** 297
    Testimonial: *Pamela's Story (Breast Cancer)*

12. **JESUS, THE RESURRECTION, THE LIFE AND THE GREAT PHYSICIAN** 325
    🌀 **Key Principle #7, Part 1:** *Spiritual and Emotional Healing*
    Testimonial: *Erin Jessica's Story (Breast Cancer)*

13. **BEHAVIORAL EMOTIONAL SPIRITUAL THERAPY (BEST)** 355
    🌀 **Key Principle #7, Part 2:** *Spiritual and Emotional Healing*
    Testimonial: *Trina's Story (Ovarian Cancer)*

14. **PUTTING IT ALL TOGETHER** 381

Afterword 396
About the Author 398
Endnotes 400
Index 411

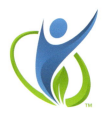

FOREWORD

By Dr. Gustavo Vilela, MD

"Why did this happen to me?"
"Doctor, please take these cells out of me!"
"Is this tumor malignant?"

The above are real questions I usually get from patients in my clinical practice. This is the image people have of cancer: something unexpected, malignant and bad that does not belong to their body.

Cancer: hearing the diagnosis strikes us like a lightning bolt of fear and worry. Even more, it is generally perceived as an "evil" that came from the outside and is inside one's body just with the purpose of doing harm. However, this is a rather symbolic and emotional picture of the situation. Understanable, but not real. Cells are not good or bad. Cells do not think, and they do not have feelings. Diseases are not enemies or spells that invade us maliciously.

Cancer cells are flesh of our own flesh.

They are just cells. They are alive, they have biological mechanisms, they simply function automatically. They do not have bad intentions.

What makes them acquire a so-called "cancerous" behavior?

When a group of cells is hit by moderate, continuous and long-term stress, be it internal, external, chemical, microbial or physical stress, cells start to suffer. They gradually head to a state of high entropy and low-grade order/information until they reach a critical survival point.

In this moment of near death, our cells adapt by turning on cellular survival mechanisms. However, this ability to adapt can backfire and make cells abnormal and potentially malignant.

In their journey through life, our cells are aided by these autonomous mechanisms to withstand a variety of genetic and epigenetic triggers. If something puts them at risk, this survival strength will be found. And we should be grateful it works like this. Otherwise, we would not thrive, and we would probably not exist. These cells would have perished along the way.

Cells are part of a whole system. And when someone has cancer, it just means the system has been put into an extreme adaptation scenario. A tumor is a sign of a cancer syndrome. A tumor is just the tip of the iceberg. Cancer is made of ill cells trying to survive in a hostile environment.

Cancer cells are victims—they are not "malignant."

In order to survive and overcome the near-death state, cells turn on genes that make them stronger, more resistant, fast proliferating, difficult to be destroyed. The only intention is to defend themselves from the risk of annihilation and to pass their genes on to daughter cells. This is part of the automatism of survival.

These survival genes that are recruited are called "oncogenes" by modern science—genes that cause cancer. Do you believe Nature makes genes with the intention to produce cancer? Again, this is a symbolic view. Obviously not!

These survival genes exist in our cells to help them defend themselves from critical situations and for tissue repair. What happens is that these genes are turned on because cells are at risk and fighting. Humans named these genes "oncogenes" as part of the human need to label things. But Nature does not think like that.

Everything in the cell is supposed to work beautifully!

Intracellular water alteration, reduced energy production, abnormal electrical activity, intracellular and extracellular pH modifications, and modified metabolism are some examples of how our cells change in order to become more resistant, invasive and proliferating.

Now imagine if you try to destroy them with chemotherapy or radiotherapy. This is an additional stress that may increase their survival potential, change them to a very resistant phenotype, and cause the cells to acquire a gene expression that is no longer the original ancient one.

This is when things get more complicated…

And this is why instead of recommending an Extermination Program, we would rather do a Cell-Care Program.

This means looking at these cells as victims of environmental stress: internal and external. In terms of external stress, one should consider: chronic heavy metal intoxication (lead, mercury, nickel, cadmium, etc.); copper and iron excess; agricultural pesticides; tobacco; fluoride; alcohol; xenobiotics; electromagnetic radiation; ionizing radiation; viral, parasite, mycobacterial and fungal chronic infections; cell wall-deficient bacterial infection; and more.

As examples of internal stress, one can include metabolic, oxidative (free radicals), and inflammatory stress.

All these stressors need to be addressed for a comprehensive therapy.

Orthodox oncology does not see things like this, since conventional cancer treatments simply aim to destroy the cell without considering the root causes that made the disease happen in the first place. I am not saying chemotherapy and radiotherapy should not be used! They are part of the strategy, since they are the fastest way to reduce the number of altered cells. But from an integrative point of view, conventional treatments should be combined with treatments that address the *causes* of the disease. Integrating strategies are the best solution for a successful outcome.

In this book, you will be guided to a full spectrum of therapies that can positively impact your cancer treatment. It can be useful for patients, families, or anyone interested in the prevention and treatment of cancer and other diseases. You will learn about all the environmental stressors that need to be considered for better health.

Do not wait until you have cancer to follow the suggestions here. Cancer is mostly an acquired disease, not a genetic condemnation. Start now by adopting good nutrition, pursuing a low toxic body load, taking care of your immune system, striving for spiritual and mental balance, and maintaining good quality of your system's microbes.

Your body is your main and only house in this world. Do not neglect it.

This book is a tribute to such an integrative approach. We should be grateful there are doctors in the world like Antonio Jimenez, who are open-minded and willing to think outside the box as they seek better solutions to help suffering people.

Dr. Gustavo Vilela, MD
Hematologist-Oncologist, University of Sao Paulo, Brazil
Fellowship in Hematology, Bone Marrow and Cord Blood Transplantation
  (Hôpital Saint Louis, France)
Cell Therapy Diploma (University of Paris, France)
Fellowship in Integrative Medicine (University of Arizona)

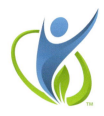

ACKNOWLEDGMENTS

First and foremost, I thank **God** for giving me the gift of being able to effectively help my patients, and for using me as His instrument of healing. In addition, I am grateful to Him for opening doors of opportunity in my life, for guiding me through the journey of helping cancer patients, and for giving me wisdom and discernment in all things.

To **Mom and Dad**: thank you for always supporting me, and taking our family out of Colombia so that we, your children, could have a better life and greater opportunities in the United States of America.

To my **wife**, Marcy: thank you for being the solid "rock" in my life, who has always stood by and supported me, which I have really needed throughout the years! You have been instrumental in helping us to get through many challenges. I am grateful for your discernment and for putting God first in all that we do.

To my **children**, Tony Jr., Josey, Whitney, Collin, and our twins, Isabella and Isaac: thank you for being such great kids, and understanding when I have had to travel and be away from home. You help me to be a better father and doctor, and encourage me to strive each day toward greatness.

To my **patients**: thank you for challenging me and teaching me so much; for honoring my philosophy and work, following the 7 Key Principles of Cancer Therapy, and realizing their value in your recovery. Thank you also for sharing with me the good as well as the bad times in your healing journeys.

To my **mentors**: thank you for guiding me into the field of complementary oncology, early on in my conventional medical training.

This led me to travel the world and become involved in work and research opportunities in the most unique places, from Africa to Asia to Latin America and Europe.

To **Dr. Subrata Chakravarty, my friend**, "brother from another mother," and Chief Science Officer at Hope4Cancer: thank you for always being there for me, and for your willingness to research until the wee hours of the night, brainstorm new ideas, and help me to develop and write new protocols.

To my Hope4Cancer **staff**: thank you for your daily efforts and dedication to your work, and for the loving, kind, professional care that you give our patients. I couldn't do what I do without you.

To **my writer**, Connie Strasheim: thank you for helping me capture my ideas, work, and what I've learned throughout my medical training and career—in a creative, easy-to-understand, comprehensive and yet scientifically accurate manner. Thank you also for your patience with me throughout this project, and for your inquisitiveness and research, which has helped to make this project what it is: a powerful, beneficial resource for others.

And finally, to **you, the reader**: I am so grateful to you for reading this book and for trusting me with the message that God has placed in my heart. Thank you for pursuing your purpose in natural healing.

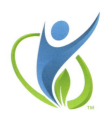

PREFACE

About Antonio Jimenez, MD, ND
"Dr. Tony"

My passion to become a doctor and treat cancer patients stemmed from my own health challenges, as well as my father's battle with cancer.

I was born blind in my left eye, as a result of congenital macular degeneration. And because I was also very thin, my mother would take me to the family doctor every month for a B-complex vitamin injection. While the injections never helped me to gain weight, my frequent visits to the doctor as a child helped me to determine early on in life that I wanted to become a doctor myself.

On one occasion in my childhood, I was really sick with a chest cold and my mother took me to a doctor who was an associate of my regular doctor—and he gave me a prescription that contained five different medicines.

I remember thinking, "Wow, this is a lot of medicine for me."

So I asked the doctor, "What are all these medicines for?"

He simply replied, "They are for the problem that you have, so take them." And then he walked away.

I followed him down the hallway of the clinic, and insisted. "Doctor, can you please tell me what all of these medicines are for?"

Again he replied, "I already told you, these are for the problem you have, so take them." Then he walked away again.

Little did I know it then, but this exchange would form the beginning of the basis of my healing philosophy later in life.

I realized that I wasn't going to get any further with the doctor, so I ripped the prescription paper up and threw it into the trashcan. I said to my mom, "Take me home. Get me some chicken soup or something, I don't want to take all of these medicines."

In that moment, I told myself that when I became a physician, I wasn't going to be like this doctor. I was going to listen to my patients, hear their concerns, and respond fully to their questions. I would treat the root cause of their illnesses, rather than suppress their symptoms with a bunch of medicines.

I have since lived out that philosophy in my work in medicine.

On another occasion, when I was a child, I asked my family physician if it was possible for me to become a doctor if I could only see out of one eye. His response was, "You can become anything that you want to, if you work hard."

This, along with my other early experiences with doctors, were turning points in my life because I realized that I could, first of all, become a doctor while seeing out of just one eye. Secondly, I could treat my patients differently than how conventional medical doctors had treated me. I wouldn't become like that doctor who had disregarded me: an inquisitive and curious 10-year-old boy who simply wanted to know what medicines he was putting into his body.

In recent years, I've also battled tinnitus and hearing loss. These challenges, combined with my vision problem, have taught me how to really be present for my patients, and listen to them. When you can only see out of one eye and your hearing has been compromised, you focus more on your patients when you're talking to them, and vice versa.

I've learned how to be a good listener. One of the first things we learn in medical school is to pay attention to how our patients walk into the room. We are taught to ask ourselves such questions as, "Are they limping? Do their faces reveal that they are in pain?" We look at their constitution.

However, most doctors today disregard that very important lesson. They do not listen to—or even observe—their patients well enough to make their primary assessment. By the time most doctors see their patients, they have already been ushered into an exam room and had their vital signs taken. As a result, we lose the opportunity to make that first impression.

Physicians must learn to listen to their patients in order to truly know what they need. We need to realize that every question they have comes from a place of needing to understand the "why's" of what we do for them.

Doctors are not gods. And because we make mistakes, I want my patients to be proactive and to challenge me and my team. However, most of us put doctors on a pedestal and believe they can't do any wrong. Yet we know that every year in the US between 210,000 and 440,000 hospital patients die from preventable mistakes made by doctors and other healthcare professionals. These are called iatrogenic causes of disease.[1]

So respect your doctors, but do your own research.

My Path to Integrative Medicine

Immediately following medical school, I did my internship at a hospital that had a complementary medicine wing. Here, they would give the patients treatments like coffee enemas, ozone, and Vitamin C, and I noticed that those who were given these treatments seemed to heal faster, better, and with fewer side effects than those who didn't receive any complementary therapies. This spurred my interest in integrative medicine, which combines both conventional and complementary medicine for a more effective approach to cancer treatment.

Today, my medical staff and I prescribe conventional therapies such as low dose chemotherapy and surgery, when it's necessary. Most of our patients, though, have exhausted conventional options, and come to us for something different. So our approach is integrative; meaning, we do everything under one roof! But more on that later.

I became interested in helping people to heal from cancer after my father was diagnosed with prostate cancer in his early 60s. One day, shortly after I completed my medical internship, he called me from Pasadena, Texas, where he had been living at the time. He was suffering terrible side effects from an injection treatment that his doctor had given him.

He wanted to find a better way to heal, so I said, "Okay, give me a few minutes and I will call you back."

After I hung up the phone, I cried. I couldn't believe that the father I loved so much had just told me he had cancer. I decided then and there that I would find a better way to get him well. So I called him back and said, "Okay Dad, let's do it!" He became my first cancer patient.

Fortunately, I was able to help him fully recover by taking a holistic approach to healing the root causes of his cancer, which included an individualized nutritional and immune enhancing plan. He lived to be just short of 83, and when he passed away, it was from heart disease, not cancer.

Treating my father was a turning point in my life: the first one that would lead me to treat other cancer patients and eventually establish the Hope4Cancer Treatment Centers.

I went to medical school in Mexico where, like in the United States, students attend class for four years, then do an internship to become doctors. However, all doctors in Mexico must also do a year of social service, which involves working in the "boonies" (rural areas where services and resources are scarce). Places where, as we say, doctors are often not just doctors, but "the doctor, the mayor and the priest!" We did not have labs, X-rays, and other modern tools, so we learned to develop our clinical skills. This is the Mexican government's way of bringing doctors to rural communities.

Following my year of service in the boonies I went back to work at the same hospital where I did my internship. Then something amazing happened.

I went to visit my parents in Texas, and while there, I attended a local church service on a Saturday night, where a guest minister had come to speak. There were about 1,000 attendees, and during the service the minister did an "altar call."

Oddly, when that happened, I found myself getting up and making my way to the front of the church, or the altar, even though part of me didn't really want to. Inside, I was thinking, *Tony, sit down!* But it was as if God was pushing me to go forward.

When I reached the front of the church, I closed my eyes and prayed. Soon, there was a crowd at the altar. Then the guest minister prophesied, saying, "There's someone here who is going to do great things in medicine, but it's not in this country. And he's going to travel the world, and is going to treat governors and famous people, but it's not in this country. And he's going to have a healing center, where people from all over the world will come to find healing."

As she spoke these words, I thought, *I'm a doctor, and I don't practice medicine in this country—could it be that she's talking about me?*

Then, as if God had heard my thoughts, the minister pointed straight in my direction and said in front of all the attendees, "It's *that* young man right there!"

I still didn't think she was talking about me because there were many people surrounding me. But then she looked right at me and said, "Yes, you in the blue shirt!"

I was wearing a blue shirt. She said to the attendees, "Let's all extend our hands toward him (me) and pray for him." And everyone prayed for me in that moment! I was about 31 years old at the time.

I now know that the prophecy I received was from God, because since that time, the events that the minister spoke of have all come to pass in my life! I've traveled to many countries to teach about integrative cancer treatments, and now have several clinics in the Americas. The prophetic word was a confirmation to me about how God was intending to use me to heal people with cancer, and how He has in fact used me for that purpose.

I worked at an integrative cancer hospital for nine years before opening up my own clinic in Tijuana, Mexico. I did this because I had new treatment ideas that I wanted to implement at the hospital, but which I couldn't, even though I worked in leadership level positions. So I opened Rapha Clinic in the year 2000. *Rapha* comes from the Hebrew term *Jehovah Rapha*, which means, "The Lord Who Heals."

We have since changed our name to the Hope4Cancer Treatments Centers. In 2015, we opened our second treatment center in Cancun, Mexico because we could no longer accommodate all of our patients at the Tijuana center. It had been my dream for a long time to open a second treatment center in Mexico, and now we have the ability to treat many more patients. That dream continues to grow in the stories of patients who have found peace and renewed confidence in our two faith-filled, healing centers.

My wife, Marcy, is the Chief Executive Officer of the Hope4Cancer Treatment Centers, and like me, she is passionate about helping cancer patients. We met years ago when she came to the treatment center with her then five-year-old daughter, Whitney, who had been diagnosed with leukemia.

Marcy came to see me because she wanted Whitney to receive natural cancer treatment. As well, Whitney had been given vaccinations some years prior to that, which, according to her ophthalmologist, had damaged her eyes and subsequently required her to have two eye surgeries. So when Whitney was diagnosed with cancer, Marcy was wary, and decided she would avoid conventional treatment.

Fortunately, Whitney recovered from both the leukemia and the eye problem. Now, at the time of this revision (2021), she is a healthy 26-year-old wife and entrepreneur, with three children!

Integrative medical doctors who treat mostly stage IV cancer patients, as we do, must have a strong work ethic, passion for their patients, and a lot of tenacity. That is because this set of diseases called cancer (cancer isn't just one disease, as you will soon discover) is a challenge, although there is also much hope for recovery.

I am thankful for the success our clinics have had with late-stage cancer patients that conventional medicine has otherwise given up on. I attribute this success first and foremost to God, who gives me wisdom. In addition, I attribute it to my personal challenges, as well as to my parents, who immigrated to the US from Colombia when I was five years old. My dad was a truck driver, and my mom worked in a factory for Avon cosmetics. Both had loving, caring spirits, and a strong work ethic and family structure. This combination of virtues greatly impacted and shaped me, and influenced me in my work in medicine today.

The Mission and Vision of Hope4Cancer

Marcy's and my mission and vision for Hope4Cancer Treatment Centers is to provide every one of our patients, wherever they come from across the world, the best opportunity to heal from cancer—or whatever diagnosis they present with—in spirit, soul and body.

Our core values are faith, hope, love and generosity. This book describes our 7 Key Principles of Cancer Therapy from the standpoint of these values. We, along with our 200-plus staff, do our utmost to implement these core values into our daily work and impart them to our Hope4Cancer family. Indeed, our approach is a fundamental reason for our success.

Patients also often praise and thank us for the love, care, personal attention and dedication they receive at Hope4Cancer. Here, they have a name and can expect to be treated as a person, not as a number. **We treat the person with cancer, not the cancer in the person.** Faith is the foundation of Hope4Cancer, and as such, we continually aim to demonstrate the love of God to our patients, in a way that is honoring and loving to people of all faiths.

The presence of God is tangible at Hope4Cancer. For instance, when Karlis, who hails from Eastern Europe, was leaving after a day of visiting, he exclaimed, "Oh doctor, when I walked into your clinic, I felt something different! I didn't understand what it was, but I felt molecules of energy . . . and it made me emotional!"

Eastern Europeans are typically very reserved, stoic people, but Karlis had experienced something profound at Hope4Cancer that had excited him—and I believe it was God!

Our Treatment Approach

We aim to continually develop and deliver cutting-edge, research-based, effective non-toxic therapies and protocols to provide our patients with the best care possible.

Unlike the perception among some within the conventional medical community, integrative treatment is not quackery. We don't do "snake oil" treatments. Our team is made up of experienced medical doctors, PhD scientists and registered nurses who have decades of experience in integrative cancer care therapies.

Our mission is to become known as the world's number one choice for integrative cancer care as well as the preferred resource for state-of-the-art complementary therapies. We work tirelessly toward a legacy that will transform the way cancer is treated today.

Finally, we are dedicated to providing the best at-home patient care program in the world, so that our patients can continue their healing journey knowing that we are there for them every step along the way.

Treatment Outcomes

Because of our integrative approach to cancer treatment, we have achieved remarkable success in helping many advanced-stage cancer patients far outlive their conventional doctors' prognoses, and/or experience a much better quality of life. These are often people whom the traditional medical community has given up on. I am happy to report that many of these patients are also now cancer-free. A retrospective analysis of our patient records between 2015 to 2019 has shown that we outperform 5-year survival data for metastatic cancers as reported by the National Cancer Institute in the United States by large margins.

Indeed, we have witnessed many healing miracles at Hope4Cancer and believe that everyone, no matter their current condition, has the ability to heal and become whole when they are simply empowered with the right tools.

With that in mind, I encourage you to believe that you too, can recover, no matter what your doctor or anyone has told you, and no matter how difficult or impossible things may seem. As the Bible says, **"With God, all things are possible"** (Matthew 19:26).

When you discover the amazing healing tools that God has made available to you, and determine to take responsibility for your health, you can recover and live longer. You can also experience a much better quality of life than what you thought or were initially told by your doctor. So read on to learn more about these tools, and how you can live a victorious, prosperous and healthy life, free from cancer!

J. J.

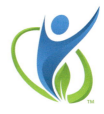

1

Healing the Whole Person: Spirit, Soul and Body

"You have cancer."

When someone hears these chilling words, they become fraught with fear. They picture their lives being cut short by a devastating illness, their bodies ravaged by chemotherapy, radiation and surgery. Indeed, how many of us have been taught to associate cancer with sad images of sickness, hair loss, and ultimately, death?

Images of sick cancer patients who have undergone conventional treatments, along with dismal recovery statistics seem to confirm our worst fears. Indeed, 1 in 3 women and 1 in 2 men are developing cancer today. A meta-analysis published in 2004 in the *Journal of Clinical Oncology* revealed that the five-year survival rate for cancers of all types and stages is only 60%, and that chemotherapy increased that by only 2%.[1] The National Institutes of Health has spent over a trillion dollars on cancer research and treatment in recent years, yet the survival rates have hardly increased.

But what if virtually everything we've been taught about cancer is wrong? What if cancer isn't a death sentence, but instead, an opportunity to be made whole: in spirit, soul and body? And what if there were treatments out there that could even heal people with stage IV cancers, or at least enable them to live full, normal lives? What if those treatments imparted life, energy, vibrancy and joy to the spirit, soul and body, rather than sickness?

Well, I have good news for you: such healing treatments do exist that have enabled many cancer patients—even those whom conventional medicine had given up on—to either fully overcome the disease or far outlive their conventional doctors' prognosis, while significantly improving their quality of life.

I know, because we use these treatments at our centers, and have witnessed many of our cancer patients recover and reclaim their lives.

Do you know that it's possible to live a long, healthy life, even with a tumor? Conventional medicine has taught us that health means the absence of a tumor, but health and lasting recovery from cancer don't happen just because we eliminate the tumor. Rather, health is realized because we remove all of the underlying factors that caused the cancer in the first place, in addition to the cancer itself.

Further, the treatments, diagnostics, and devices I will be sharing with you in these pages are very effective, life-giving and gentle. In addition, they don't just heal the body, but rather, the whole person. This is because we are all tripartite, or three-part beings, with a spirit, soul and body, and our parts are interconnected and affect one another, for better or worse.

The spirit is the highest part of our being that helps us connect and communicate with God; our soul includes our mind, will and emotions. Our body is the "container" for our spirit and soul and operates under the influence of the latter two. God desires not only for our body to be healthy, but our soul and spirit, as well, because we heal from cancer when our entire person is made whole.

What's more, the human spirit, in cooperation with the Spirit of God, was designed to be in charge of the soul and body, and as such, can affect the soul and body. So when your spirit is renewed and connected to the Spirit of God, your soul and body will often heal more profoundly, effectively and rapidly.

In fact, numerous studies show that people who pray—or are prayed for—often heal more completely and faster than those who don't pray or receive prayer. One of the most famous of these studies was conducted by cardiologist Randolph Byrd and published in 1988.

For this study, more than 393 coronary care patients were either admitted to a prayer group (192 patients) or a control group (201 patients). Christians outside of the hospital prayed for the prayer group, and over time, those patients who received prayer showed much better recovery rates than those in the control group. They were five times less likely than the control patients to require antibiotics and three times less likely to develop pulmonary edema. While twelve of the control patients needed intubation to help with breathing, none of the prayed-for patients did.[2]

One reason that healing statistics in conventional oncology are typically poor is because treatments don't usually take into account the health of the soul and spirit. Even in functional, integrative or complementary medicine, healing the soul and spirit are sometimes treated as secondary aspects of recovery, rather than its cornerstone and foundation.

I believe, however, that we are all designed to be in a relationship with our Creator. And when your spirit is aligned with His, and you use tools to address the healing of your spirit and soul, then the healing of your body will naturally and more easily follow.

I'm not talking about religion, which may conjure up images in some people's minds of following a set of rules or traditions to please man or appease God. Although God is certainly found within religion, He is also found within our heart, mind, and day-to-day activities.

I believe the Bible provides insights into His nature and character. For instance, 1 John 1:5 says, "God is light, and there is absolutely no darkness in Him." On a scientific level, we know that without light, life cannot exist. Even more, light lives in anyone who looks to Him and trusts in Him for their healing.

The God that I know is all-good, all-loving, all-knowing and all-powerful, and an ever-present help in our time of need. In essence, there is no evil in Him, and it is not His will that you, or anyone you know, should suffer or be sick. While He can use all circumstances for your good, He did not give you cancer to make you a better person!

Instead, He created you to enjoy life, be healthy, and prosper in all of your ways: relationally, physically, spiritually. When you get to know Him, He will give you faith to believe Him for these things (if you don't already!). Consider 3 John 1:2, which refers to God's will for our lives: "Dear friend, I pray that you may prosper in every way and be in good health physically just as you are spiritually" (HCSB).

When I picture prosperity, I think of how I wake up in the morning and say, **"Thank you, God, for the gift of life today!"** Imagine a tree planted by the riverbank, bearing fruit each season, having leaves that don't wither (see Psalm 1:3).

True prosperity, then, is not about financial wealth or material gain. At its foundation, it is about our spiritual health. I love this passage from the New Testament, which talks about the benefits of living in spiritual prosperity: "The Holy Spirit produces this kind of fruit in our lives: love, joy, peace, patience, kindness, goodness, faithfulness, gentleness, and self-control" (Galatians 5:22-23, NLT).

I recall once writing in my high school yearbook a favorite quote that I believe is still relevant and true today: "God heals and the doctor takes the fee!"

I realize that you may not have the same spiritual philosophy or beliefs as mine, and if so, that's okay. I simply want to share about the God I know and invite you to get to know Him as well. I think you'll find that He's a good friend, counselor, healer and confidant who can help you, no matter where you are in your spiritual journey, or what you believe. He not only wants you to know Him and His tremendous love for you, but He wants you to be healed and whole. He can and will help you to get there, faster and more effectively than if you simply used medicine alone, because He is in fact, the Great Physician!

In Chapter 12, I'll share more about how you can develop a personal relationship with Him, enabling you to live whole in Him throughout your days. In addition, I'll also explain how you can be sure it is His will for you to be healed, and how He can help you to receive that healing for your spirit and soul, trusting His timing for completion of bodily healing.

Many scientifically minded people believe in the Big Bang theory of evolution, and indeed, every biology book I know of begins with the theory that every atom comes from a pre-existing atom. But where does the first atom come from? Nobody knows. Rather, I believe that God created all things, He exists outside of time, and He created every atom that exists now and which has ever existed.

Consider Hebrews 11:3, which says, "By faith we understand that the universe was created by God's command, so that what is seen has been made from things that are not visible" (*HSBC*). In other words, God created the physical realm from the invisible realm.

The accomplished healer understands that healing is an art, and that at the foundation of healing is an innate knowledge that all wisdom comes from the Divine. When a doctor is stuck and doesn't know what to do with a patient, that is when that innate knowing, which comes from the Holy Spirit, comes in and becomes useful. It doesn't come from the mind or the doctor's training.

What's more, humankind can accomplish many things through science, but there are some things that only God can do, such as heal people from the most advanced diseases, and create life. Following is a personal story to illustrate that.

My wife, Marcy, and I have surrogate 9-year-old twins who were fertilized in vitro. For the in vitro fertilization, we sought out one of the best in vitro doctors in the world. My sperms and her eggs were placed in a petri dish, which was set to a specific temperature and appropriate conditions for fertilization. The doctor timed Marcy's cycle precisely, harvested her eggs at just the right moment, and did everything that he was trained to do to ensure a positive outcome.

Despite this, the doctor couldn't ensure that fertilization between my sperm and her egg would occur, because the fertilization process is an act of God. No human can create that. Man can create all of the right conditions for the fertilization to happen. For example, he can make sure that the nutrients and temperature in the petri dish are just right, but when a human being is conceived as a result of a sperm and egg coming together, God does it.

Interestingly, there is a light show of sorts that occurs during conception. An article entitled, "Scientists Witness 'Flash of Light' During Conception," published on April 26, 2016 on *Fox News Health*, seems to confirm this. The reporter said, "For the first time, researchers have witnessed the exact moment conception occurs—and have recorded the ensuing explosion of sparks that form when sperm meets an egg."

I believe that we are all conceived in a "spark of joy" from God!

In my career, I've observed that anyone who has been close to death, even the most fervent atheists, will say in their darkest hour, "God help me!" I believe this is because innately, our human spirit knows that there is *a* creator. But if you don't know *the* Creator, I encourage you to keep your heart and mind open to the possibility that He exists, that He loves you and is good. He is only half a turn away and is more than willing and able to help you. And He will meet you wherever you are at in your faith walk.

Consider this: in ancient Greek and Egyptian civilizations, whenever people were sick, the first person in the community that they would be sent to was a spiritual leader; a priest or rabbi. After that, they were sent to the equivalent of a psychological counselor, and only lastly, to the medical doctor. In those societies, healing was focused first and foremost upon the spirit. Secondarily, they treated the mind and emotions, and only lastly, the physical body.

Now, in Western society, that order has been reversed and most doctors focus primarily upon healing the body. Few practitioners and patients pay much attention to the spirit and soul, yet I don't believe that this is the highest and most effective way to be healed. **We must return to a whole-body approach to wellness that focuses on the spirit and relationship with God as the cornerstone to recovery.** From that foundation, we employ tools to heal the soul and body. In this book, I will share those tools with you.

If you still aren't convinced that healing your spirit and soul are foundational for recovery, know that an abundance of research has shown a direct correlation and connection between stress and/or trauma, and disease.[3] Some astute practitioners have even observed that certain cancers are caused by specific emotional conflicts. When those conflicts are removed, healing occurs—sometimes spontaneously!

In addition, through my many years working as an integrative cancer doctor, I've observed that God uses medicine to heal, but He also heals people supernaturally. Healing miracles are more common worldwide than some of us may believe, yet tend to occur most frequently in places where people believe in them. The good news is that God's healing is for everyone, including you. Throughout the book, I will share with you why this is true, and then show you how you can receive that healing.

In the meantime, just know that with God, all things are possible. As Ephesians 3:20 says, "Now to him who is able to do immeasurably more than all we ask or imagine, according to his power that is at work within us."

That means that for those of us who look to Him for help, we can expect better outcomes than if we were to simply try to heal ourselves or our patients with just medicine.

Vanessa had a brain tumor and was told that she had only weeks or perhaps a month to live. By the time I met her, she had already gone through surgery, chemotherapy and radiation. When she came to Hope4Cancer, she was stuttering due to the tumor.

While she and her husband, John, were at the clinic, he said, "Vanessa, tell Dr. Tony your favorite verse in the Bible."

To which Vanessa replied, "With Dr. Tony, a-a-all things are possible!"

I then said, "Vanessa, it's 'with God all things are possible!'"

Yet the statement was a powerful demonstration of her faith; and I believe that because of her faith, she far outlived her original prognosis.

At our treatment centers, we've seen many healing miracles in people who have survived and recovered from cancer, despite tremendous odds. These are people who have been transformed and/or healed, either through a miracle of God or with medicine. Yet when we have faith in God, He makes even medicine miraculous!

For example, a few years ago, a pastor came to us for three weeks of treatment. He was a leader of a mega-church in the Midwest, and had been diagnosed with stage IV prostate cancer and extensive bone metastasis.

When he arrived at the clinic I ordered several tests, including a high-resolution color power ultrasound and PSA, a standard blood test for prostate cancer. To our surprise, all of his scans and tests came out clear.

How could this be? We had reviewed his past medical records that confirmed his diagnosis of terminal and advanced prostate cancer, which had failed to respond to conventional therapies.

I ordered more detailed tests, including a bone scan and MRI, and still, the results were negative, revealing no signs of cancer. So I said to him, "Go home, there's nothing that we need to treat here."

Remarkably, even though this man was a minister who knew about the power of God to heal, and had taught thousands of people about Him, he could not believe that his God had just performed a miracle on him.

Instead, he asked me, "Well, what do you think happened?"

I replied, "God healed you on your way over here!"

So he returned home and his urologist said to him, "These tests from Mexico can't be right."

The pastor called me again, and I told him that the MRI, CT scan and bone scan devices that they used in his hometown clinic to test him were the same machines that are used all over the world to look for abnormalities that could indicate cancer.

Still, I encouraged him to do the tests again—and once again, they all came out clear. Finally, he was convinced that God had in fact healed him.

These stories of divine healing are not uncommon at Hope4Cancer. Perhaps it is because we pray for and with our patients that we see miraculous healing. God performs miracles, but He also gives us the wisdom we need to treat each person medically in the best possible way, with treatments that are given strength and anointed by Him.

Healing the Body at the Energetic Level

We are all energy beings. This isn't just a New Age philosophy, but a scientifically demonstrated principle. Scientist Albert Einstein first proved this when he discovered that energy equals matter times the speed of light, or $E=mc^2$. What this means in layman's terms is that all matter, including the physical body, is made up of energy.

Healing happens when our cells vibrate within a certain, higher energetic frequency range, while disease occurs when the cells are in a lowered energy state. For instance, the cell is healthy when the trans-membrane potential of a cell (which refers to the difference in electric potential between the interior and the exterior of a cell) is around -90 mV, while cancer occurs at around -30 mV.[4]

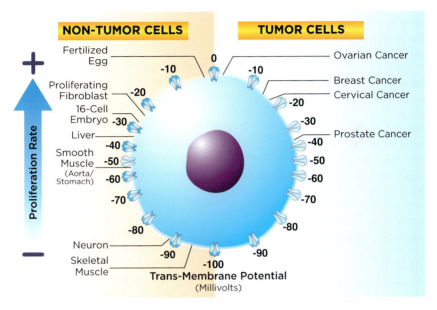

Figure 1. Relationship between the electric potential difference of cells across their membrane and their ability to multiply rapidly. Cells in rapidly growing environments (e.g., embryos) are characterized by less negative potential differences, while more mature cells have more negative values. Not surprisingly, tumor cells show values in the less negative range.[4]

In addition, we all have an innate energy that keeps our organs and systems functioning and alive. Some call this energy the "vital force," or in Eastern medicine, "qi" or "prana." The inherent vital force of the body is often subdued due to cancer, but God's Spirit can ignite our vital force so that we can heal.

Many other influences affect the energy of every cell, tissue, organ and system in our body, including our emotions, thoughts, environment, and medical treatments such as herbs and homeopathic remedies.

For example, when you have hope, the frequency of that positive emotion gets "downloaded" into your cells, which is conducive to healing. Hope is a powerful healer, and yet it also transcends your physical body. Whenever you have hope, it impacts your spirit, and once you are healed on the spiritual level, then your soul and body will tend to follow. This is because healing occurs first on the spiritual level, then on the mental and emotional levels, and finally, on the physical level.

What's more, I believe words that come from God, or which are anointed by the Holy Spirit (such as words from Scripture), have a higher energy frequency than just commonly spoken positive words. As such, these higher-frequency words may heal the body more quickly and effectively.

Consider Hebrews 4:12, which states, "For the word of God is living and effective and sharper than any double-edged sword, penetrating as far as the separation of soul and spirit, joints and marrow. It is able to judge the ideas and thoughts of the heart" (HCSB).

Further, words that come from the Spirit of God are supernatural, living entities that can heal not only your soul and spirit, but also your body.

John 6:63 says, "The Spirit gives life; the flesh counts for nothing. The words I have spoken to you—they are full of the Spirit and life."

Here, the author is referring to the words that God has spoken throughout the Bible. While not every Scripture may be relevant for your life today, I believe that if you ask Him, God will highlight certain Scriptures for you to speak and meditate on, which can bring life to your spirit, soul and body.

Japanese scientist Masaru Emoto, author of *Hidden Messages in Water*, has demonstrated how words and thoughts can even affect elements like water. According to Emoto's observations, frozen water crystals that had positive, loving thoughts directed toward them, showed more brilliant, complex and symmetrical patterns than water crystals that had negative thoughts directed at them.[5] While Emoto's observations remain unsubstantiated, there is gathering scientific evidence that our thoughts may indeed affect our cells.

Most of us can probably recall a time in our lives when we or someone we know prayed for another person and they were spontaneously healed! Or perhaps it's even happened to you.

Healing the Root Causes of Disease at the Cellular Level

In the physical realm, we treat cancer at the level at which it starts, which is at the cellular level, because the basic unit of life is the cell. We all have trillions of cells, and many cells, taken collectively, make up tissues. These tissues make up organs, and organs make up the various systems of our bodies, such as the digestive system. Then the systems, when taken together, make up the body.

Conventional medicine, on the other hand, treats cancer as an isolated entity that affects certain tissues or organs, rather than a systemic disease that starts at the cellular level. For instance, if you have a tumor in your colon, you might have it surgically removed and if the tests show no cancer elsewhere in your body, then your doctor may tell you that you are in remission.

However, you can seldom completely cut out all cancer from the body. So when doctors tell patients that they "got it all" (referring to the tumor), they really haven't. That is because some tumor cells can break off from the original tumor and remain circulating in the body, where they can later form new tumors.

Further, the underlying processes that caused the cancer in the first place still haven't been dealt with, which can cause the cancer to re-emerge.

To heal the root causes of illness, we must address all the factors that caused "dis-ease" in the spirit, soul and body. As you will soon discover, research shows that cancer is primarily caused by environmental toxins, both chemical and electromagnetic. Chronic infections, a poor diet, an unhealthy lifestyle, and emotional factors all affect the expression of our genes.

The science of how the environment affects our genes is called epigenetics. And each of these epigenetic factors must be dealt with, along with the cancer, in order for long-lasting, full recovery to occur. As we have discussed, we must expect God's healing miracles as well! I discuss each of these factors more in depth in Chapter 2. For now, know that healing from cancer isn't just about removing a tumor or eliminating cancer cells.

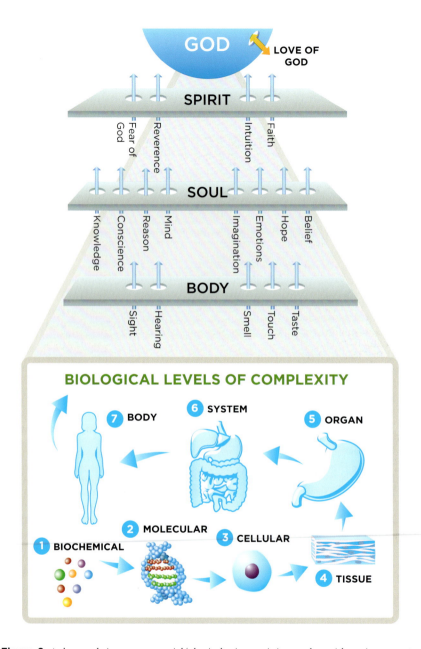

Figure 2. As human beings, our material/physical existence is incomplete without its transcendent interactivity with our higher planes of existence—the soul (mind, will and emotions) and the spirit (the eternal part that is connected with God).

Thus, we must first work on healing the cell, and as we do this, we will restore the voltage, or energy of the cell, and with that, the cellular communication pathways. As these are restored, the body will move more toward healing and away from disease.

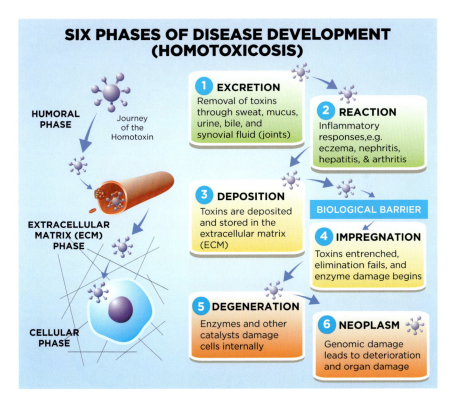

Figure 3. The disease symptoms that we observe are only the end result of an underlying disease process that evolves over time. The concept of homotoxicosis seeks to explain this transition. Homotoxicology is the foundation of medical philosophies such as biological medicine.

To heal the cell, we do many things, including: increase the uptake of nutrients into it; hydrate it; and detoxify it of heavy metals and other environmental toxins. This is the first stage of treatment that's required to bring a patient from disease to health. By doing this, we help create an environment in which cancer cells can't thrive and ultimately no longer have a reason for "being."

We bring order to the chaos of cancer. Cancer cells exhibit a noisy, disorganized energy or motion, while healthy cells are organized and balanced. When the cells are acting in an organized and balanced manner, we are living in harmony with our Creator and our environment.

We use many tools and therapies at Hope4Cancer to restore the energy and functionality of the cells, which we will share with you throughout the book. I believe that these methods will help you to heal more deeply and profoundly than perhaps you ever thought possible. Some of the tools and therapies must be done in a clinical setting, so we encourage you to share them with your doctor.

What Do Health and Wholeness Look Like?

Health and wholeness aren't just about having a healthy, functioning and thriving body, although that too is important. It's about having peace, and waking up in the morning and realizing that because you have another day ahead of you, you are blessed. It's about having gratitude toward God for who He is and all that He has given you and the blessings that will happen to you that day.

A healthy life is about knowing you aren't alone and that you will get through every trial and problem you have to endure. It's about integrating simple things, like laughter, sunshine and healthy food into your daily life. It's about avoiding negative influences like inappropriate media and unhealthy relationships.

Healing is also about having a balanced life and being able to live well, and prioritizing the most important things that you need to do for the day. It's about evaluating yourself every morning and reviewing the previous day, and then thinking about what you can do to make today better.

Planning is particularly important for cancer patients, who have so much to do but often see themselves as having a short life span. Many operate out of sympathetic mode, or "fight or flight," which causes high cortisol ("stress" hormone) levels and is contrary to healing. Learning to live and operate out of a spirit of rest, knowing that it's okay if you can't get everything done that you need to get done, is conducive to and essential for recovery and health.

Healing is also about letting go and surrendering control of your life to God. Trying to maintain control in this life is a bit like trying to maintain control on a roller coaster. The ride has its own logic and is going to go its own way, regardless of how tightly you grip the bar. There is a thrill and a power in simply surrendering to the ride and fully feeling the ups and downs of it, letting the curves take you rather than fighting them.

When you fight the ride, resisting what's happening at every turn, your whole being becomes tense and anxiety is your close companion. When you go with the ride, or with God, accepting what you cannot control, freedom and joy will inevitably arise.

One of my favorite things to say aloud every morning is, "The Lord (God) is my shepherd, I shall not want." There's nothing more powerful than knowing and trusting that God will provide for all of your needs for the day.

In summary, health transcends the physical body, and is about so many other things: what we believe and think, how we live, our day-to-day attitude toward life, and our connection to God.

Speaking of attitude, I've observed that those who overcome cancer are people who never give up. They tend to be positive, proactive optimists who see the glass as half full rather than half empty. They are connected to their spirit and soul (or their mind, will and emotions). Their faith is unwavering, even when they have a setback, a bad scan or blood test result. They are the patients who are able to change their future and heal because they have faith and hope. Ultimately, they "know" that they will be healed.

If this doesn't describe you, though, don't worry—many people who have a positive attitude about their healing didn't become faith-filled optimists overnight. Later in the book, we will give you strategies that can help you change your perspective and outlook on life. Even more importantly, once you get to know God and His perspective on your life, you may automatically find it easier to have faith and positivity about your recovery.

Sometimes, people with cancer ask me, "What did I do to deserve this? Why did I get this disease? I am a vegetarian, I go to church, pray, meditate" (and so on). Emotions such as fear, blame, guilt, shame and anger are common in cancer patients. These emotions get embedded in the cellular memory, which can then make every cell of the body toxic.

This is another reason why any plan of care must include work at the emotional level, because the cells retain the energy and information of all our emotions. At our centers, we have tools for helping patients remove the effects of such negative emotions from their conscious and subconscious minds (more on this later as well).

Be encouraged—there are better answers for cancer than what your doctor, the media or society may have taught you. I'm talking about answers that have brought many patients into remission and enabled them to live longer, happier and more vibrant lives than what some believed possible. Let go of what society and conventional medicine have taught you about cancer treatment, the recovery process and cancer outcomes. **Cancer doesn't have to be a death sentence, recovery doesn't have to be grueling or painful, and treatments don't have to weaken your body.**

Instead, I encourage you to embrace the recovery process and see it as an opportunity for self-discovery, restoration and redemption. In turn, you can uncover and heal those areas of your life that were unhealthy and causing you trouble, even long before you had cancer. In doing so, you just may find yourself emerging from the shadows of cancer stronger, happier and healthier than you ever were before!

SUMMARY

- Cancer is not a death sentence. A full recovery is possible, especially when healing is addressed on all three levels: spirit, soul and body.
- Your spirit oversees the soul and body; when your spirit is made whole through relationship with God, your soul and body can more easily heal.
- Conventional medicine has taught us that health means the absence of a tumor, but healing from cancer is about removing

all root causes of illness: spiritual, emotional, environmental and infectious.
- The body must be healed at the cellular level, which involves hydrating and detoxifying the cells, and giving them the right nutrition.
- The right attitude and lifestyle foster healing; you can learn to cultivate these by implementing the tools and ideas presented throughout this book.
- We are energy beings. Our food, medicine, emotions and environment all affect our energy, for better or worse.

QUESTIONS FOR FURTHER REFLECTION

1. What is the difference between your spirit and your soul? Which is the higher level of your being and can command the healing of your body?
2. Why is healing from cancer possible, even if you have failed all conventional treatments?
3. What makes the Hope4Cancer approach different from that of conventional medicine?
4. What are some of the root causes of cancer?
5. Describe the role of God in healing.

ADRIANA'S STORY

Adriana is a happily married 51-year-old from Sardinia, Italy, who was diagnosed with pancreatic cancer in 2015. She lives with her husband in Newport Beach, California. When she's not spending time with her family and/or friends or traveling the world, she enjoys exercising in the outdoors. Formerly a corporate executive for a Fortune 500 company, she now works as a life coach from home.

I was diagnosed with a slow-growing pancreatic cancer in July 2015, at age 48. At that time, the doctors told me that I had a 1.7 centimeter-sized mass in the body of my pancreas. I was shocked, because I didn't have any symptoms whatsoever.

I was devastated by the diagnosis, as my lifestyle, diet and exercise habits were extremely healthy. I had also just married the man of my dreams and was very fulfilled in my career. I felt like I was on top of the world, so I wondered how this could happen.

I did not have any tumor markers in my lab reports that indicated a cancer diagnosis. The only evidence of the diagnosis was scans and ultrasounds, which showed that there was an uninvited guest taking up residency in my pancreas!

The first surgeon that I met with described the best and worst scenarios that could happen to me. She didn't really know though, because they hadn't yet done an endoscopy, so she wasn't sure what type of cancer I had. She told me that I might have anywhere from several months up to five years of life left!

Up until the diagnosis I had always considered myself to be the perfect picture of health with an endless zest for life. Everything from my diet and supplements, to my exercise routine, mental balance, relationships and outlook on life, was geared toward a strong immune system and disease prevention.

I'm the youngest child in a big Italian family of eight kids and no one in my family has ever had cancer, and nobody recalls cancer in our lineage. Most of my siblings are still alive and my mom is 94 years old and still in great health for her age.

So I was shocked about my diagnosis for two reasons: first, because I didn't look sick and didn't have any symptoms; and secondly, because what the surgeon had told me was so devastating. I had been "flying high" in life, and now here I was, just a moment later, down on the floor!

Needless to say, I was in disbelief about the diagnosis, although I was also certain that if my body had produced the cancer, with the right help, it would also expel it.

The surgeon told me that I needed to do an endoscopy to find out exactly what we were dealing with. On reviewing the results, she wanted to schedule a surgery. I told her that I needed to get a second opinion, because I didn't really want to do surgery.

I began to research, and came across some people on Facebook who had had surgery for a PNET (Pancreatic Neuroendocrine Tumor). I even met a man who had done what's called the Whipple procedure, 20 years earlier, and who was now in his 80s or 90s, and healthy.

I figured that because he'd had such great success, maybe I should go see the surgeon that he had seen. So I did, but the second surgeon told me that instead of doing the Whipple procedure, he was going to do a distal pancreatectomy, and cut out my pancreas from the middle to the end. He was also going to remove my spleen.

Shocked, I said, "Why do you have to cut out so much if the tumor is less than two centimeters in size? That seems so drastic!" I thought, *What about the endless complications following surgery that no doctor speaks of?*

I was still really bewildered about things at this point. I immediately began to ponder the "quality versus quantity" of my life: the benefits of having a better quality of life versus a longer life. And the more that

I researched, the more that I realized that it wasn't going to be a peaceful ending for me if I did surgery!

I didn't go back to the first surgeon because her whole attitude toward the diagnosis and treatment process wasn't very reassuring. She was granting me, at best, five more years of life.

I thought to myself, *five years of life!* I can probably squeeze at least a couple of more years out of life just by doing nothing! I then envisioned myself unable to eat anything, being in excruciating pain, and unable to do all of the things that I loved most.

The second surgeon had been more reassuring. Yet, I was still not convinced that surgery was the right route to go. So several weeks later, I consulted with one of his colleagues, who told me that they could do a laparoscopic surgery. I then recalled that the first surgeon had said not to do a laparoscopic surgery, because it was risky. If something bad were to happen to me during the surgery—if there was a problem—they would not have time to open me up to fix the problem. I could even bleed to death!

Yet it was confusing because this surgeon seemed to be assured that my outcome and prognosis following the surgery would be good. He didn't put an expiration date on me like the first surgeon had.

I decided to schedule a surgery for the following month, as a friend of mine was getting married the following week. My husband thought that I was just procrastinating my healing to have a "good time," although truthfully, I feared losing my health and well-being forever.

After this, I traveled from California to New Orleans to see a surgeon who specialized in treating the kind of tumor that I had.

I told the oncologist, "I'm confused about the results of my endoscopy; some of the wording regarding the position of the tumor is contradictory. I'm not a doctor so I could be missing something."

He looked at me like I was crazy.

I continued, "When you read my paperwork, you'll see that some of the doctors say that the cancer is in the body of my pancreas, while others say that it's in the tail, and they all have a different opinion about what surgery to perform."

The surgeon replied, "Well, if you read here (on the paperwork) you'll see that it says the tumor is in the body-tail of the pancreas! But we won't know exactly what it is until we open you up. Then we'll know if it's benign or malignant."

I met with the reconstructive pancreatic surgeon, who was a bit more reassuring. He recommended a tumor resection with a possible splenectomy. A friend from Facebook told me that he and his group of doctors were the best out there. She knew, because her husband had had a PNET (pancreatic neuroendocrine tumor) cancer and had gone to these doctors, so I agreed to the surgery.

I ended up canceling both surgeries, however, because a force inside me seemed to say, *This is not the way to go. This is not the answer!*

It had now been three months since my initial diagnosis, and I had consulted with many top specialists in Western medicine from all over the country. I concluded that their approaches were all either going to kill me or at least make me very sick. None of it aligned with my way of thinking and living. It just made no sense that in order to stay alive, I had to give up my well-being.

I started doing intense research and investigations on alternative therapies and non-conventional treatments. I spent countless hours reading and consulting with alternative and integrative doctors. I visited endless numbers of clinics and spoke with many people who were in remission. Finally, I discovered Dr. Tony and my reality started changing.

My brother had suggested that I contact the Hope4Cancer Treat-ment Centers, so I had a telephone consultation with Dr. Tony, the leading physician there.

He told me that he could offer me a multi-faceted approach to healing that wasn't just "cut and dried." It encompassed physical, mental, psychological, and spiritual therapies, which would all be given to me as part of the program. He said that the therapies were all non-toxic and would not harm me.

When I asked him how effective his protocols were, he didn't promise me anything. He didn't say, "You will be cancer-free," but neither did he tell me that the cancer would spread.

Instead, he basically said, "One of three things is going to happen: Your tumor will either disappear, it will continue growing, or it will remain the same. I can only offer you what I can offer you." He was very straightforward and forthright.

I still wasn't one hundred percent convinced that I wanted to go to Hope4Cancer. Time was passing, and my husband said, "You need to make a decision. You can't procrastinate this any longer."

However, the tumor was only at a stage I, and it was apparently a slow growing one, so I thought, *If it's slow growing, then why is there all this pressure to go through surgery?*

I told my husband that we had put a lot of effort and energy into researching conventional treatment options, so now we needed to do the same for the alternative non-conventional options. He was very supportive and did his best not to impose his beliefs onto me.

However, he was very scared as he is more "old school" and his beliefs are more aligned with those of Western medicine.

I watched Ty Bollinger's documentary, *The Truth About Cancer* and began to make changes to my daily life, based on what I was learning from the series. I began to take additional cancer-fighting supplements, changed my diet, and started doing coffee enemas; I also started juicing and undergoing IV treatments at a local holistic cancer clinic. I didn't stay long at that clinic, though, because the environment wasn't very comforting or nurturing for me.

Then, in November 2016, I visited Hope4Cancer, just to get to know the treatment center and see the patients there. I also wanted to find a patient who had decided not to go to Hope4Cancer as a last resort, after they had failed surgery and chemotherapy. I wanted to meet somebody who had intentionally chosen it as a first approach to treatment.

So I went and met with the staff, and with Dr. Tony again, this time in person. He patiently answered all my 100-plus questions as honestly and authentically as he could. Not once did he rush me through the process of making a decision, or treat me as someone who just didn't understand. He was sympathetic, but also realistic and straightforward.

What's more, the treatments his center offered were in line with my beliefs on how to heal, and his staff was welcoming and nurturing. It was a family-like environment.

While there, I also met an older woman, who, just like me, was very health conscious, and still developed breast cancer. She had decided to go to Hope4Cancer as her first approach to treatment, so meeting her and hearing her story solidified my decision to go.

I stayed at the clinic for three weeks, and did most of the therapies they had to offer, and which Dr. Tony suggested. My regimen included intravenous Vitamin C, chelation therapy, ultraviolet blood irradiation, and sauna therapy—among many others.

In addition, I decided to eliminate all animal-based products from my diet. I also cut out soy and any foods that I knew would turn into sugar in my system, including flour and grains. So during my first year of treatment, I ate mostly raw or steamed vegetables, and supplemented my diet with protein from quinoa, nuts, chia and other seeds. I also prepared shakes with almond and coconut milk and juiced organic, sugarless veggies up to three times daily. I also added fasting into my regimen as a way to reset my immune system.

Once home, I did Sonodynamic Therapy, sauna and infrared lamp therapy, and grounding. I did a variety of exercises, from yoga to walking on the beach, and spent lots of time in the sun to get my Vitamin D for the day. I also meditated and prayed daily.

In addition, I went back to my local holistic clinic for additional IVs and hyperbaric chamber treatments. Everything that Dr. Tony suggested I do, I did, including Recall Healing, which I have now been doing for a year.

Finally, I reduced all sources of environmental toxins in our home. We exchanged our water filtration systems for better ones. I also exchanged my toxic chemical makeup and personal care body products for natural ones, and did the same with our household cleaning supplies.

I pretty much did everything, or about 99% of everything Dr. Tony suggested I do to get well! I am still a work in progress, but the good news is, three years after my diagnosis, the tumor in my pancreas is stable and has not changed in size according to my MRI. My blood work and other tests show that my immune system is strong, that I am extremely healthy, and I have no elevated tumor markers.

Not only that, but I feel great, and my health and emotional state are back to what they were before I was diagnosed with cancer. And I continue to get stronger and stronger.

Dr. Tony transformed my fear, chaos and confusion into a comforting and hopeful journey to recovery. Thanks to him, today I am on top of the world again, and truly feel like I'm living the best years of my life. For this and so much more, I am so blessed and beyond grateful.

When I think of Dr. Tony, there are many adjectives that come to mind, which describe him as a doctor, individual, and friend. Some of these include: patient, knowledgeable, trustworthy, reliable, optimistic, compassionate, and a true pioneer.

What I really love about Dr. Tony's approach is that it's not just about him being the expert and the doctor; it's about him helping you make the best choice for yourself, and he allows you to ultimately do that. You don't find many doctors like that, who empower their patients, even in many alternative clinics.

I'm not really concerned that the MRI is still showing a tumor. My philosophy has always been that if the mass is not causing any pain, then perhaps it just needs to stay right where it is. And given that it has not grown, hasn't injured me, and I'm strong and healthy, then perhaps it's actually there to protect me from something. Maybe that's what my journey is about—discovering why it's there, and to teach me the true value of life.

If you have just been diagnosed with cancer, I encourage you not to rush into making any decisions. Instead, do your research, and don't allow fear to take your decision-making power away from you. "Cancer" is just a name; a label that somebody has given to the problem or thing that you have in your body.

Regardless of what treatments you pursue, choose the journey that is most aligned with your lifestyle and who you are as a person. Don't allow others to make decisions for you, and don't rush decisions. Take all the time you need to make an informed decision—your illness didn't just happen overnight, so why should you be pushed to make an overnight decision?

It's also important that you sit down with yourself and reflect upon what's going on in your body, and how you are responding to the news of your diagnosis. Silence and time with yourself is sometimes more important than talking to another doctor, family member, friend or other survivor, or even going to another specialist. When you are quiet and reflective, the answers you need will come.

So do what suits you most. If you are religious, pray. If you like to meditate, then meditate. If you like to take walks in nature or at the beach, then do it. And if you don't think the advice other people are giving is right for you, don't accept it. Learn to set boundaries with people that don't support you or your decision; after all, it's your body and your life.

It's also important to remember that even if you have surgery, and you remove the tumor, it's not the end of the treatment road. You must do other therapies to prevent a reoccurrence. And please, do all the emotional work necessary to heal and release any emotional issues that are holding you back, so you can set yourself free to experience abundant health, joy, and balance.

Living a preventative lifestyle isn't a guarantee that you won't get an illness. But again, your diagnosis is just a name to call whatever it is that you are dealing with. It's not a death sentence and it doesn't have to define you or your healing journey.

It has been three years since my original diagnosis, and I am thriving and triumphing. I feel more alive than ever, and you can too!

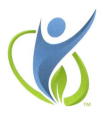

2

About Cancer and Its Causes

Cancer is a scary word for many of us. When we hear it, we might envision deformed, invasive and angry cells that have "gone rogue." We envision a malevolent force with an agenda to take over and destroy the body. But what if we saw cancer as groupings of cells that simply got confused and didn't get the message that they were supposed to stop dividing and spreading? Cells that did not know they were supposed to remove themselves from the body when it was time to do so?

Because cancer is really just that: a group of cells that divide and multiply unchecked in the body and don't die when they are supposed to. **It is an opportunistic disease that occurs whenever the terrain of the body, along with the spirit and soul, become greatly imbalanced.** Yet often, cancer can be reversed—or at least managed—once these things are balanced and restored, and the factors that caused the cancer are removed.

The 10 Biological Hallmarks of Cancer

While cancer cells may be confused, they are not purposeless proliferators. Rather, they display an innate intelligence and certain characteristics that must be accounted for while treating the cancer.

There are 10 biological hallmarks of cancer. These include its ability to:[1]

1. Send out growth signals that lead to uncontrolled cell growth.
2. Bypass the body's normal growth-suppressing signals.
3. Resist normal programmed cell death, or apoptosis.
4. Multiply indefinitely.
5. Stimulate angiogenesis, or new tumor blood vessel formation, from which tumors get their nutrients and eliminate waste.
6. Activate invasion processes to spread and cause metastases.
7. Create inflammation.
8. Deregulate the body's metabolism.
9. Evade the immune system.
10. Destabilize DNA in healthy cells.

In addition, cancer cells:[2]

- **Are intelligent social entities -** They exhibit rudimentary forms of social intelligence, and have the ability to act collectively in ways to adapt to the prevailing conditions of the body.
- **Get smarter -** They learn from experience and solve existential problems. This makes them unpredictable.
- **Can alter their own genes -** Research shows that they can alter their own genes to change their behavior and susceptibility.
- **Wear a "cloak of invisibility" -** They can hide from the immune system by blocking recognition by the immune complement system.
- **Use healthy cells to help them achieve their goals -** They employ healthy cells as decoys to fool the immune system.
- **Learn to rapidly resist drugs -** Cancer cells communicate with each other to rapidly develop drug resistance incredibly faster than one would expect through the process of natural selection. This is one reason why chemotherapy and radiation are often ineffective strategies (more on this in the next chapter).

- **Display a primitive, back-to-basics intelligence -** Cancer cells exhibit the innate intelligence of primitive life forms such as bacteria that are able to survive, communicate, colonize, and work together better in community.

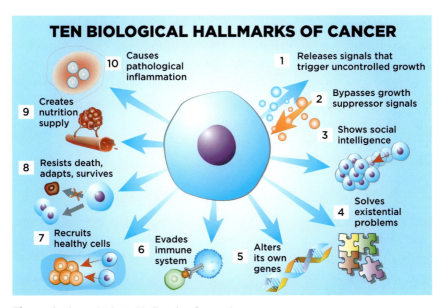

Figure 4. The ten biological hallmarks of cancer.[1]

How Tumors Form

Cancer cells become tumors through a very purposeful, calculated process. First, they actively recruit other cancer cells as well as healthy cells as they extend a "cable" toward them and "lasso" them into a group of cells. The cable may be made up of proteins from the cell membrane wall of the cancer cell. This lassoing is not a passive effort caused by the chance collision of cancer cells with others; but rather, purposeful growth.[3]

Just a few cancer cells are needed to become a tumor: only 5% of the original, or initial grouping of cancer cells. These cells multiply and exercise their mastery over the other "recruits"—mainly healthy cells—to drive cancer growth.[3]

Tumor formation is an intelligent act. Cancer cells seem to know what they are doing when they create a tumor. Tumorigenic cells are not highly sophisticated cells and function more out of an instinct to survive. This is in contrast to normal, healthy cells, which are more evolved and possess more highly developed, complex processes.

What's more, tumors are built to survive and grow by creating favorable microenvironments and specific defense systems within the body. Perhaps even more surprisingly, cancer cells can transform normal cells into cancerous tumor cells. Researchers at Harvard, Bellvitge and MD Anderson have shown that tumor cells secrete mRNA and microRNA-containing exosomes (which are fluid-filled sacs that are involved in cell signaling and intercellular communication). These have the capacity to transform healthy cells into malignant ones, revealing a new key to cancer cell propagation.[4]

Researchers and doctors are still learning how to overcome cancer's survival mechanisms. Our long-term success against cancer will be determined by treatment approaches that not only selectively target cancer cells and their survival tactics, but which also create a cancer-disfavoring environment. On a physical level, we must treat the cancer as well as the terrain of the body, using novel, non-toxic cancer therapies.

What Causes Cancer

We all form cancer cells daily, but we have a powerful immune system that normally keeps the development of these cells "in check" and does not allow tumors to form or metastasize. God has created us with an amazing defense system, but sometimes the influences of the broken and toxic world in which we live cause it to malfunction. As a society, we have violated the natural laws that God created for our well-being, and it has resulted in a myriad of toxic stressors that have left us susceptible to cancer and other diseases.

Yet God knew in advance that our lives and the earth would become toxic. The Bible foretold many events that have already occurred, and also foretells events that are yet to come.

Revelation 21:6 tells us that God is eternal, the Beginning and the End of all things. As such, He is outside of time and space, and knows what will happen in the days to come. And because God knew in advance what would happen to the world, He also provided us with tools in both the natural and supernatural realms, such as plant-based foods and herbs, to heal our bodies from the effects of these toxins.

Factors That Create a Favorable Terrain for Cancer

Many factors create a favorable environment in the body for the development of cancer. They include, but are not limited to:

- Spiritual brokenness, or separation from God.
- Emotional trauma, and harmful beliefs, thinking patterns and behaviors.
- Inflammation.
- A compromised immune system.
- Poor dental work and dental problems, such as mercury amalgams, and infected root canals.
- Poor acid-alkaline balance.
- Pre-existing genetic factors.
- Chemical and electromagnetic environmental toxins.
- Hypoxia, or a low-oxygen environment in the body.
- Mineral deficiencies.
- Microbial imbalances, such as chronic infections, or not enough beneficial bacteria in the gastrointestinal tract.
- Excessive free radical production.
- Deficiencies or excesses of nutrients.
- Metabolic factors, such as thyroid and other hormonal imbalances.

All these factors, especially when taken cumulatively, create an environment in which abnormal cells can grow, proliferate and form tumors, and ultimately, spread to distant organs.

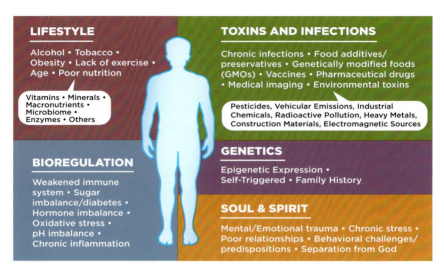

Figure 5. The biological terrain that influences cancer.

So, cancer doesn't just happen; rather, it is an opportunistic process that occurs because our spirit, soul and body are imbalanced. In turn, this creates an altered "terrain" in the body that is favorable to cancer growth. Terrain-altering factors that set the stage for these imbalances include: separation from God; unhealthy beliefs, thinking patterns and behaviors; environmental toxins; nutritional imbalances; and chronic infections.

In this chapter, I will share some of the environmental instigators of cancer, and in later chapters I will give you tools to address these and the other factors that lead to its development.

Spiritual Brokenness and Soul Wounds

Because we are spirit-soul-body beings, when one part of us suffers and is disconnected from God, the other two parts suffer too, for they are all interconnected. Our human spirit is the head of our whole person, not the tail, and we were created first and foremost for relationship with our Creator.

In John 14:23 Jesus says, "If anyone loves Me, he will keep My word. My Father will love him, and We will come to him and make Our home with him" (HCSB).

So if we are disconnected from God, because we don't know Him, have a distorted view of Him, or don't believe in Him, we can't thrive in the fullness of who and what He's created us to be.

For example, if you believe God desires you to be sick in order to teach you a lesson, then it can be difficult to believe that He loves you. And if you doubt His love, then it can be difficult to have faith that He can heal you.

When we aren't connected to God, or have suffered traumas in our lives (especially in childhood), it can create soul wounds that cause us to habitually entertain lie-based or harmful beliefs and thoughts. These lies, in turn, can affect our cellular behavior.

For instance, if you had a parent who knowingly (or unknowingly) communicated that you are worthless or unlovable, then that belief can result in toxic thoughts that affect your cells and over time, cause cancer or another disease.

We once had a patient with leukemia, Donny, whose father used to compare him to his older brother and tell him that he was worthless. The father would constantly brag that his older son was faster, stronger, and more intelligent than he was.

Interestingly, we've found that a common emotional conflict behind leukemia is having a lack of self-worth or identity. When Donny came to the clinic, he had been given only a month to live, and had already failed prolonged chemotherapy.

Well, we helped him change his mind set and heal the lie-based beliefs that were making him sick. This included forgiving his father. While he didn't fully recover, he ended up living a year and a half beyond his original prognosis. I believe that it was because of the emotional healing that he received at our center.

When you have a strong spirit-soul-body connection, including a strong relationship with God, and a positive, truth-based mind set, disease processes become disfavored in your body.

Early on in my career, while working at a big hospital and during a visit with one of my patients, the patient excused herself to go to the bathroom. While she was in there, the patient that was in the bed next to hers said to me, "You know, Doc, I'm going to do better than your patient."

Somewhat startled, I said to her, "Excuse me?"

She replied, "I am going to do better, because I have God in my heart, and your patient doesn't."

While her comment may have sounded unkind, it was a lesson that helped to solidify my belief that having a relationship with God fosters recovery.

Many studies confirm that trauma and stress can lead to disease. For example, a study review published in the *Journal of Analytical Science and Technology* in 2015 states, "Psychological or psychosocial stress has been emerging as one of the key factors associated with cancer initiation, growth, and metastasis."[5]

One way that harmful beliefs and thoughts lead to disease is by causing us to live in perpetual "fight or flight" mode, or fear. Fear-based living fosters an environment in which cancer can occur, because our immune system shuts down when we are in this mode.

In addition, we find that our patients' inherent bodily constitution and personality type play a role in how they are affected physically by emotional stress.

In the end, we may still not know for certain all of the reasons why people get cancer, although we do know that cancer is caused by multiple factors. For some people, lie-based thinking or toxic relationships may be the primary causative factor, while for others, pathogenic infections or environmental toxins may be primary. At our centers, we address all potential factors so our patients have the best chance for a full recovery.

As well, you will want to **find a doctor who understands that cancer is a multifactorial problem, and treats every root cause.**

The Role of Environmental Toxins in Cancer

We are awash in a sea of environmental toxins, the likes of which did not exist decades ago. Every year, thousands of new chemical and electromagnetic toxins are released into the environment, many of which have been linked to cancer and other diseases. They are found in our household and personal care products, our food, water, air, soil, cars, buildings, houses, furniture, clothes and other places.

Many studies and many clinical findings have proven that we store these toxins in our bodies and that they can cause disease. For example, a 2009 study by the Environmental Working Group found that babies are born with an average of 287 chemical toxins in their bodies![6] Those of us who have been around, 40, 50 or 60 years most likely have many more toxins inside of us.

The incidence of cancer has skyrocketed in recent decades, in part due to these toxins. A century ago, 1 in 100 people got cancer. Now, in the United States, that ratio has increased to 1 in 2 men and 1 in 3 women. Even the National Institutes of Health and The National Cancer Institute estimate that at least **two-thirds of all cancer cases are now caused by environmental factors.**[7]

Our world today is not the same as that of our ancestors, and our lifestyles have exposed us to cancer-causing agents that humans never had to deal with before the Industrial Age. God did not create our bodies to thrive on a daily diet of toxic pollutants. However, knowing what would happen in the future, I believe He gave us resources that would help lessen these toxins' impact upon our bodies and reverse the cellular conditions that lead to cancer in the first place.

We are no longer living in the Garden of Eden, but in Chapter 8, I will share with you some strategies that will help you eliminate these toxins from your home and body. For now, I'd just like to briefly share some major toxins that have been associated with cancer, according to scientific research:

Cancer-Causing Toxins[8]

- **Mold toxins -** These are ubiquitous in the environment. Chronic exposure induces cancer through a variety of mechanisms. Not everyone is susceptible to sickness from mold, but mold expert Ritchie Shoemaker, MD, estimates that 25% of all people cannot adequately detoxify mold,[9] which means that mold toxins, or mycotoxins, can accumulate in some people and cause symptoms or disease. Some molds, like aflatoxin, have been linked to cancer.[10,11]

- **Heavy metals -** Including mercury, arsenic, lead, cadmium and others.[12] These are found in our air, water, food and soil. Mercury is found in dental amalgams.
- **Pesticides (including herbicides) -** Ubiquitous in our food supply, even in some organic foods.[13]
- **Polycyclic aromatic hydrocarbons -** Products of fossil fuel combustion, especially petrochemicals, and are found in polluted air.[14]
- **Bisphenol A** (BPA) - A chemical used to make many plastics and resins, including water bottles and food storage containers.
- **Dioxins and dioxin-like chemicals such as polychlorinated biphenyls (PCBs) -** Industrial chemicals that are found in contaminated water, soil and food.[15]
- **Heterocyclic amines -** Chemicals that form when food is cooked at high temperatures, especially via grilling or broiling.[16]
- **Ultraviolet radiation -** Can be healthy for the body in moderation, and when it comes from the sun, but which in excess, can cause cancer.[17]
- **Electromagnetic field (EMF) Radiation -** Produced by microwave towers, cellular phones, Wi-Fi, smart meters and many other sources. Man-made EMF radiation is associated with DNA damage that can cause cancer.[18]

This list is not exhaustive, but should give you a general idea of some major toxins that have been associated with cancer. You can't completely avoid being exposed to these toxins, but you can do things to lessen their effects upon your body. Even praying for God to protect you from their effects, and blessing your food and water is important!

Toxins cause malignancies in a variety of ways, such as by damaging DNA, impairing hormonal and immune function, as well as liver detoxification. They also have been found to stop apoptosis, or natural programmed cellular death. More information on each of these mechanisms follows.[19,20,21]

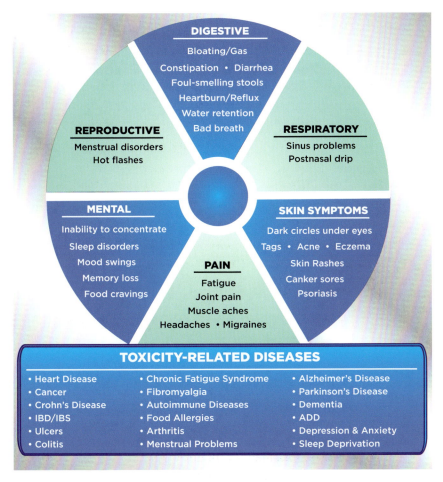

Figure 6. Symptoms of chronic toxicity and associated diseases.

First, environmental toxins may break DNA strands. Damage to DNA is a major initiating factor in causing cells to mutate and become cancerous.[22,23]

Secondly, when the liver's detoxification mechanisms are compromised, and it has too many toxins to process, this can cause an overactivity of what are called phase I liver enzymes. These enzymes normally convert toxins into harmless substances, but if the liver is exposed to a too-heavy toxic burden, the enzymes may turn them instead into cell-damaging carcinogens.

A third way that environmental toxins cause cancer is by suppressing the immune system's ability to recognize cancer.[24]

In addition, toxins can cause hormonal imbalances, which create a setup for cancer in a myriad of ways. For instance, imbalances in sex hormones like estrogen and progesterone have been found to promote certain cancers, like breast and prostate cancer. Many hormonal imbalances can create conditions in the body that favor cancer development, but it is beyond the scope of this book to describe every mechanism. Suffice it to say that balancing the hormones is essential for recovery.

Finally, toxins can switch off genes that tell normal cells when to die. This process, called apoptosis, is absent in cancer cells, which allows them to reproduce essentially without limit.

Microbial or Infectious Causes of Cancer

According to the American Cancer Society, infections are linked to 15-20% of all cancers, or 1.2 million cases per year worldwide, and are suspected to cause cancer via the following mechanisms: [25]

1. By directly affecting genes that control cellular growth and apoptosis.
2. By causing long-term inflammation and the release of cytokines, which over time leads to changes in the cells and immune system and ultimately, cancer.
3. By causing suppression of the immune system and the immune cells that protect the body from cancer.

There are other theories about how pathogens cause cancer. Among these are that they produce toxins that disturb the cell cycle. The cell cycle is sort of like the cell's "life" cycle. A disturbed cell cycle results in altered cell growth and DNA that is similar to that caused by carcinogenic, or cancer-causing agents.

The International Agency for Research on Cancer (IARC) has discovered a number of cancer-causing infectious agents,[26,27] each of which has been linked to the development of specific cancers, and include:

- **Epstein-Barr virus -** cancer of the nasopharynx, stomach and others
- **Kaposi's sarcoma-associated herpes virus (KSHV/HHV8) -** Kaposi sarcoma, lymphoma, multiple myeloma, among others
- **Human papilloma virus (HPV) -** Cancers of the cervix, anus, skin and aerodigestive tract
- **Hepatitis B and C virus (HBV) -** Hepatocellular carcinoma
- **Human T-cell leukemia/lymphoma virus (HTLV) -** adult T-cell leukemia/lymphoma
- **Helicobacter pylori -** Gastric and esophageal cancers
- **Chlamydia trachomatis -** Cervical and ovarian cancers, ocular lymphoma
- **Salmonella typhii -** Gallbladder, hepatobiliary, pancreatic, lung, colorectal cancers
- **Streptococcus bovis -** Colon cancer
- **Chlamydia pneumoniae -** Lung cancer
- **HIV-1 virus -** Kaposi sarcoma, cervical cancer, non-Hodgkin's and Hodgkin's lymphoma, anal cancer, lung cancer, cancers of the mouth and throat, skin cancer, and liver cancer
- **Merkel cell polyomavirus -** Skin cancer
- **Simian virus 40 -** (Mesothelioma, brain cancers, bone cancers, lymphomas)

The discovery that microbes can cause cancer is not new. Throughout history, researchers have shared their theories about how microbes cause cancer, even before modern studies began to substantiate it.

For instance, late American Royal Raymond Rife, the inventor of an electromagnetic frequency device called the Rife machine, believed that cancer was caused by a virus. He also discovered that every pathogen had a unique energetic frequency, and that you could kill any pathogen by treating it with a specific frequency, using a Rife machine.

The late Hulda Clark, a renowned Canadian naturopath, believed that parasites caused cancer by taking advantage of a weakened immune system and further undermining it. Dr. Clark developed herbal and other protocols to reverse cancer, which involved removing parasites.

Tullio Simoncini, MD, an Italian medical doctor who today practices medicine in Europe, believes that cancer is caused by fungi, specifically Candida. He wrote a book called *Cancer Is a Fungus* based on this theory, and developed a sodium bicarbonate protocol, which he now uses as part of his healing process for patients with cancer.

Renowned integrative doctor Dietrich Klinghardt, MD, PhD, who practices medicine in the United States, believes that parasites are involved in most chronic diseases, and that the metabolism of cancer cells resembles that of parasites. He has found that prescription and herbal anti-parasitic medications can also have strong anti-cancer effects.

Other researchers and medical professionals have observed correlations between certain cancers and specific pathogenic microbes, as well as correlations between certain cancers and specific emotional conflicts.

At Hope4Cancer, we have observed that many patients with cancer have pathogenic microbes. For example, I once had a patient who came to the clinic with an unspecified type of cancer, and her medical workup revealed that she had cytomegalovirus, Epstein-Barr virus and *Toxoplasma gondii*. When we treated her for all three of those infections, she had a dramatic recovery from not only the infections, but also the cancer.

The late German physician Ryke Geerd Hamer, MD, the creator of German New Medicine, observed that certain cancers seemed to be linked to specific unresolved, acute and severe emotional conflicts, which created shocks in the brain that he called "Hamer Herds."

He found that often, once those conflict shocks were resolved, the patient's cancer would also resolve. His work has become recognized worldwide within the integrative and naturopathic cancer communities, and some practitioners within these communities have found German New Medicine to be useful for helping their patients to heal from the emotional causes of cancer.

In summary, throughout history many researchers have developed different theories about what causes cancer. Yet in my experience, cancer is caused by many factors, and treatment must address all of these, including eliminating the cancer and restoring the terrain of the body. We do this using our 7 Key Principles approach, which forms the foundation of our treatment philosophy.

The Role of Environmental and Lifestyle Factors in Gene Expression

Many of us have been given the impression that cancer is caused largely by genetics, because much emphasis in conventional medicine has been given to the genetic causes of cancer. Yet few cancers are truly genetic in nature: perhaps 2.5-5% of all cancers.

Researchers such as Bruce Lipton, PhD, author of *Biology of Belief: Unleashing the Power of Consciousness, Matter and Miracles* have found that our environment, including our thoughts, largely affect how our genes are expressed, and that the expression of our genes determines our health, more than the genes that we were born with.[28] The study of how our environment, lifestyle and other factors affect our genes is called epigenetics.

Gene expression, and turning genes on or off, is a bit like turning on or off a light switch. You have the ability to press the light switch to turn the lights on or off, but if you don't do that, nothing will happen. Genes are similar in that you have to turn them on or off in order for them to express themselves properly.

Typically, when you go into a room, you find that the light switch is by the door. But what if the light switch is in a corner of the room or some other obscure place? If you don't know where it is, you may find yourself fumbling around in the dark room, looking for the switch, and it may take time for you to turn on the lights.

Similarly, if you are not eating well and living an unhealthy lifestyle, it may take a while for you to switch on the healthy genes and switch off the bad ones in your body. That's because, with all the chaos out there, the mechanisms that normally turn genes on and off have been disabled. But, you can switch the healthy genes on again, and switch off the bad ones, by making the right diet and health choices.

The fact that we can alter our genetic expression by our lifestyle choices is great news for those of you who may have been told that you have a cancer caused by genetic factors.

For example, even if your mother or grandmother had breast cancer, this doesn't mean that you have to be a victim of breast cancer, too! Further, your relationship with God and the health of your spirit and soul can affect your genes, just as much as any medicine, detoxification program or diet.

Final Thoughts

Cancer has a certain intelligence, but our bodies also have a powerful innate intelligence and can overcome cancer's survival mechanisms. This is especially true when we are guided by God and competent, integrative-minded doctors, and are given the proper tools and treatments.

God knew about cancer and what was going to happen to our planet before the first tumor ever manifested itself. And as I mentioned, I believe He has made provision for us to overcome the toxic factors affecting our environment and consequently, cancer. So while it may seem dismal to ponder the barrage of things that can cause cancer and the strategies that cancer uses to thrive in the body, we can be encouraged. God is the creator of all things, and is greater than the forces that are against us.

He is greater than our fears, the environment, and the cancer itself.

What's more, He operates above the physical or natural realm, and His power and ability to heal you is infinitely greater than cancer's ability to damage or destroy you.

The Bible tells us, "I am able to do all things through Him who strengthens me." (Philippians 4:13). And in Matthew 19:26, Jesus said, "With man this is impossible, but with God all things are possible." These Scriptures are relevant for your life today, too.

God has also created our bodies with an amazing ability to overcome the toxic onslaughts of the world and to self-repair when they are given the proper tools. If you have cancer, you may find it difficult to see your body as capable and strong, but consider Psalm 139:13-14, which says, "For it was You who created my inward parts; You knit me together in my mother's womb. I will praise You because I have been remarkably and wonderfully made" (HCSB). That is how God sees you—as fearfully and wonderfully made!

Further, Proverbs 3:6 says, "...in all your ways submit to him, and he will make your paths straight." God will show you the way to wellness, if you look to Him and ask for His help. It is inherent in us to be healthy and whole. God did not make human beings sick, and He therefore does not want you to be sick. He did not make you that way!

In addition, God has created us in His image, or likeness. Genesis 1:27 says, "So God created mankind in his own image, in the image of God he created them; male and female he created them." Yet how many of us see ourselves as made in the image of God, rather than as victims of disease?

You are a reflection of God, who created you with an innate ability to heal. He gave you a remarkable immune system that was designed to overcome disease, with His help—whether that help comes as a supernatural manifestation of His touch, or as medicine.

Now that you know a little more about cancer and what causes it, you can be more empowered to overcome it. So, read on to discover more about how He can work through you and the medical practitioners He has put in your path to help heal you. His desire is for you to thrive and live the best life that He has envisioned for you.

SUMMARY

- Cancer is caused by spiritual, emotional and physical factors, each of which affects the others.
- When the body's "terrain" is damaged or unhealthy, cancer can gain a foothold and flourish. When the terrain is healthy, cancer cannot live there.
- Soul wounds caused by trauma create lie-based beliefs, thoughts and behaviors that can, over the long term, create an environment in which cancer can occur.
- Environmental factors are estimated to cause two-thirds of all cancers. Chemical and environmental toxins are among the most important of these.
- Emotional issues are a factor in all cancers. The degree to which emotions cause or foster cancer varies from person to person.
- Infections are estimated to cause 15-20% of all cancers.
- Genes are responsible for only 5% of all cancers. We can influence the expression of our genes by positively altering our lifestyle and environment.

- Cancer has an innate intelligence and has developed many survival mechanisms. An effective treatment plan must address all of these mechanisms.
- God is greater than cancer and the environmental factors that cause it. With His help, you can be more strongly empowered to overcome it.

QUESTIONS FOR FURTHER REFLECTION

1. Why must healing be addressed first and foremost on a spiritual and emotional level?
2. What are some of the terrain problems that can create a favorable environment in the body for cancer to develop?
3. What are the most important causes of cancer, on a macro level?
4. What are some environmental toxins that have been linked to cancer?
5. Why don't we have to be victims of our genes?
6. Describe some of cancer's survival mechanisms.

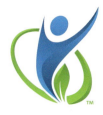

3

Novel and Safe Methods to Screen, Diagnose and Track Cancer

While cancer can be screened, diagnosed and tracked using a variety of tools, no one single exam or lab test can, by itself, tell you whether or not you have cancer. The only sure-fire way is from a biopsy, which, as you will later learn, can be unsafe and at times inaccurate.

Your doctor must personally evaluate you and your symptoms, do a physical exam, and review your medical history in order to create a comprehensive, effective healing plan.

This may all sound obvious, but medicine has become impersonal; you may be surprised to discover that many oncologists don't have an opportunity to get a good first impression of their patients. This is because they often don't see them until long after they have been admitted to the hospital. Or, they meet the patient only after a medical consultation, vital signs having been taken, and with them already lying down on the exam table!

Years ago, after my dad had quintuple bypass surgery, he had to go to the cardiologist every month for routine checkups. During one checkup, the doctor did little more than listen to his heart with a stethoscope, and then give him a prescription. When my dad went to the pharmacy to fill the prescription, he realized that he had been given a prescription that he didn't recognize.

So he called me and said, "Son, the doctor hardly examined me. He checked my heart and then the nurse gave me a prescription—Prozac. What is this?"

Because Prozac is an anti-depressant medication I said, "Dad, are you depressed?" To which he replied, "No."

His case represented a perfect example of a situation in which the doctor had missed important clues about what the patient, my father, needed.

Today, medical visits are rushed and doctors often miss important physical and interpersonal clues that would give them profound insights into the condition of their patients.

At Hope4Cancer, our approach to patient care is very personalized and thorough. We believe it's important to look each patient in the eye, get an initial impression of them when they first come into the office, and discern their emotional and physical well-being. We ask them such questions as, "How are you feeling, emotionally and physically? How is your appetite, your bowel habits and energy levels?"

We also carefully evaluate their medical history. It's important for you to work with a doctor who does the same, and who takes a personal interest in not only your physical, but also your emotional, well-being.

In addition, we evaluate our patients' symptoms. Symptoms that may indicate cancer include, but are not limited to:

- Unexplained weight loss.
- Not feeling quite like "yourself."
- Fatigue or being overly tired.
- Sores that don't heal.
- Unusual bleeding or discharge.

- A lump or mass that isn't painful. Painful lumps or masses generally indicate infection or another disease process. Cancer doesn't usually hurt in the beginning stages; only after it has become advanced does it cause pain.
- Persistent cough.
- Persistent hoarseness in the voice.
- Changes in bowel habits; constipation or diarrhea.

All of these symptoms can indicate other illness as well, but if you have any of them, you may want to ask your doctor to rule out cancer, just to be safe—even if he or she suspects another illness to be the cause.

Nobody knows your body quite like you do, though, and if you listen to God, He will give you wisdom about which doctors to see and what tests and treatments to pursue.

Proverbs 3:6 says, "In all your ways submit to him, and he will make your paths straight." If you aren't comfortable with a physician, it may be that God is telling you to move on until you find one with whom you will feel comfortable and at peace.

As a society, we tend to think that our doctors have all the answers, when in reality, they don't. You can help your doctor make an accurate diagnosis, however, by giving him or her as much detail as possible about how you are feeling and your symptoms.

Even more, the communication between you and your doctor should be bi-directional. In conventional medicine, patient-doctor visits are often rushed, and based more upon the doctor telling the patient what to do. But it's important that doctors learn to listen well to their patients and for the interaction to be two-way.

Perhaps you haven't yet been diagnosed with cancer, but suspect that you have a serious problem based on your symptoms. If your doctor doesn't know for certain what's wrong, insist on getting more tests done until you find out what the problem is. And if your current doctor can't help you, keep looking until you find one who can.

On occasion, my patients will say to me, "My doctor said my symptoms were caused by a cold, or a respiratory infection like bronchitis, so they basically ignored them." While most colds and cases of bronchitis are just that, they can, on occasion, indicate a more serious underlying illness.

For this reason, the doctor's priority should be to rule out the worst-case scenario, and not assume that a lump or persistent issue is due to a benign problem. Many of my patients had symptoms for months before they were diagnosed with cancer. But because their primary care doctors told them they had bronchitis or some other relatively benign problem that would eventually go away, they lost valuable treatment time.

The bottom line is that their doctors were not thorough enough in evaluating them.

Patients also need to take responsibility for their health, and not wait until their symptoms become serious before seeing a doctor. I once had a patient with a tumor in her breast, but waited until the tumor became the size of a cauliflower before she sought medical help. These kinds of mistakes cost patients and doctors valuable treatment time.

When you're sick or have symptoms that just won't go away, it's always better to rule out the worst-case scenario from the beginning. This is particularly important if you have cancer in your family or have been living an unhealthy lifestyle (e.g., if you are sedentary, not getting enough sleep, or have unhealthy nutrition).

Also take caution if you live near facilities or construction sites that emit cancer-causing chemical, electromagnetic or radiation-related toxins, such as a nuclear power plant or power lines. For instance, studies have found that children who live within 600 meters (1,968 feet) of a power line have an increased incidence of leukemia.[1]

In Southern California where I used to live, my family and I had moved into a house that had well water. About three years after we moved in, the former tenant called to tell us that his wife had passed away from kidney cancer. I suspected that her cancer was somehow linked to the quality of the water, so I immediately sent a water sample to a reputable laboratory for analysis. We discovered that it contained high levels of arsenic, cadmium and uranium—all of which have been linked to cancer! And even though we put filters in the water system, they still did not remove all of the heavy metals. So, we had to find a new source of water.

It's important to know about the chemicals and toxins that you are being exposed to in your environment, and to mitigate their effects as much as possible. Some basic strategies for cleaning up your home and body are found in Chapter 8 on detoxification.

Cancer Diagnostic Tests

At Hope4Cancer we do a variety of tests, including blood and imaging tests, to evaluate our patients before they start treatment. This enables us to determine the current status of their health as well as of the cancer, and what treatments they may need. We also do tests throughout their treatment process, to evaluate how well they are responding to the therapies. We use some of the same tests as conventional oncologists, along with many others, since no single standard blood test or imaging test is adequate to diagnose cancer.

Imaging Tests

PET and CT scans are arguably among the best scans for detecting solid tumors, and are most commonly used in conventional oncology. According to the American Cancer Society, however, both PET and CT scans emit 250 times the amount of radiation of just one X-ray![2]

A 2007 study, published in the *New England Journal of Medicine*, estimated that overuse of CT scans alone is responsible for 1.5-2.0% of all cancers. Based on the latest incidence rate, that would amount to approximately a million new cases in the next 30 years.[3]

If patients do these tests frequently enough, they become exposed to very high levels of radiation. In and of itself, such exposure can worsen cancer or even create new cancers in the body by causing healthy cells to mutate.

For this reason, we don't perform these tests at Hope4Cancer and I recommend avoiding them or minimizing their use. Other imaging techniques can be just as effective for detecting solid tumors, which I will discuss later in this section.

Now, if you or your doctor really want to do a PET or CT scan, I advise taking high amounts of toxin binders beforehand, as well as afterward. The best agents to use for this are chlorella or spirulina, which are natural substances that will help to "mop up" the radiation toxins.

In addition, you may want to do a detoxification therapy such as an infrared sauna, and drink ample amounts of purified water, which will help to minimize the effects of the radiation. To learn more about these detoxification approaches, see Chapter 8.

Another reason why PET scans aren't ideal is because patients must take radioactive glucose for the test, which cancer cells not only preferentially uptake, but also feed on. In fact, this type of glucose is their favorite food! (Radioactive glucose is given to patients before the PET scan because it lights up the tumor, so that when the scan is run, the tumor can be easily identified.)

Some of the imaging tests that we prefer, and which we use to detect solid tumors, include the ultrasound and magnetic resonance imaging (MRI). Both of these tests are used in specific situations, and are much safer than PET, bone or CT scans.

Sometimes, it's a struggle to get conventional doctors to recommend an MRI, but I have found it to be a good scan for detecting tumors. That said, all imaging tests can miss tumors, which is why a comprehensive testing approach is always best.

Again, no one particular test can definitively diagnose cancer, except for a biopsy. But unfortunately, a biopsy can be dangerous because it can spread cancer. A biopsy is a procedure in which a needle is inserted into a tumor or area of the body where cancer is suspected, and cells are collected for analysis.

During this process, cancer cells often become disturbed and dislodged from the tumor or area in question. They then can end up migrating to other areas of the body, either via the bloodstream or lymphatic system and interstitial fluid. This allows them to set up camp elsewhere in the body.

That biopsies spread cancer has been confirmed by multiple studies. For example, a 2014 study published in *Journal of International Society of Preventive and Community Dentistry* stated, ". . . several case studies have shown that after diagnostic biopsy of a tumor, many patients developed cancer at multiple sites and showed the presence of circulating cancer cells in the blood stream on examination."[4]

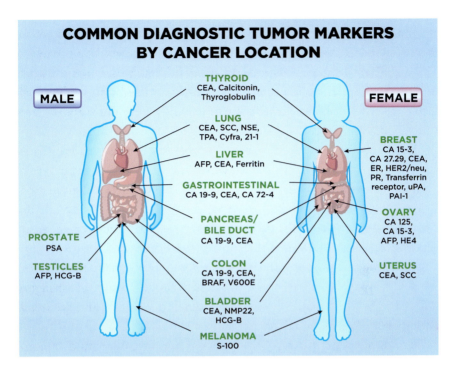

Figure 7. Common diagnostic tumor markers.

Biopsies aren't really necessary, though, unless you are going to do chemotherapy. When you do all the other tests that I share with you here, and receive a good clinical evaluation, they will give you a good indication of whether cancer is present in your body, and to what degree.

Cancer Marker Tests

Blood tumor marker tests are another integral part of our testing process, and are commonly used by conventional oncologists. Tumor markers are proteins or antigens that are produced by cancer cells or other cells of the body in response to cancer.

By themselves, positive blood tumor marker tests do not always indicate cancer, or how advanced the cancer might be. That is because cancer proteins—or antigens—don't always show up in the blood; or conversely, they may show up in excessive amounts relative to the total body burden of cancer.

In addition, some cancers don't secrete antigens or tumor proteins. As a result, doctors who rely solely upon this type of testing may be falsely led to believe that a person with cancer is in remission when in reality they are not. Yet, the test is generally useful for helping to substantiate a diagnosis, and for tracking treatment response.

Some examples of cancer antigen tests you may have heard of include: the PSA, which is a standard marker for prostate cancer; the CA 15-3 and CA 27.29, which are breast cancer markers; and the CA 125, which is an ovarian cancer marker. There are many others; these are just a few examples.

Circulating Tumor Cell (CTC) Test

It is not the tumor itself, but the spread of the cancer, or the metastasis, into vital tissues and organs that typically becomes a threat to the patient's life. CTCs are types of cancer stem cells (CSCs) that are key to the metastatic process. They break off from the original tumor and adapt to survive for long periods of time as they circulate in the blood looking for the next place to establish themselves. Testing for the presence of CTCs can provide valuable information regarding the presence and relative metastatic potential of the patient's cancer.

Most CTCs are mesenchymal cells that are formed from epithelial tumor CSCs through a cellular change known as the epithelial-to-mesenchymal transition (EMT).[5] As epithelial cells convert to mesenchymal cells, they lose identifying cell surface markers that make them even more invisible to immune surveillance. They also become more mobile, easily detaching from the tumor and entering the circulatory system. Once it reaches a potential target site, the mesenchymal CTC reverts to its epithelial form via a mesenchymal-to-epithelial transition (MET) and becomes the seed for the metastatic tumor.

CSCs can't be killed by conventional treatments such as chemotherapy or radiation; only by natural agents. This is one reason why conventional treatments can fail to eliminate cancer, and why cancer recurs in some patients who have only done conventional therapy.

The good news is, God has given us natural treatments that are effective at removing CSCs. I will share some of those with you in the following chapter.

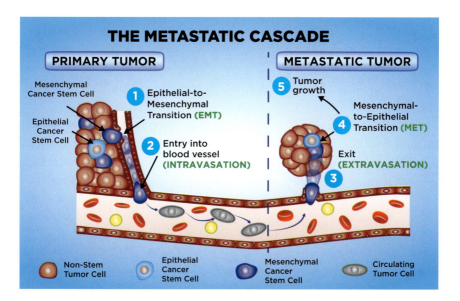

Figure 8. Circulating tumor cells and how they cause metastasis.

Finding a CTC is like finding a needle in a haystack because they exist in low numbers in the presence of billions of other cells in the circulatory system. In general, there are two approaches to testing for CTCs: the biochemical (or immunoaffinity-based) and the biophysical (label-free) methods.[6]

The biochemical methods rely on the identification, through laboratory tests, of specific biomarkers on the surface of the isolated CTCs that are indicative of the parent cancer. The two best-known laboratories that do CTC testing of this type are Cell Search, which is in the United States, and Maintrac, a laboratory in Germany. For the test, you simply go to your local lab, have some blood drawn and then send for processing.

Biochemical methods suffer from some major drawbacks. They are reliant on the identification of specific biomarkers that limit them to identifying only epithelial CTCs. As we discussed above, the majority of CTCs are mesenchymal, which cannot be detected with these methods. They rely on testing only a small sample of the blood, which adds to their poor sensitivity. They also require several hours to process the blood samples.

Biophysical methods leverage the physical properties of the CTCs such as density, electric charge, and size. These methods are "label-agnostic," which means that they do not rely on the presence of specific biomarkers on the cells, opening the possibility of identifying mesenchymal CTCs, the real culprits behind metastasis!

The finding of sensitive and accurate biophysical methods has been an enormous challenge for scientists. In the next section, however, I will describe an innovative method called Photodynamic Infrared Spectroscopy (PDIS). This is a method in development that has good potential to overcome many of these challenges. All in all, the CTC count is a good overall indicator of how much the cancer has progressed. Still, every single test that is used to detect cancer and patients' treatment progress must only be considered as a single data point in the overall picture. It must be evaluated along with other tests, to determine whether cancer is present and to what degree.

Photodynamic Infrared Spectroscopy (PDIS)

PDIS is a technology in development that can detect both epithelial and mesenchymal circulating tumor cells (CTCs) within the bloodstream; even a single one! It involves giving the patient a photosensitizer such as indocyanine green (ICG) or chlorin e6, which is infused into the bloodstream, and then preferentially taken up by cancer cells.

Subsequently, the blood is non-invasively screened for the presence of CTCs using a highly sensitive infrared spectrometer, which operates at a wavelength range of 400-1100 nm and picks up cells marked by the photosensitizer.

While PDIS is a breakthrough screening tool, the principles upon which it is based have been established in medicine over many years. These principles include photodynamic diagnosis and spectroscopy as established means of cancer testing.

PDIS has many advantages:

- It is very safe and minimally invasive.
- The photosensitizers that are used for the procedure are well-tolerated by patients.

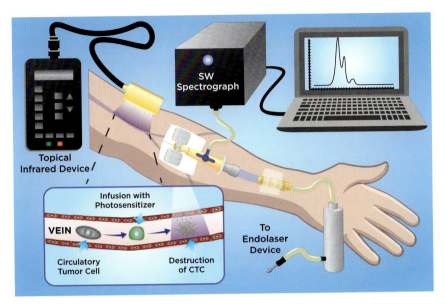

Figure 9. The Photodynamic Infrared Spectroscopy (PDIS) screening and treatment process.

- It scans the entire volume of blood flowing through the patient in real-time, not just a small sample sent to a laboratory.
- Importantly, patients aren't exposed to ionizing radiation, as is the case with other screening methods (CT and PET scans).

It is a truly remarkable screening tool; one that will be able to quickly establish metastatic potential, as well as monitor a patient's progress. Because it measures CTCs in the blood, it establishes more defined prognoses for our patients, and detects cancer cells before they form a tumor. In addition, PDIS is a useful tool for routine cancer screening, especially when there is a strong family history of cancer.

CTCs are often referred to as "silent metastatic disease," because they can lead to tumor metastases.[7] As cancer cells that are circulating in the blood, however, they aren't detectable on routine tests. Silent metastatic disease is associated with reduced survival in cancer patients, so being able to detect CTCs will enable us to achieve optimal outcomes with our patients.

Finally, PDIS is not only a screening procedure, but also a powerful treatment modality: if CTCs are detected, we can immediately administer Photodynamic Therapy to the patient, which will then destroy the marked CTCs in their bloodstream. See Chapter 4 for more information.

Indirect Cancer Marker Tests

While some tests directly indicate whether cancer cells are present in the body, other tests can indirectly indicate the potential presence of cancer, or whether conditions in the body favor their development down the road.

The following are additional tests that I recommend and encourage you to share with your doctor:

- **Lactate dehydrogenase, or LDH or LD.** This is an enzyme that is elevated under certain conditions, such as when a child's bones are growing; when elevated it can reveal liver problems or inflammation, or cancer.
- **High sensitivity C-reactive protein, or CRP.** When cancer is advancing, this marker is consistently elevated on lab tests.
- **Monocyte and lymphocyte counts.** These are cancer fighting cells that, when their numbers are low, can indicate cancer. Low white blood cell counts in general also indicate immune system suppression and potential cancer.
- **Hemoglobin or hematocrit.** Low numbers of either of these indicate anemia. Most cancer patients are anemic, so these are two important markers that can help to establish whether and how much the cancer is progressing.
- **Albumin.** This is the body's most abundant protein and an indirect marker for prognosis. The higher the albumin, the better the cancer patient's prognosis tends to be. I like for the patient's albumin to be at or above 4 mg/dl because my colleagues and I have found that those who have these levels fare better in their recovery.

Again, none of these lab markers alone can predict whether you have cancer, but when taken together, they can reveal whether cancer is likely to be present. Only a biopsy can tell you for sure if there is cancer in your body (but again, biopsies also spread cancer).

The Cancer Profile

The Cancer Profile© test is another valuable indicator that measures indirect markers for cancer, or other biochemical imbalances in the body that could indicate cancer. American Metabolics Laboratories and Metabolic Research, Inc., which were founded by Emil Schandl, PhD, created this test. The Cancer Profile also can be used as a tool for the early detection of cancer, as well as to monitor disease reduction or progress on cancer treatments.

The Cancer Profile includes a number of direct and indirect tumor markers. Among the most important of these is HCG, or human chorionic gonadotropin. HCG is a hormone that's elevated in women during pregnancy, as well as in people with cancer. Most cancer patients have an HCG range of 1-5; less than 1 is considered normal, while 1-3 is considered a gray zone. Dr. Schandl states on the American Metabolics Laboratories website that HCG is a broad-spectrum tumor marker that is found to be elevated in 70-80% of all people with cancer.

Another important marker that the Cancer Profile measures is the phosphohexose isomerase (PHI) enzyme. PHI plays an important role in causing healthy cells to become cancerous, and affects cancer cell division and growth, motility, and metastasis, among other functions. It also promotes angiogenesis, or new tumor blood vessel formation.

PHI may be elevated in patients with gastrointestinal, kidney, breast, colorectal, and lung cancers, and is an excellent marker that can be elevated in developing or existing cancers.

Normal results are <34.0 U/L (less than 34), with a gray zone of 35-40. That said, if there is an established malignancy, a change even within the normal range could be significant.

Other Tests

Other tests that are commonly used in conventional medicine (but which I don't generally recommend) are bone scans and mammography which, like PET and CT scans, expose patients to a lot of radiation.

According to the American Cancer Society, mammography exposes patients to 0.4 mSv of radiation,[2] the equivalent of about seven weeks of background radiation from the earth and space. While that may not seem like much, women may get anywhere from 25 to 50 mammograms over their lifetime, and the effects of radiation exposure are cumulative.

What's more, the results of mammography are not always accurate, and there is no research that proves that mammography prevents cancer or extends the patient's life. In fact, one landmark study published in 2014 in the *British Medical Journal* found that 22% of breast cancer patients evaluated were overdiagnosed based on their mammography tests, and survival rates are the same in women who do mammography versus those who don't.[8]

Mammography is purported to detect cancer early, before it becomes a problem. But the truth is, mammography only detects a cancer after it has reached 5 mm in size, when there are already many cancer cells in the breast and the cancer is fairly advanced.

Thermography is a better alternative to mammography for assessing abnormalities in the breast tissue that could indicate breast cancer. Thermography is a non-invasive test that looks for heat changes in the breast tissue and can detect an abnormality in the breast five years before it actually develops into a cancer. Our experience has shown it to be much safer and more accurate than a mammography! Many integrative doctors do thermography tests. To learn more about this type of testing, see: ALFAthermo.com.

In the end, the tests you need to do will depend on the type of cancer you have and where it's located in your body, among other factors. For instance, an MRI is used to detect brain cancer. A colonoscopy is used to detect colon cancer. A high-resolution pelvic MRI may be used to locate prostate cancer. A thermography test, along with an ultrasound and MRI, are used to detect breast cancer. All of these imaging tests would then be used, along with the appropriate blood marker tests.

Problems with the Conventional Approach to Cancer

Chemotherapy and radiation sometimes have their place in cancer treatment. One problem with these therapies, however, is that they are focused on eliminating cancer where it manifests in the organs, rather than removing the root causes of disease.

For example, if a person has colon cancer, the conventional approach is to remove the tumor, followed by chemotherapy and radiation, rather than focusing on healing the cellular dysfunction that caused the cancer in the first place. By removing the tumor, doctors only remove the manifestation of the disease, rather than the disease itself.

Consider this: the cell is the basic unit of life. Cells are used to make up tissues, while tissues make up organs, and organs comprise systems. All of these systems then make up the entire body. Cancer is a disease that starts at the cellular level, yet conventional medicine targets only the end organ where the cancer presents itself, rather than addressing it at the level of the cell.

Of course, we need to target the cancer in the organ that it shows up in, but for maximum benefit and outcome we need to heal cancer where it starts—not simply remove it from the organ(s) where it manifests.

Another problem with chemotherapy and radiation is that they are toxic to your body and weaken your immune system—which is what you most need to fight cancer! They also harm healthy cells as well as cancerous ones, and can potentially create new cancers in your body. Often, patients die not from their cancers, but from these treatments themselves. Whenever possible, it's best to look for alternatives to chemotherapy and radiation, but do listen to God and a good integrative doctor when making decisions about what to do!

At Hope4Cancer, most of our patients have already undergone and failed chemotherapy and radiation treatment. Yet in many cases, and with the help of God, we've been able either to help them completely recover, greatly extend their lifespan or, at least improve their quality of life. So healing, even in late-stage cancers, *is* possible without chemotherapy and radiation, especially when you have a faith-based approach to healing, coupled with determination.

That said, there are instances when chemotherapy and/or radiation are appropriate and necessary. For example, they can be the right course if a patient has a pancoast tumor, which is a tumor that presents itself in the apex or top upper lobe of the lung. In this case, it is crucial to give that patient radiation therapy right away as this is a very aggressive type of tumor that can lead to an array of symptoms. These symptoms include Horner's Syndrome or severe arm and/or hand pain.

As another example, chemotherapy is necessary whenever a patient has leukemia and white blood cell counts (WBCs) within the 80,000-100,000 range, because only chemotherapy can lower those numbers quickly enough. After that, it's best to follow up with natural therapies.

Other types of cancer that have shown to respond well to chemotherapy include lymphoma and testicular cancer. But even those cancers need to be treated at the root level using the 7 Key Principles outlined in this book, or you will only be treating the branches of the tree, not the roots!

Overall, though, chemotherapy and radiation have not been found to be very effective for most cancers. A meta-analysis, or combined analysis of clinical trials on more than 15,000 patients with 22 types of cancer that were studied from 1990-2004 revealed that the contribution of chemotherapy to the five-year survival rate of these cancer patients was only 2%.[9]

At our centers we do insulin potentiation therapy (IPT or IPTLD) in certain situations. This is low-dose chemotherapy that works in conjunction with insulin to more effectively target cancer cells. And because it does so with less medicine, there are fewer side effects. IPT is described in greater depth in Chapter 4.

Many doctors have had positive clinical outcomes using IPT, but not many studies have been done on it to date, so it is difficult to compare its effectiveness to full-dose chemotherapy. That said, most integrative doctors follow a multifactorial approach to cancer treatment, using IPT in conjunction with other treatments. So, it would be hard to isolate each treatment and evaluate how effective each one is individually.

IPT, however, has many benefits over traditional chemotherapy. First, it is much less toxic than full-dose chemotherapy because it requires anywhere from 20-40% of the full drug dose. As well, cancer cells don't become resistant to it as quickly as they do to traditional chemo.

Second, the quality of life of those who do IPT is much better than those who do full-dose chemotherapy, since it is less damaging to the gut, where 75% of the body's immune system resides. It may also be more effective than full-dose chemotherapy because it uses insulin to drive the treatments deeper into the cancer cells. I explain this concept in greater depth in Chapter 4.

Finally, and perhaps most importantly, you must know that chemotherapy doesn't kill cancer stem cells! In fact, an article published on August 15, 2017 on the National Cancer Institute website shared the results of a study **in which chemotherapy was actually found to increase the numbers of circulating tumor cells!**[10] It's imperative, then, to do natural therapies concurrently with chemotherapy and radiation, if you or your doctor decide that this therapy is best for the type of cancer you have.

Even surgery leaves behind CSCs. You can't cut cancer away. You can de-bulk a tumor mass through surgery, and this is sometimes important, especially if the tumor is obstructing an organ, but you will always want to do complementary therapies after doing any conventional treatment, to help eliminate CSCs. Remember, **cancer is rarely a local disease**.

In the end, though, I am a medical doctor, which means I'm not 100% anti-chemo or anti-radiation. Treatment must always be about what's best for the patient, which sometimes means chemotherapy and/or radiation. Sometimes, physicians need to take drastic measures with their patients.

Regardless of the therapies you and your doctor choose, however, you must always rebuild your immune system, since this is what you most need to overcome cancer. But you don't want to wait until you've failed chemo and radiation to do that!

Finally, as you know by now, cancer has many causes and represents a multifactorial problem. Therefore, it's going to require a multifactorial treatment approach that may include—but which always goes beyond—chemotherapy and/or radiation.

Final Thoughts

No single test by itself can be used to diagnose cancer, except for a biopsy, which has been shown to spread cancer. Unfortunately, conventional oncology often relies on dangerous tests such as this, along with PET and CT scans, when we have so many safer options available.

At Hope4Cancer, we utilize blood and other tests like thermography, in combination with safe imaging tests like the MRI, along with careful review of our patients' symptoms, to assess cancer. By doing things this way, we are able to effectively detect cancer and what it's doing in the body, without harming our patients in the process.

DIAGNOSING/MONITORING CANCER

Table 3.1.

Diagnostic Tests	Study Type	What It Measures	Advantages	Disadvantages
Positron Emission Tomography (PET) Scan	An imaging scan that uses a special dye that has a radioactive tracer. This tracer is either swallowed, inhaled, or injected into a vein in the arm, depending on what part of the body is being examined. The abnormal cells then absorb the tracer.	Pinpoints cancerous activity within the body, and can identify disease in its earliest stages, as well as the patient's immediate response to treatments. It reveals how the body is functioning and uncovers areas of abnormal metabolic activity. Cancer cells have a higher metabolic rate than noncancerous cells. Because of this high level of metabolic activity, cancer cells show up as bright spots on PET scans.	May yield more precise information about the cancer than exploratory surgery; provides unique information, including details on both the function and anatomic structure of the body that is often unattainable using other imaging procedures.	A PET scan can show how an organ is functioning, but without a CT or MRI image, it can be difficult to pinpoint the exact location of any cancerous activity within the body. It can also cause allergic reactions, and exposes patients to high levels of radiation.

continued on page 89

Diagnostic Tests	Study Type	What It Measures	Advantages	Disadvantages
Computerized Tomography and Computerized Axial Tomography (CT/CAT) Scan	An imaging procedure that uses special X-ray equipment to create detailed pictures, or scans, of areas inside the body.	Analyzes the internal structures of various parts of the body. It is used to diagnose muscle and bone disorders, such as bone tumors and fractures. It can pinpoint the location of tumors, infections and blood clots, and can be used to detect and monitor disease, as well as to evaluate the effectiveness of treatments.	A major advantage of the CT/CAT is its ability to image bone, soft tissues and blood vessels, all at the same time.	Some patients may have an allergic reaction to CT/CAT contrast materials that contain iodine. Soft-tissue details in certain areas can often be better evaluated with an MRI.
Photodynamic Infrared Spectroscopy (PDIS)	Screening test in which a photosensitizer is infused intravenously and preferentially taken up by cancer cells, to reveal the presence of circulating tumor cells in the blood.	Detects circulating tumor cells and can provide an estimate of treatment efficiency.	Minimally invasive, very accurate, and the results are obtained in real time. It is not only for screening but can also be used to see if a sensitizer was absorbed in tissue and to evaluate the efficacy of a treatment. Patient isn't exposed to radiation.	Sensitizer absorption limitations; may not be absorbed by all cancer cells.

continued on page 90

Diagnostic Tests	Study Type	What It Measures	Advantages	Disadvantages
Ultrasound (High-resolution Power Color Doppler)	A test that uses sound wave frequencies to create an image of tissues, lymph nodes and/or tumors.	Provides imaging and information regarding pathologies in the abdomen, breast, heart, lymph nodes, blood vessels, pelvis and musculoskeletal system.	Is a non-invasive procedure that can be used alongside CT, MRI and PET scans. It is an excellent tool for invasive procedures such as venipunctures, biopsies and resections. Can also be used to guide interstitial Photodynamic Therapy procedures.	It doesn't have the ability to penetrate bone; images may not be clear, due to the patient's body composition. Also, it may be more difficult to identify possible cancers in certain situations; for instance, if a person has gas or the lesions are hidden or deep in the body.
Magnetic Resonance Imaging (MRI)	A radiology technique that uses magnetism, radio waves, and a computer to produce images of body structures.	Useful for showing soft tissue structures and organs, and blood flow through organs/tumors.	Does not involve exposure to harmful radiation, and is useful for evaluating soft tissue, blood flow, swelling and inflammation.	Results can be affected by movement and can't be used if patients have metal implants.
Bone Scan or Scintigraphy	A type of nuclear radiology procedure in which a radioactive substance is used to assist in examining the bones. The radioactive substance, called a radionuclide, or tracer, will collect within the bone tissue in areas of abnormal physical and biochemical change.	A nuclear imaging test that helps to diagnose and track several types of bone disease, including bone cancer. It is very sensitive to any changes in bone metabolism. The ability to scan the entire skeleton makes a bone scan very helpful in diagnosing a wide range of bone disorders.	Provides details on both the function and anatomic structure of the body often unattainable using other imaging procedures.	Allergic reactions to the radioactive contrast medium may occur, but are extremely rare.

continued on page 91

Diagnostic Tests	Study Type	What It Measures	Advantages	Disadvantages
Mammography	An X-ray test that uses ionizing radiation to see inside the breasts.	Produces an image of breast tissue on film and reveals both normal and abnormal structures within the breasts. Therefore, it can help to identify cysts, calcifications, and tumors.	It can be used to detect earlier stage cancers; however, once a lesion is detected, it may already have spread.	Uses radiation, so there is a risk of side effects. Also, 22% of all mammograms give false positive results[8] so further testing such as additional testing with MRI or ultrasound may be required to verify results.
Thermography Two types: 1. Contact Regulatory 2. Digital Infrared	A probe or camera detects radiation in the long-infrared range of the electromagnetic spectrum and produces images of that radiation, called thermograms.	Is used for the early pre-clinical diagnosis of cancer, as well as to monitor the patient during treatment. Thermography is completely safe and uses no radiation.	It can detect vascular changes in breast tissue, even dense tissue and breast implants, many years in advance of other screening methods. Hormonal changes do not affect the results.	Can have false-positive and false-negative results, and is rarely covered by medical insurance. Does not detect cancer but an abnormality in the tissue.
Biopsy	For this procedure, a piece of tissue or sample of cells from the body is analyzed in a laboratory. This is the only way to definitively diagnose cancer.	Cancer cells in tissue.	The patient should receive a definitive diagnosis, recovery time is brief, and patients can soon resume their usual activities.	Bleeding, infections, and accidental injury to adjacent tissue structures can occur. Also, the amount of tissue obtained from a needle biopsy may not be sufficient and the biopsy may have to be repeated. Can spread cancer.

continued on page 92

Diagnostic Tests	Study Type	What It Measures	Advantages	Disadvantages
Tumor Marker Examples: 1. PSA (prostate) 2. CEA (GI tract) 3. CA 15-3 (Breast) 4. CA 27.29 (Breast) 5. CA 125 (Ovarian) 6. CA 19-9 (Pancreas)	Blood test.	A tumor marker is a biomarker found in blood, urine, or bodily tissues that can be elevated by the presence of one or more types of cancer. There are many different tumor markers, and they are used in oncology to help detect cancer.	Potentially useful in cancer screening, as well as in aiding in diagnosis; assessing prognosis; predicting the likelihood of a positive response to therapy; and monitoring patients with diagnosed disease.	There has been no evidence to prove that tumor markers are 100 percent reliable for determining the presence or absence of cancer. Many circumstances can contribute to elevated tumor marker levels. The main weakness of tumor markers is that they are not sensitive nor specific enough to detect cancer.
Circulating Tumor Cells (CTC)	Blood test and Photodynamic Infrared Spectroscopy.	Cancer stem cells circulating in blood.	Minimally invasive, and can play an important role in diagnosis as an adjunct to imaging. Studies suggest that the CTC is able to detect tumor recurrence in metastatic breast cancer patients before imaging tests detect it.	Expensive, is not regulated, and the blood test can have false positives, and is not accessible to all patients/clinics.
Cancer Profile	Blood/Urine test.	Based on the premise that detectable biochemical changes occur in the human body during its transformation into a cancerous state. It is composed of six tests: 1) HCG (human chorionic gonadotropin);	Measures a combination of six biomarkers which, when taken together, correlate with the development and progression of cancer. Three of these markers are tumor markers, and the other three evaluate the downstream effects of cancer on the organs and immune system.	There is insufficient clinical data to prove its accuracy. It is a useful tool but it needs to be correlated with the results of imaging studies. Can only be done at American Metabolic Labs in Florida.

continued on page 93

Diagnostic Tests	Study Type	What It Measures	Advantages	Disadvantages
Cancer Profile (cont.)	Blood/Urine test (cont.).	2) PHI (phosphohexose isomerase enzyme); 3) CEA (carcinoembryonic antigen); 4) GGTP (gamma-glutamyl-transpeptidase); 5) TSH (thyroid-stimulating hormone); and 6) DHEA-S (dehydroepiandrosterone sulfate).		
Monocytes and Lymphocytes	Blood test (Complete Blood Count- CBC).	Immune cells, the numbers of which are suppressed in cancers, especially those that affect the blood and bone marrow.	Simple test that can be done in any lab, and gives a quick assessment of the immune system.	Blood cell counts can be altered by many conditions, so imaging studies are needed to confirm the cause of abnormal values.
Lactate dehydrogenase (LDH)	Blood test.	Lactate dehydrogenase (LDH) can be a good indicator of cancer development and progression. LDH levels become elevated when cells and tissues are damaged, and are particularly high during active tumor progression into various internal organs.	Represents a very valuable enzyme in patients with cancer, with the possibility for easy, routine measurement in many clinical laboratories.	Patients with malignancies, but there are not enough clinical trials to prove it can be an accurate tool.

continued on page 94

Diagnostic Tests	Study Type	What It Measures	Advantages	Disadvantages
C-Reactive Protein (CRP)	Blood test.	Measures inflammation. With the discovery that cancer is strongly related to the body's overall inflammatory status, there has been a growing interest in CRP as a predictor of prognosis in people with a variety of cancers.	When CRP is measured at the time of diagnosis, high levels consistently predict poor survival, whereas normal levels (especially the lower-end of normal) predict good outcomes.	It is a general inflammatory marker, but is not specific for cancer. Therefore, imaging studies are needed to correlate/confirm the cause of high levels.
Hemoglobin (Hb)	Blood test.	Measures whether a patient has anemia, as well as the blood's ability to transport oxygen. Inflammatory cytokines such as TNF-alpha and IL-6, among others, play a major role in the possible causes of anemia in people with cancer.	Simple and accurate.	Further testing is needed to find out why the anemia exists.
Albumin	Blood test.	Measures one of the most important proteins in the body that can be correlated with the cancer patient's prognosis.	Is easy to do and part of a complete blood chemistry panel.	There are many reasons why albumin can be high or low.

SUMMARY

- Cancer is diagnosed using a variety of tools. No one exam or lab test can, by itself, tell you whether you have cancer.
- Imaging tests are used to diagnose solid tumors. MRI, ultrasound and thermography are among the safest tests used for this purpose.
- Direct and indirect blood tumor marker tests help to establish a diagnosis but must be used in combination with other tests.
- A circulating tumor cell (CTC) test can screen for the presence and metastatic potential of the cancer and monitor for success of treatments, and how advanced it is in your body.
- The Cancer Profile measures indirect markers of cancer and can be used to monitor progress on treatments.
- Chemotherapy and radiation sometimes have a place in cancer treatment but have side effects, cannot kill cancer stem cells, and weaken the body.

QUESTIONS FOR FURTHER REFLECTION

1. Why are PET and CT scans and mammography not the best diagnostic imaging tests for cancer?
2. What test is used to find cancer stem cells, and why are these cells the most dangerous?
3. What are some potential symptoms of cancer?
4. Why can't you rely upon just one testing method to diagnose cancer?
5. Why is a holistic, or integrative approach to cancer superior to the conventional one?

RIVI'S STORY

Rivi was diagnosed in 2012 with pancreatic cancer in her late 60s. She is a Bible scholar, author and public speaker whose teachings have been distributed internationally in nearly 30 countries. She has three daughters, including one named Tova, who was instrumental in helping with her treatment decisions. Despite many challenges, she is now cancer-free and doing well.

I was initially diagnosed with bile duct cancer in 2012, although at first, my doctors didn't agree on what type of cancer it was. Some claimed that it was pancreatic cancer; others said it was bile duct cancer. Eventually, they agreed on pancreatic, although on some level it didn't really make a significant difference, because pancreatic and bile duct cancer behave similarly in the body. Neither of them are promising diagnoses.

My journey into cancer started with a physician's assistant who assured me that I did *not* have cancer and that I could be healed with a simple operation. Later, at the hospital, as the doctors ran endless tests on me, we began to suspect that my healing was not going to be simple at all. The assistant's words seemed irresponsible.

The truth was that for three weeks leading up to that day, I had had the feeling that something terrible was about to happen to me, but I didn't know what it was. I believe in God, and I chose to trust that He would deal with it.

I never thought it would be cancer.

So when the doctors told me, I went numb. It didn't feel real. I wasn't afraid at that point, though. I was more in shock than anything else. It's hard to explain. Looking back, there were moments in which I felt like I was playing out the role of a robot, simply functioning and doing what I needed to do to get well.

The fear didn't come in until after I started my healing journey. It was only then that I realized I had been standing at death's door. So it was only when the real threat was pushed away from me that I actually began to feel the fear.

When I first met cancer, I was told that it was around a stage II or III, and that I would need a Whipple operation, which is one of the most complicated surgeries in medicine. The operation took 11 hours, and I was "under" (or sedated) for just over 13 hours.

During the operation, they cut out portions of my pancreas, liver and intestines, and took out my gallbladder and bile ducts. They then "re-plumbed me" so that everything could "work" again.

The surgery necessitated removing small parts of all these organs since they share a blood supply, and the cancer can easily migrate between them.

What I didn't know at the time was that the operation was risky, and there was a real chance that I would not come out of it.

Again, though, I trusted God that I would, and here I am today—alive as ever. Honestly, though, I'm glad I didn't know everything that was involved in the procedure and how dangerous it was beforehand.

Following my surgery, the doctors wanted me to do chemotherapy and radiation, to mop up any remaining cancer cells. I refused. They told me that I didn't need to be afraid of it, and pointed out how severe the Whipple had been, insinuating that the hardest part was over. What they did not know is that I have always had an aversion to chemo and radiation, even long before I was ever diagnosed. So I stood my ground.

My recovery following the surgery was long; almost four months. It was insane. It was difficult. It was a slow and painful recovery because it's such a horrendous operation. Four agonizing months passed before I could walk down a hall without assistance, or even sleep in my own bed. I had to sleep in an armchair in the living room for months. I was in major pain all the time.

My surgeon was still insisting that I do chemotherapy and radiation, saying that if I didn't, I'd end up with metastasis. So during the time when I was stuck in the armchair, I did a lot of research. My children and I thought that the cancer would probably come back unless I continued with some type of treatment, and decided that we'd better know what we were doing, so we looked into everything out there. I do research for a living, so it came naturally to me, and what I found confirmed my gut feeling: there was no way I was going to do chemo.

When I went back to be tested, for the first time following the surgery, the tests revealed that I in fact already had metastasis to my liver. The cancer was now at a stage IV. The surgeon insisted that I absolutely had to do chemotherapy or radiation or else I would die within six months.

All of this happened within the first four months of my diagnosis.

At this point, it was "all systems go." My kids and I decided that we needed to make some major changes in our lives. We had already changed our lifestyle and diets and removed all of the cancer-causing toxins from our home. I had done some Vitamin C IVs, based on research that I had found which showed that Vitamin C in large amounts could kill cancer. But with this new diagnosis, it became apparent that the cancer was too aggressive and that we needed more help. Fast.

My surgeon said I needed treatment immediately. I had two weeks to decide what to do. During those two weeks, my family and I aggressively researched all of the alternative cancer clinics we could find.

As a cancer patient, when you start looking at clinics, it's all extremely confusing. You don't know who (if anyone) is telling the truth, and how to differentiate between all the options you are learning about. Luckily, I knew what type of treatments I wanted to do, and we focused on finding a clinic that would do those.

We visited several clinics in Mexico, and decided on the Hope4Cancer Treatment Centers. Dr. Tony was a big part of why we chose Hope4Cancer. The first day we met, he sat me down and patiently answered all my questions, explaining everything I wanted to know, even taking the time to draw out diagrams. He seemed kind and genuinely caring, as well as knowledgeable, and I appreciated the fact that he had answers for every question and concern that I brought up to him.

I also discovered that his work at the treatment center was on the cutting edge of medicine, and appreciated that he frequently traveled to check out new treatments and bring back what he learned to the center.

There was a lot that I appreciated about the treatment center. They spoke English, unlike some of the other places we had visited. They offered all the therapies I was interested in, unlike many of the other clinics and treatment centers, which did not have such extensive options.

Another thing I liked about Dr. Tony and Hope4Cancer was the fact that they offered a follow-up, at-home treatment program. This was important for us, as my family was very concerned about what would happen when I arrived home. It was overwhelming to think that we might have to do it all ourselves. Unfortunately, many cancer clinics have programs that leave patients confused in the aftermath, once they are at home alone.

During my stay at Hope4Cancer, I did a number of treatments, including Dr. Tony's Sono-Photo Dynamic Therapy, high dose intravenous Vitamin C, coffee enemas, a detoxification protocol, lots of supplements, and much more.

When I first arrived, they ran a lot of tests, one of which measured the amount of activity in the tumor's blood vessels. Tumors get their nutrients through blood vessels, so eliminating the blood vessels that feed them is important.

After just two weeks of treatments at the center, there was a 60% reduction in the blood vessels around the tumor. It was good news. I knew we were doing the right thing. When I went home, I did all the at-home treatments that the Hope4Cancer staff gave me. They also showed me what to do.

I returned to the clinic a month later for a follow-up visit, and then for another one two months after that.

Four months after I first went to Hope4Cancer, I no longer had any tumors.

I no longer had cancer.

This was astounding. Dr. Tony told me to go back to the hospital to have an MRI so we would know for sure that the tumors were gone, so I did. I went back to the surgeon and sure enough, the MRI showed no cancer.

My surgeon was dumbfounded. He rechecked the results. The odds of something like this happening were below 1%.

When the results came back the second time, they revealed the same thing. There was no cancer in my body.

The surgeon sat down with me, took a paper and pen, and wanted to know everything I had done. Everything. So we went over the details and everything I had done to get well. I truly believe that it changed how he now looks at cancer.

The truth is, I was supposed to be dead six months after my diagnosis, according to the doctors.

Instead, after two weeks of treatments at Hope4Cancer, and four months of treatments at home on my own. . . I was now cancer-free.

It was a miracle.

We were very happy when we got the news. It was right before my daughter's birthday, and it made for an extra-special celebration.

I was so grateful that the treatments worked, though I know in my heart that it was not just the treatment that had miraculously healed me. It was also the hand of God, as well as the prayers of many people around the world.

Today, it has been more than eight years since my diagnosis, and almost eight years since the cancer disappeared. Dr. Tony and I have remained friends; he is a genuinely wonderful person.

I am healthy and grateful to still be here to speak to other people who are—or have been—in my situation. I tell them that no one can tell you when you are going to die, and there are always possibilities available to you. I truly pray my story brings hope to those of you who feel like there is none.

4

Effective Integrative Cancer Therapies

KEY PRINCIPLE #1
NON-TOXIC CANCER THERAPIES

Did you know that some of the most powerful and effective cancer treatments are made from plants and other elements that God created, such as light, water, oxygen and sound? It's as if God knew when He created the world that one day we would be facing an epidemic of cancer. As a result, He provided us with an environment rich in anti-cancer compounds that would meet our other survival needs, as well.

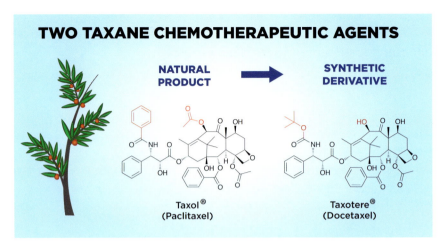

Figure 10. Most of our drug "ideas" derive from the natural world. Plants and animals create a variety of chemical and biochemical compounds designed to protect themselves from invading pathogens. Many of these substances have been leveraged, because of their toxicity, to be used as drugs. Taxol® is a prime example of a popular chemotherapeutic agent obtained from the bark of the Pacific Yew tree. Subsequently, laboratory alteration of its structure led to another popular chemotherapeutic, Taxotere®.[1] Nature is our grand designer and provides us the resources we need to survive—as long as we choose wisely.

Remarkably, many of these compounds are more effective than chemotherapy drugs and radiation at eliminating cancer, and at the same time, are gentler and safer for the body. Further, God designed them so they would be toxic to abnormal cells, but harmless to healthy ones. Moreover, that they would not only kill cancer, but also support the body on multiple levels.

Which would you prefer, treatments that knock out cancer cells but are toxic to the body and don't address the root causes of disease, or those that are non-toxic, effective for eliminating cancer, and heal the body's terrain? At our treatment centers, we have many healing solutions that don't involve harming the body, and are more comprehensive than treatments that simply kill cancer cells.

As well, we believe that the effects of these natural therapies are potentiated and made supernatural when we pray over them, as well as when we pray over our patients. Consequently, prayer improves our patients' outcomes.

KEY PRINCIPLE #1 | EFFECTIVE INTEGRATIVE CANCER THERAPIES

We have developed 7 Key Principles[2] that form the foundation of our cancer treatment program. They include:

1. Non-Toxic Cancer Therapies
2. Immunomodulation
3. Full Spectrum Nutrition
4. Detoxification
5. Oxygenation
6. Restore the Microbiome
7. Emotional and Spiritual Healing

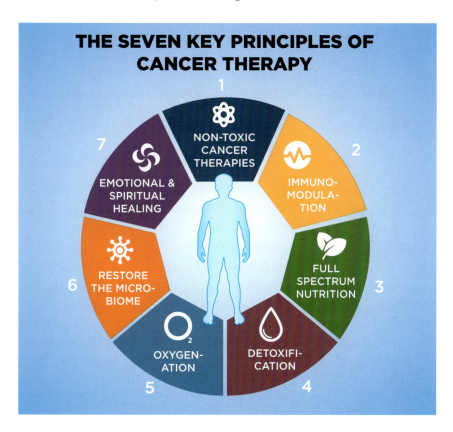

Figure 11. The 7 Key Principles of Cancer Therapy form the bedrock of our treatment philosophy and have guided the healing process for our patients for more than 25 years. These principles were first published in a peer-reviewed journal in 2012.[2]

103

No single therapy or key principle by itself is sufficient to heal from cancer. But when we design a protocol for a patient based on the 7 Key Principles, we are able to not only heal the cancer in the person, but the person with the cancer! And because we are multifaceted beings with a spirit, soul and body (if you'll recall, our soul encompasses our mind, will and emotions), our approach addresses all aspects of who we are.

In this chapter, I will share with you the first Key Principle of Cancer Therapy, which is Non-Toxic Cancer Therapies. These therapies have cytotoxic, or cancer-killing properties, but also strengthen the immune system and heal the body in other ways. Some of these overlap with the immune therapies that comprise Key Principle #2 and which I share about in the following chapter, but are also mentioned here for their cytotoxic benefits.

You may find that other integrative cancer doctors prescribe some of the treatments that I share with you here. A few are relatively well known and widely utilized within integrative medicine, while others are unique to Hope4Cancer.

Therefore, if you are unable to come to Hope4Cancer, you may be able to find a doctor in your area that uses some of these approaches. For best results, though, I recommend visiting Hope4Cancer so that you can take advantage of the synergistic effect that the therapies provide when you do them all together.

On that note, no single therapy I share with you here is a standalone solution for cancer. Each one must be combined with others to effectively address all of the cancer's survival mechanisms and heal the body. You may find that a number of integrative oncologists do some of the following therapies in combination with others that we do not offer at Hope4Cancer, and their approach may or may not be as effective or beneficial as ours.

In any case, I recommend thoroughly researching the treatment approach of any doctor or clinic that you consult with, and talking to their former patients. And of course, do your research before determining whether a different treatment program using only some of the following therapies or others is best for you. Either way, you will want to find a program that incorporates all of the 7 Key Principles that we describe here.

I do not recommend doing any of the following therapies as a stand-alone approach to cancer. As I mentioned in Chapter 2, **cancer has many survival mechanisms that can only be addressed through a comprehensive, multifaceted healing program.**

In addition, because we do all of the following therapies together, we cannot say which are the most beneficial for any one particular person. However, we do know that in combination, they have cancer-fighting and immune-boosting properties; they function in synergy with one another; and their effects are enhanced whenever they are administered together.

When the treatments are done collectively as part of our 7 Key Principles approach, we have seen remarkable outcomes in many of our patients. About 75 percent of our patients have metastatic cancers and approximately 70 percent have a history of prior toxic conventional treatments. But with God's help, they are often healed or their lives are significantly extended, and/or their quality of life is greatly improved!

Core and Foundational Therapies

Our cytotoxic, or cancer-killing therapies are divided into two categories: core and foundational. Our core therapies are the most powerful and are diagnosis-specific; that is, they are prescribed according to the type of cancer patients have, and are based on the first Key Principle of Cancer Therapy. The foundational therapies enhance the benefits of the core therapies, are based on the other six Key Principles, and are given to everyone.

At the time of writing, some of our core therapies include: Sono-Photo Dynamic Therapy (SPDT), Photodynamic Therapy Plus (PDT Plus), Sunivera and Helixor (or mistletoe), all of which are powerful anti-cancer treatments that also enhance immune function. The foundational therapies also have anti-cancer properties and include many treatment options, such as hyperthermia, ozone, intravenous Vitamin C and Vitamin B-17, or Laetrile—among others.

Once we start treatment, we periodically monitor our patients with objective tests such as labs and scans, as well as subjective tests that clinically evaluate their physical and emotional symptoms.

Sono-Photo Dynamic Therapy (SPDT)

Sono-Photo Dynamic Therapy (SPDT) involves using sound and light, in combination with a sensitizing substance called SP-Activate, to target cancer cells. Photodynamic Therapy (PDT) uses light, while Sonodynamic Therapy (SDT) uses sound. Since 2004, Hope4Cancer has treated more than 4,000 patients with these signature therapies, making us the most experienced clinic in the world in this therapeutic area.

For both of these therapies, the patient first takes SP-Activate, which is a natural, non-toxic derivative of chlorophyll, which is given sublingually (or under the tongue). It is dosed based on the patient's body weight, and is absorbed mostly by cancer cells in a ratio of 70:1; meaning, that for every 70 cancer cells that absorb it, only one normal cell uptakes it.

After giving the patient the SP-Activate, we then wait 24-36 hours. During this time, the cancer cells continue to absorb the substance, while any normal cells that initially absorbed it, end up releasing it (rather than retaining it). This effect has been documented extensively not only for photosensitizers, but also other drugs, and is known as the Enhanced Permeability and Retention (EPR) Effect.[3]

The EPR Effect is usually attributed to the poorly developed and disorganized vasculature and lymphatic drainage of the tumor. These features allow for easier accumulation but harder elimination of surrounding photosensitizers and other macromolecules.

Now, SP-Activate has no chemically or biologically active properties—until it is "awakened," or activated by specific sound or light wavelengths and intensities. But once it is activated by sound and/or light, it produces reactive oxygen species (ROS), which are free radicals, or negatively charged oxygen molecules, that kill cancer cells upon contact.

Another essential benefit of SPDT is that it decreases angiogenesis, the process by which new blood vessels form in and around tumors. Tumors get their nutrition via these blood vessels, so by stopping the

KEY PRINCIPLE #1 | EFFECTIVE INTEGRATIVE CANCER THERAPIES

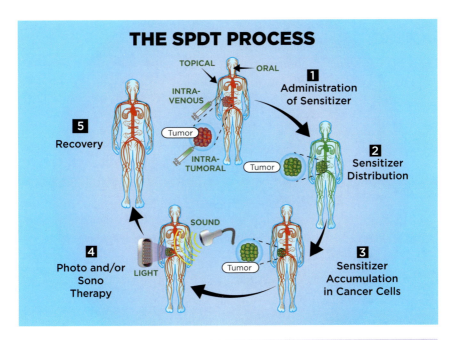

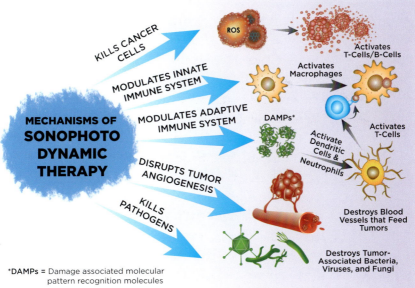

Figure 12. (a) Representation of a typical Photo or Sonodynamic Therapy treatment process. **(b)** The multiple mechanisms of Sono-Photo Dynamic Therapy.

creation of new ones, we can effectually deprive them of their food source and reduce the flow of nutrient-rich blood to them. We can also reduce the tumor's ability to eliminate toxins and metabolic waste.

Further, SPDT activates the immune system and recruits immune cells to migrate to the site of the tumor. In addition to destroying cancer cells, SPDT has also been effective in eliminating tumor-associated pathogens.

Finally, given the non-toxic nature of the components, SPDT is very useful as a long-term treatment for the tumor, without the side effects of other conventional approaches.

SPDT is very useful for all types of cancer except brain tumors, because it doesn't penetrate through bones such as the skull. Also, the SP-Activate sensitizer only absorbs into solid tumors, so it isn't effective for blood cancers like leukemia. However, new developments in PDT technology, described in the next section, allow us to address cancers in ways that were not possible before.

Why do we need both light and sound activation? While photodynamic light activation is backed by decades of research, it has been notoriously difficult to get light to penetrate past the superficial layers of the skin (however, see PDT Plus section below). Sound, on the other hand, can travel through water very successfully. Since the body is made of 75-80% water, sound waves use that leverage to travel to tumor sites located deep in the body.

Depending on the type and location of the tumor, we can determine the best way to apply the two methods. By combining IV Photodynamic Therapy with Sonodynamic Therapy, we can:

1. Stop the tumor's growth.
2. Reduce its size.
3. Eliminate any circulating tumor cells.

Photodynamic Therapy Plus (PDT Plus)

Photodynamic Therapy Plus (PDT Plus) uses advanced multi-wavelength laser light technology that delivers specific wavelengths in the ultraviolet,

LIGHT AND SOUND TECHNOLOGIES USED IN SPDT AND PDT PLUS

We use a variety of sound and light technologies for SPDT, including:

- **Light beds,** which provide either full spectrum or infrared and red laser lights across the patient's entire body, therefore targeting cancer cells throughout the body, including all tumors and metastases.
- **Advanced pulsed LED light technology,** which delivers LED light to the body and penetrates it more deeply than other types of light.
- **Fiberoptic laser technologies that can deliver light intravenously, topically, or directly into the tumor (interstitially).** An upgraded form of this technology delivers laser light endoscopically to target cancers in different internal organs.
- **Topical light technology devices including a laser watch,** and intranasal and intraaural devices that deliver light to the body via the blood vessels in the wrist, sinuses, and ear canal, respectively.
- **Ultrasound technology,** which delivers a specific sound frequency and intensity to the body that can activate absorbed sensitizers.

visible, and infrared regions of the spectrum. PDT Plus uses fiberoptic technology to deliver laser light through catheters that can be applied intravenously, topically, or directly into the tumor. By employing this technology, PDT Plus has overcome one of the most significant drawbacks of prior PDT technology—its poor depth of penetration.

Each of the laser light wavelengths is capable of activating photosensitizers specific to that wavelength, significantly increasing the range of effectiveness of the PDT methodology. For example, curcumin, hypericin (St. John's wort), and indocyanine green (ICG) administered intravenously, are three photosensitizers that are activated by blue, yellow and infrared wavelengths, respectively. SP Activate, which is given sublingually, is activated by red light. Activated by the deeply penetrative infrared wavelengths, ICG has even been used to treat bone metastasis.

In addition to their role as photosensitizers, some of our photosensitizers have well-researched and useful anti-cancer (and other) health benefits of their own. Curcumin is an excellent example, with extensive health benefits. According to a study published in April 2017 in *The Journal of Traditional and Complementary Medicine*, curcumin stops angiogenesis, suppresses inflammation, stimulates immune function, quenches free radicals that cause cellular damage, halts metastases and stops tumor cell proliferation.

After administering the photosensitizer, we then use fiber optic lasers to deliver specific light wavelengths depending on the photosensitizer used either through a vein or directly into the tumor. Sometimes we also inject the photosensitizer directly into the tumor.

Specific light wavelengths individually have profound therapeutic benefits and can be used by themselves for health and wellness applications. This type of therapy is known as "photobiomodulation" or "low-level laser therapy" (LLLT). I describe the benefits of photobiomodulation in more detail in Chapter 9.

PDT Plus is one of the state-of-the-art technologies at Hope4Cancer Treatment Centers that can be used alongside PDIS technology (described in Chapter 3), when available, to not only detect but also destroy CTCs. By screening for the presence of CTCs in blood, PDIS allows us to determine the potential for metastasis in a patient, and at the same time, destroy the identified CTCs.

The benefits of PDT Plus include the ability to: 1) deliver light directly into or close to the tumor location; 2) treat freely circulating tumor cells (CTCs) that are responsible for metastasis; 3) maximize the use of different photosensitizers and their corresponding light wavelengths.

It is possible to effectively treat blood vessels close to the surface of the body with laser light technology entirely non-invasively.

The PDT Plus Watch delivers laser light wavelengths directly to activated cancer cells via the blood vessels in the wrist. These blood vessels are very close to the surface of the skin. To activate the cancer cells, the patient first takes an oral photosensitizer. It's a fantastic way to accomplish the results of intravenous laser therapy without even having to use a needle!

Also, we use intranasal and intraaural lasers to deliver light directly into the brain, ears, or sinuses, all of which are used as pathways to target tumors in the brain. The nose is the best access point to the brain; light travels very well there.

Light therapies don't just have cytotoxic properties. Like many things that God has given us in nature, they serve a multitude of purposes. Among these, they:

1. Increase oxygen uptake to the blood.
2. Enhance metabolic processes.
3. Decrease and remove bad proteins like LDL lipoproteins (or cholesterol) from the blood.
4. Stimulate the mitochondria and ATP, or energy production.
5. Stabilize healthy cell membranes.
6. Help increase the release of melatonin.
7. Demonstrate antimicrobial effects.

Measurable Effects of SPDT

Before and after treating our patients with SPDT, we perform a high-resolution, color ultrasound on and around the tumor area and affected lymph nodes, to evaluate the vascular flow. This enables us to see how the therapy has affected the tumor blood vessels. Studies at Hope4Cancer have consistently shown that our patients have anywhere from a 48-54% decrease in vascular flow to their tumors or lymph nodes after just three weeks of SPDT therapy, as compared to their baseline ultrasound.

Formally published studies also confirm the effectiveness of SPDT. For example, one study, the results of which were published in *Ultrasonics Sonochemistry* in March 2015, showed SPDT to markedly inhibit tumor

HEALTH BENEFITS OF DIFFERENT LIGHT WAVELENGTHS AND ASSOCIATED PHOTOSENSITIZERS USED FOR PDT PLUS

Table 4.1.

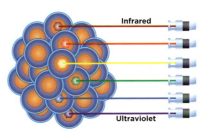

Color	Wavelength	Associated Photosensitizer
INFRARED	810 NM	INDOCYANINE GREEN
• Photodynamic and photothermal effects • Treats metastatic lesions in deep tissues as well as in bones • Used for cancer cell imaging, as well as circulating tumor cell detection and destruction		
RED	658 NM	CHLORIN E6
• Improves blood flow and blood cell characteristics • Activates macrophages • Improves proliferation of lymphocytes (B- and T-cells) • Stimulates production of immunoglobulins and cytokines • Improves oxygenation and energy metabolism • Improves micro-circulation		
YELLOW	589 NM	HYPERICIN
• Improves antioxidant enzymatic system • Antidepressant and pain-relieving benefits • Improves serotonin and Vitamin D production • Improves hormonal function		
GREEN	532 NM	NONE
• Improves function and elasticity of red blood cells • Improves oxygenation, reduces lactic acid formation • Reduces blood viscosity (thickness) • Regulates mineral balance and overall homeostasis • Increases cellular energy production		
BLUE	405 NM	CURCUMIN, RIBOFLAVIN
• Releases nitric oxide which dilates blood vessels, promotes cellular regeneration, and modulates immune system • Lowers blood pressure • Activates telomerase with potential anti-aging benefits • Reduces pro-inflammatory cytokines		

continued on page 113

KEY PRINCIPLE #1 | EFFECTIVE INTEGRATIVE CANCER THERAPIES

Color	Wavelength	Associated Photosensitizer
ULTRAVIOLET	375 NM	NONE

- Strengthens immune system and detoxifies
- Increases tissue oxygenation
- Destroys pathogens
- Improves circulation and dilates blood vessels
- Improves Vitamin D synthesis

growth and cancer cell migration in lab mice with breast cancer metastases to the lungs. The researchers also found that when Sonodynamic Therapy and Photodynamic Therapy were combined, they were much more effective than when either therapy was used alone.[4] A review published in 2014 concluded that SPDT is a promising new treatment for a variety of cancers.[5]

We have found that SPDT, when used as part of the 7 Key Principles of Cancer Therapy, is effective for treating solid tumors that are located in organs such as the pancreas, prostate, breast, bladder, colon, esophagus, lymph nodes, spleen, kidneys and liver. SPDT has also been found effective in the treatment of melanoma, head and neck cancers, lymphomas, and sarcomas. Intravenous Photodynamic Therapy can be used to target leukemias and brain cancers.

In summary, Sono-Photo Dynamic Therapy:

- Targets cancer cells both locally and systemically.
- Reduces tumor burden.
- Reduces tumor vascularity.
- Activates/modulates the immune system.
- Destroys pathogens.
- Improves patients' quality of life.

Vitamin C

Vitamin C may be one of God's most powerful natural cancer-fighting substances. It has antioxidant and pro-oxidant effects, depending on the dosage that's used and how it's administered, so it not only heals the body and strengthens the immune system, but can also eliminate cancer cells and pathogenic microbes.

Incidentally, **humans are one of few mammals that don't synthesize their own Vitamin C.** In the wild, when an animal becomes injured, its body's production of Vitamin C increases by a thousand-fold, which activates wound healing. Yet in humans, this doesn't happen. When we are sick or injured and our bodies require much more Vitamin C, we must obtain it externally, from supplements and food, since we can't make it ourselves.

In cancer recovery, Vitamin C is needed to support both the body's immune function and repair processes, and is also extraordinarily useful for killing cancer cells, including cancer stem cells.

When it is given in lower doses of up to 12.5 grams daily, Vitamin C acts primarily as an antioxidant. It strongly supports proper immune system function and scavenges DNA-damaging free radicals that can cause cancer.

It activates natural killer (NK) cells, which are among the most important immune cells involved in fighting cancer. It also boosts interferon, a signaling protein that is involved in immune function—among other things. Vitamin C is involved in a number of the body's repair processes, such as connective tissue repair.

When given intravenously and in doses above 12.5 grams daily, Vitamin C acts as a pro-oxidant and causes hydrogen peroxide to form inside cancer cells. Hydrogen peroxide is very toxic to cancer cells, yet doesn't harm normal ones. This is because normal cells produce high amounts of an enzyme called catalase, which neutralizes the peroxide. A few cancers produce catalase, but many (or most) don't.

The late Linus Pauling, PhD, one of the most influential biochemists in history and a two-time Nobel Prize winner, was the first researcher to prove that high doses of Vitamin C were lethal to cancer. In the 1970s, he and British cancer surgeon Ewan Cameron, MD, used 10 grams (or 10,000 mg) of intravenous Vitamin C, followed by 10 grams of oral Vitamin C daily, to treat terminal cancer patients. Many of these patients apparently went into remission, or experienced dramatic improvements to their well-being as well as increased longevity, as a result of the treatment. Dr. Pauling's book, *Vitamin C and Cancer*, provides a history of some of these patient cases.

What's even more exciting is that studies at the University of Salford in the UK have recently proven something that we at Hope4Cancer have hypothesized for years: Vitamin C can destroy not only tumors, but also cancer stem cells,[6] which, if you'll recall, cannot be eliminated using conventional therapies. It does this by inhibiting energy production at the cancer cell's mitochondrial level.

According to an article published on June 12, 2017 on the university's website, researchers showed Vitamin C to be up to 10 times more effective at stopping cancer cell growth than pharmaceutical drugs that are used for that purpose, such as 2-Deoxyglucose (2-DG). Yet they say that when Vitamin C is combined with an antibiotic, it is up to 10 times more effective, making it nearly 100 times more effective than 2-DG.[6]

Patrick B. Massey, MD, PhD, Medical Director of Complementary and Alternative Medicine at Alexian Brothers Hospital Network, and President of ALT-MED Medical and Physical Therapy, confirms the powerful anti-cancer effects of Vitamin C. In an article published on April 29, 2017 in the *Daily Herald*, he cites studies from the University of Manchester (England), University of Calabria (Italy), and the Albert Einstein College of Medicine (United States), which have demonstrated that Vitamin C interrupts the Krebs cycle in cancer stem cells. The Krebs cycle is a metabolic pathway used by cancer cells to generate energy, in addition to glycolysis.[7]

According to Dr. Massey, one large study published in *Cancer Epidemiology, Biomarkers and Prevention* demonstrated that taking Vitamin C reduces the risk of mortality as well as the recurrence of cancer in breast cancer patients, because of how it affects cancer stem cells. For this study, nearly 5,000 women who took oral Vitamin C were followed for four years and found to have an 18% reduced risk of mortality and a 22% reduced risk of cancer recurrence.[7]

Many other studies demonstrate the multifaceted benefits of Vitamin C in cancer treatment. For instance, one analysis of 15 studies, published in *Neuroepidemiology* in 2015, showed that oral Vitamin C intake was associated with a lower risk of developing glioma, a deadly brain cancer.[8] In another analysis of 17 studies that included 4,827 pancreatic cancer cases, oral Vitamin C intake was associated with a decreased risk of pancreatic cancer.[9] Many other studies show similar positive benefits of Vitamin C for other types of cancer.

We administer 25 grams of Vitamin C intravenously to our patients, slowly over a period of two hours, three times per week. We recommend that our patients continue taking Vitamin C orally after they return home, for its antioxidant and immune-supportive benefits.

To determine your ideal Vitamin C dosage for immune enhancement purposes, start by taking 1,000 mg daily and increase by 500 mg daily until you reach bowel tolerance, or start having loose stools. This is called the "C-flush" dose. Non-corn, non-GMO sources of Vitamin C made from cassava or beets may be the best tolerated and safest for the body. I also prefer buffered forms of Vitamin C (sodium ascorbate) as well, because most people's stomachs tolerate them better.

Laetrile, Amygdalin, Vitamin B-17

Laetrile, amygdalin and Vitamin B-17 are three terms used interchangeably to refer to a natural, yet powerful cytotoxic compound found in the seeds of certain foods. "Amygdalin" in Greek means almond, since bitter almonds are one principal source of this compound, in addition to apricot, peach and plum seeds, and a handful of fruits. For cancer treatment purposes, however, the main source of amygdalin (or Laetrile and Vitamin B-17) comes from apricots.

Like many other natural treatments that we use, amygdalin is selectively toxic to cancer cells. Again, it's as if our Creator made these wonderful substances in nature that were designed to benefit normal cells, and at the same time, remove any harmful ones.

Ironically, mainstream medicine has argued that amygdalin is dangerous because it contains cyanide, a compound that they contend is toxic to normal cells, as well as to cancerous ones. What they don't understand, though, is cyanide is only released inside the cancer cells, not the normal, healthy ones!

I have been using amygdalin since 1988 and to this day, I've never had a patient experience any toxic reactions from it. This is because cancer cells contain an enzyme called beta-glucosidase, which is what triggers the release of cyanide from amygdalin, which can kill the cells. Normal cells don't have this enzyme. So while amygdalin penetrates both types of cells, cyanide is only released selectively into cancer cells.[10]

Actually, when beta-glucosidase comes into contact with amygdalin, it breaks into not one, but two entities, cyanide and benzaldehyde—both of which are toxic to cancer cells.

A study review published in the *Journal of Cancer Research and Therapeutics* in August 2014 summarizes the pharmacological activity, toxicity and antitumor activity of amygdalin.[11] The researchers say, "It (amygdalin) has anticancer function by decomposing carcinogenic substances in the body, killing cancer cells, blocking nutrient source of tumor cells, inhibiting cancer cell growth, and could also reduce the incidence of prostate, lung, colon and rectal cancers."[11]

The researchers go on to say that amygdalin has been manufactured and used to treat cancer in more than 20 countries, including Mexico, the United States, Germany, Italy, Japan and the Philippines.

We give amygdalin to our patients both orally and intravenously. The ideal therapeutic dose when it's given orally is 500 mg, 30 minutes before each meal, and 500 mg before bedtime, for a total of 2,000 mg daily.

Amygdalin is a very powerful remedy, but like all of our treatments, it is not a standalone solution for cancer. It is also very safe and effective, with no side effects. Some practitioners give their patients amygdalin intramuscularly, but it's painful when done this way, so I prefer oral or intravenous methods of administration.

Unfortunately, decades ago the FDA banned doctors' ability to prescribe amygdalin in the United States or Canada. However, any citizen of the world can come to Mexico or another country where it is legal, such as Germany, or other parts of Europe and Asia, purchase it, and then bring it back to their home country legally. Currently, it's used most extensively in Mexico, home to its main manufacturing facilities.

Amygdalin has an auspicious history and reputation for being a powerful anti-cancer agent. When I started working as an integrative cancer doctor in 1988, we would give our patients coffee enemas and amygdalin, and put them on a good nutritional program. Oftentimes, that was enough to get them well. Now, our environment and bodies are more toxic, and we are surrounded by more negativity, spiritual darkness and bad news than ever before. This is part of the reason why we maintain our focus on improving our treatments to serve our patients better.

I also believe that cancer cells have mutated more in recent years. Like many types of microbes, they have adapted to their environment. As a result, we now have to be more aggressive and comprehensive in our treatment approach. Amygdalin continues to be a powerful workhorse in our treatment arsenal, however, and a fundamental component of our recovery program.

Sometimes I see people with cancer taking amygdalin on their own in the form of apricot kernels. While taking kernels can be a good preventive strategy, it is difficult to get enough of the amygdalin compound in the seeds for cancer treatment purposes. To do that, you'd have to ingest ½ to 1 pound of kernels daily! But for cancer prevention purposes, taking 20-40 kernels per day may be sufficient, depending on your history.

If you have a stage III or IV cancer, I recommend doing amygdalin treatments intravenously. If you have a stage I or II cancer, oral amygdalin supplements may be adequate.

The beauty of amygdalin is that it can access and reach all areas of the body, including all the organs. Thus, it is even useful for cancers of the brain, where not all treatments reach. Another great benefit of amygdalin is that it affects all types of cancer (unlike other natural treatments) because all cancer cells contain beta-glucosidase.

Again, though, every day cancer treatment becomes more complicated, and there are many intangible factors involved in healing from cancer. These include such things as removing environmental toxins, toxic relationships, and undue stress from the person's life. We can't adequately quantify the effects of these factors, so amygdalin is just one element of our treatment program.

Amygdalin takes time to work in the body. Initially, patients can expect their quality of life to improve and the disease to stop progressing, and over time, their tumor burden to diminish.

Finally, another nice benefit of amygdalin is that it has analgesic properties and can alleviate pain; some patients report a general feeling of overall well-being from taking it.

Helixor (Mistletoe)

Helixor is an aqueous solution of fresh plant extracts that come from the white-berry mistletoe. This type of mistletoe is mainly found on three types of trees: the apple, fir and pine. Ironically, mistletoe is a plant that's called "a cancer on a tree," and at the same time, it's a remedy that treats cancer!

Long revered for its history as an effective cancer treatment, mistletoe has been studied for more than 40 years, and used around the world in many integrative cancer clinics, especially in Europe. Over 7,000 scientific publications confirm the benefits of mistletoe.

Mistletoe plant extracts are cytotoxic and eliminate cancer through a variety of mechanisms. They also enhance immune function, and improve patients' quality of life, by reducing fatigue and other symptoms.

Some of the most important cancer-fighting compounds in mistletoe include, but are not limited to:

Glycoproteins - These mistletoe "lectins" as they are called, cause apoptosis, or cancer cell self-destruction. They activate macrophages, which are a type of immune cell involved in fighting cancer, and release other chemicals that increase immune response.

Polypeptides - These cause cancer cell membranes to leak. They also activate macrophages and increase the activity of granulocytes. Granulocytes are a type of immune cell that "engulfs" cancer cells.

Oligo- and polysaccharides, arabinogalactans, galacturonans -These compounds indirectly suppress tumor activity. They also stimulate T-helper cells, which play a role in immune function, and increase natural killer (NK) cell activity. NK cells play a major role in directly killing cancer cells.

Flavonoids - These help to induce apoptosis, and have antioxidant and anti-inflammatory effects, the latter of which indirectly help the body to fight cancer.

Mistletoe extracts are therefore multifactorial in their effects, and their compounds work synergistically to disable cancer and heal the body. It's amazing that God has created plants like mistletoe, which not only kill cancer cells through a variety of mechanisms, but also support the immune system and heal the body at the same time!

In short, mistletoe does all of the following (see Figure 13):

- Modulates the immune system, and in so doing, reduces the body's susceptibility to infections
- Indirectly inhibits tumor growth via immune modulation
- Stimulates apoptosis, or cancer cell self-destruction
- Lowers angiogenesis, or tumor blood vessel formation
- May regress tumors
- Stabilizes the DNA of normal cells
- Increases a patient's tolerance to chemotherapy and traditional treatments
- Improves a patient's quality of life as it reduces fatigue, increases appetite, and provides them with a greater sense of well-being

Hundreds of laboratory studies and clinical trials on humans validate the immunomodulatory and life-enhancing effects of mistletoe. Many of these studies are also summarized in the Physician Data Query (PDQ - Health Professional Version) in the National Institute of Health's National Cancer Institute website which can be accessed at: https://www.cancer.gov/about-cancer/treatment/cam/hp/mistletoe-pdq.

Mistletoe therapy should be done for at least six months to a year, sometimes longer, because its effect on the immune system builds with time. Fundamentally, mistletoe is used for all types of cancers, and has beneficial systemic effects, and so creates an unfavorable environment in which cancer cannot survive.

Different types of mistletoe are indicated for different types and stages of cancer. According to the Helixor company, mistletoe's tumor-inhibiting effects are strongest in people with carcinomas (mainly in elderly persons) and when given in high doses in close

KEY PRINCIPLE #1 | EFFECTIVE INTEGRATIVE CANCER THERAPIES

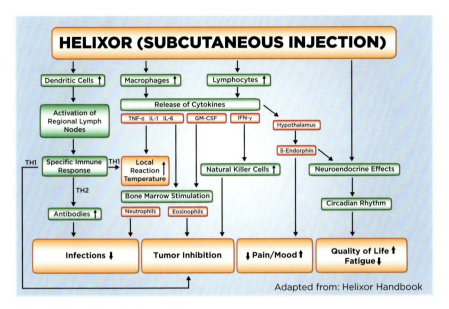

Figure 13. The effect of Helixor mistletoe treatment.

proximity to the tumor. When mistletoe is given along with other treatments, its effects are often potentiated and enhanced.

Tumor-inhibiting effects are less likely to be observed in people with sarcomas, malignant systemic disease, and primary brain tumors.

Also, the more the disease has progressed, the higher the dosages of mistletoe that are required for treatment. Mistletoe is dosed according to the stage of disease and the degree of tumor malignancy.

Hyperthermia

Give me a chance to create a fever, and I will cure any disease.
PARMENIDES, GREEK PHYSICIAN, 500 BC

Heat and fever therapy have been used for centuries in Ayurvedic, Traditional Chinese Medicine (TCM), and other traditions to treat ailments such as cancer and arthritis. Hippocrates, the Father of Medicine, also used it to treat inflammatory diseases and cancer.

Over the centuries, science and medicine have proven that whenever you can raise the temperature of the body by inducing a fever, you will stimulate both the innate and adaptive immune systems, increase tissue detoxification, and kill pathogenic infections. In addition, cancer cells are intolerant of heat and will break open, or lyse, once the body reaches a certain temperature. Higher temperatures affect cancer cells, but leave healthy cells unharmed.

Indeed, when you get the flu, what happens? Your body naturally produces a fever to eliminate the pathogens that cause the flu, right? Well, inducing a fever in your body when you have cancer can stimulate your immune system to go after the cancer, as well.

Hyperthermia is one type of heat therapy that we use to induce a fever reaction. We use two kinds of hyperthermia: full-body hyperthermia, which heats the entire body, and localized hyperthermia, which we use to target specific regions of the body.

Full-Body Hyperthermia

Full-body hyperthermia systemically targets abnormal cells and pathogens by raising the temperature of the entire body. For the procedure, patients enter an insulated chamber that uses carbon-derived heat to elevate the body's temperature. Our goal is to raise the patient's oral temperature to 101.4° Fahrenheit (or 38.6° Celsius) for the greater part of a 45-minute cycle. The core body temperature rises to about 1.5°-2.0° Fahrenheit above that. At this temperature, cancer cells lyse, or start to break apart.

The patient's head is kept outside of the chamber during the treatment, because it must be protected from excessive heat. In addition, we administer oxygen during the procedure, which is delivered to the patient's body through a nasal cannula. This creates a synergistic effect between the oxygen and hyperthermia, and allows us to deliver a "double whammy" to the cancer.

Even more, full-body hyperthermia is safe, painless and does not harm healthy cells. Our patients typically receive this therapy every other day during their stay at Hope4Cancer.

Local Hyperthermia

Local hyperthermia involves applying heat locally to tumors, at temperatures of 104°-113° Fahrenheit, or 40°-45° Celsius. This therapy functions differently than whole body hyperthermia in that rather than creating a fever in the body, it functions solely by heating up the tumor.

Yet its effects upon cancer are otherwise the same as full-body hyperthermia; the sustained elevated temperature deprives cancer cells of their ability to absorb substances needed for their survival, by destabilizing the blood vessels that feed the tumor. It also causes them to lyse, as in full-body hyperthermia. The surrounding healthy tissues remain unharmed.

Local hyperthermia is painless and harmless; it can be applied using a number of energy devices or technologies, depending on the tumor location. The method that we utilize involves placing two electrodes between two ends of the tumor area and then delivering a radio frequency current to the area. The low frequencies generated by local hyperthermia allow for it to be applied to even sensitive areas of the body.

There are contraindications to local hyperthermia, so you want to be monitored by a healthcare practitioner if you do this therapy.

Benefits of Hyperthermia

Hyperthermia impacts the body at many levels. Among these, it:

1. Restricts tumor blood flow. Since tumors get their nutrition from blood vessels, hyperthermia deprives them of nutrient-rich blood. This results in the collapse of the tumor's vascular system.
2. Causes tumor cell lysis, or breakdown.
3. Creates a heightened immune system response so that immune cells can more effectively go after the cancer.
4. Increases tissue oxygenation and detoxification. Cancer doesn't just perish in the presence of heat, but also when it's exposed to oxygen.
5. Increases energy and promotes cellular repair and regeneration.

A handful of studies have demonstrated the anti-cancer effects of hyperthermia. For example, one trial on 50 sarcoma patients, the results of which were published in *European Journal of Cancer* in 2001, showed that hyperthermia doubled the five-year survival rate of those that used it in addition to conventional therapy.

We have also tracked the progress of some of our patients who have been treated with hyperthermia. For example, one 52-year-old woman with stage III breast cancer with metastases to her sternum and lymph nodes had a 90% reduction in blood flow to her breast tumor just six months following her first treatment.[12] Similarly, a 78-year-old man with prostate cancer had a 90% reduction in blood flow to his tumor a year following his first treatment. Additional patient studies have shown dramatic reductions in tumor blood flow, as well.[12]

Hyperthermia also kills many cancer-causing pathogens, and we've found it to potentiate the effects of other therapies we pursue, such as Sono-Photo Dynamic Therapy.

Hyperbaric Oxygen Therapy (HBOT)

Oxygen sustains life, except when it comes to cancer and many pathogenic infections, which do not survive well in its presence. This means that any therapies that increase oxygen to your cells are extremely valuable in helping you to heal from cancer. Not only because they aid in destroying cancer cells, but also because they improve the functioning of your normal, healthy cells.

We do a number of diverse therapies that increase oxygen to the cells, tissues and organs, including hyperbaric oxygen (HBOT) and ozone, both of which I will share more about with you here.

First, HBOT involves delivering oxygen to the body under high pressure. For HBOT, the patient is placed in a chamber where the pressure of oxygen can be increased and controlled. Under normal circumstances, oxygen is transported throughout the body only by red blood cells. With HBOT, oxygen is dissolved into all of the body's fluids including those of the plasma, as well as the central nervous, lymphatic and skeletal systems, and can be carried to areas of the body where the circulation is diminished or blocked.

This matters because tissue damage or cancerous growth occurs in places where there is a low supply of oxygen. HBOT can make inroads into these areas and supply them with much needed oxygen. Consequently, the cancer is more susceptible to apoptosis not only from the oxygen, but other treatments as well, the effects of which are enhanced by oxygen.

HBOT is simple, painless and non-invasive. It is used as an adjunct treatment for many different conditions in addition to cancer, and is extremely safe when performed under medical supervision. The most common side effect is reversible barotrauma to the ears and sinuses, which is caused by the change of pressure that occurs during the therapy. Sometimes changes in vision may also temporarily occur.

HBOT penetrates the body more effectively than many other oxygen therapies, as the pressure involved in the therapy allows the oxygen to go deep into the organs and tissues. HBOT is beneficial for all types of cancers.

Many studies support HBOT's benefits in cancer therapy. For instance, one review published in 2016 in *Medical Oncology* concluded, "HBO (hyperbaric oxygen) can provide many clinical benefits in the treatment of tumors, including management of highly malignant gliomas (a type of brain cancer)."[13] Further, the researchers stated that it can enhance the effects of conventional therapies, and we have found it to enhance the benefits of our natural/integrative ones, as well.

This review focused on brain tumors, but similar studies and reviews on HBOT have shown it to affect other tumors, as well. For instance, a study published in *BMC Cancer* on January 30, 2007 showed HBOT to stop angiogenesis in lab rats with breast tumors.[14]

Ozone Therapy and Its Administration

Ozone (O_3) is a gas that's found naturally in the atmosphere, but which also has been used worldwide for many years in integrative clinics to treat a variety of conditions, including cancer. When ozone enters the body it breaks down into oxygen, and provides some of the same healing benefits as HBOT, although the oxygen generated by ozone generally does not go as deep into the body as HBOT.

However, ozone's benefits go beyond oxygenation. In the presence of biological fluids, adequate doses of ozone generate conditions of acute, yet mild, oxidative stress through the production of transient reactive oxygen species (ROS). This ROS triggers the cellular defense mechanisms that are capable of preventing cellular damage through nucleic acid, protein, and lipid oxidation.[15]

In chronic diseases associated with oxidative stress, destructive quantities of reactive oxygen and nitrogen species are formed, which leads to cellular damage and biomolecular oxidation. The use of ozone can decrease the chronic oxidative stress in these pathologies by activating cellular defense mechanisms.

Thus, ozone has a twofold effect upon cancer cells: it floods them with oxygen, which disfavors their survival; and activates antioxidant cellular mechanisms in the cells, which counters oxidative stress conditions in the diseased cell.

But that's not all! Ozone provides a multitude of other benefits to the body, which include:

1. Helping to eliminate xenoestrogens and other carcinogenic—or cancer-causing—toxins via oxidation.
2. Increasing levels of immune-stimulating and cancer-fighting cytokines, or chemicals.
3. Increasing levels of superoxide dismutase (SOD).
   SOD is an enzyme that is involved in the body's antioxidant defense system.
4. Optimizing white blood cell counts, which are immune system cells that help to ward off cancer.
5. Increasing microcirculation to healthy cells.

Ozone also improves the function of healthy cells, and jumpstarts their mitochondrial function. The mitochondria are the cell's powerhouses that provide energy to the cell. Recent research by Thomas Seyfried,

PhD, author of *Cancer as a Metabolic Disease: On the Origin, Management, and Prevention of Cancer* suggests that cancer is caused by mitochondrial dysfunction,[16] and provides evidence that healing the mitochondria with various modalities can help the body to overcome cancer.

By improving the functioning of healthy cells, ozone enables normal cells to better eliminate cancer-causing contaminants and pathogens, which cause inflammation and damage the body in a variety of ways.

Thousands of studies have demonstrated that ozone is both a safe and beneficial adjunct therapy for cancer and many other disease conditions. It has been used for over 50 years; the International Ozone Association reports that more than 7,000 doctors in Europe safely use medical ozone.

We also use cold plasma ozone therapy, which involves using a generator with a blue-tinted glass tube to deliver high concentrations of ozone directly to the skin. It is primarily used to treat external tumors of the breast and lymph nodes; since the liver is very close to the surface of the body, this therapy can be used to treat liver tumors as well.

Like some of our other treatments, we recommend that our patients continue ozone treatments at home after they have finished their therapy at Hope4Cancer. You can find information on purchasing affordable, home-use ozone generators at hopeforcancerbook.com.

At-home ozone treatments are simple to do; you just need to purchase an oxygen tank and tubing to use along with the generator, and then follow the instructions that come with the device. Companies that sell ozone equipment can also often direct you to videos and resources where you can learn how to use the generators.

I have found rectal and vaginal ozone, along with drinking ozonated water, to be very safe and beneficial ways to get ozone into the body. We have also found that it doesn't create toxic oxidative stress in the body.

Insulin Potentiation Therapy (IPT or IPTLD)

Insulin Potentiation Therapy (IPT or IPTLD) is a method that uses insulin to effectively transport cytotoxic treatments into cancer cells. For IPT, low doses of chemotherapy drugs or natural remedies are used, although chemotherapy drugs are most commonly used.

For the procedure, the patient comes to the treatment center in the morning, after fasting from 12 AM onward. Before we begin the therapy, we check his or her vital signs and initial blood glucose levels to get a baseline reading. We then lower the patient's blood sugar to 40-50 mg/dl, using insulin, and then administer the chemotherapy or cytotoxic agent.

Cancer cells have seven times the amount of insulin receptors on the surface of their cell membranes, and 10 times as many insulin growth factor (IGF-1) receptors as normal cells. Think of the insulin and IGF-1 receptors as windows and doors on the cancer cell. When we give patients insulin, these windows and doors open, so that they become more receptive to the chemotherapy. The effects of the chemotherapy are therefore potentiated, targeted and enhanced.

After we lower the patient's glucose level, we start administering the chemotherapy. Normally, IPT is done using only 10% of a full dose of the chemotherapy, but we've found that we get better results by using a higher dose than that—anywhere from 25-35%. Using one tenth of a dose "teases" the cells, but causes them to become more resistant to the chemotherapy, whereas our clinical experience has been that using 20-35% of a full dose is effective and yet still relatively safe for the body.

Using IPT effectively targets cancer cells and allows you to get a greater effect with less medicine and fewer side effects.

Another benefit of IPT is that it prompts cancer cells to divide, which is when they are most vulnerable to being destroyed by cytotoxic treatments.

In addition, there is less collateral damage to healthy cells with IPT than with full-dose chemotherapy. That's because healthy cells have fewer insulin and insulin growth factor receptors on the surface of their cell membranes, so most of the chemo goes to the cancer cells. Consequently, patients experience much fewer side effects (if any) with IPT than with full dose chemo. They don't lose their hair or have diarrhea or nausea, or get other significant side effects from the treatment. Whatever side effects they may get, are easy to mitigate. And, if they are going to get side effects, these usually occur within the first 24 hours following treatment, but then quickly go away.

Using IPT in integration with our other therapies tends to mitigate any side effects from the chemotherapy, and even potentiate its benefits. For example, intravenous Photodynamic Therapy works synergistically with IPT because some chemotherapy drugs act as photosensitizers, which means that the effects of the chemotherapy are potentiated when it is given along with Photodynamic Therapy.

Despite its low dose, IPT still involves the use of chemotherapy that can decrease blood cell counts. That is why we monitor our patients' red blood cells, hemoglobin, white blood cells and platelets before and after the therapy. So if any of the cell counts become too low, we have to correct those before we can do the next IPT treatment.

Usually, IPT treatments are done every 7-10 days, depending on our patients' blood cell counts and how they are feeling. We do 6-8 treatments per cycle. Like all of our other therapies, IPT is always done as part of a 7 Key Principle-based protocol.

We don't use IPT on all of our patients, or even a majority, because in most cases, we don't have to. We use it selectively, whenever we need to "buy more time" and are waiting for the other therapies to start working. We also use it in acute situations; to quickly shrink a tumor that may be obstructing an organ or critical function of the body. For instance, there could be a tumor in the esophagus or lungs that is blocking the airways, or affecting the patient's ability to breathe or swallow.

IPT isn't a new therapy. It was invented by Donato Perez Garcia, MD, a Mexican doctor who first pioneered the use of insulin to treat other illnesses such as syphilis in the 1920s, and further developed it for use in cancer treatment in the early 1930s. He used it for decades to treat a wide variety of cancers, including cancers of the breast, lung and prostate. His son, Donato Perez Garcia Bellon, MD, and grandson, Donato Perez Garcia, Jr., MD, adopted their father's and grandfather's IPT approach and used it on their patients, as well.

From 1946 onward, other doctors began to use IPT; but it never gained mainstream traction, since it was backed only by a few formal studies. Today, IPT is a popular approach in the treatment toolbox of many integrative doctors worldwide. These doctors' clinical experiences with their patients have demonstrated that it is both a safe and effective cancer treatment therapy.

IPT is beneficial for treating many kinds of cancer, and we have found it to be a valuable treatment for some of our patients, when strictly indicated.

Studies confirm the benefits of IPT. For instance, in one study on breast cancer patients at George Washington University, IPT was found to increase the killing effects of methotrexate, a breast chemotherapy drug, by a factor of 10,000.[17] In another, it was found to potentiate the effects of chemo drugs used for esophageal and lung adenocarcinoma cells.[18]

Poly-MVA

Poly-MVA is a powerful nutritional supplement that we've been giving our patients for a long time. It provides energy to compromised body systems by changing the way that the cells produce energy, and by facilitating proper cellular metabolism. It also works to heal the cells by repairing damaged or altered DNA, and by supporting the body's antioxidant processes.

As such, it can also alter the metabolism of cancer cells so that they begin to act as healthy cells again. Further, it boosts the body's immune response by replenishing key micronutrients and supporting cellular metabolism.

Finally, Poly-MVA functions as a photosensitizer that's activated by red and near infrared light, which means that it can also be used in Photodynamic Therapy.

The inventor of Poly-MVA, Merrill Garnett, DDS, PhD, developed a lipoic acid mineral complex, which is the key ingredient of Poly-MVA, and mimics an energy pathway that's present in normal cells but missing in cancer cells. Once inside a cell, this compound increases the production of ATP, or energy, in normal cells. However, when it enters cancer cells, it disrupts their preferred glycolytic energy pathway, and causes them to die.

According to the Poly-MVA website, Poly-MVA may do all of the following:

- Assist in preventing cellular damage and enhance proper celluliar function
- Support cellular and tissue oxygenation
- Help the body to produce energy for proper cell function
- Support the liver in removing harmful substances from the body
- Work as a powerful antioxidant
- Support nerve and neurotransmitter function

All of these effects help the body overcome cancer by supporting healthy energy production, detoxification and metabolic processes.

Poly-MVA contains a proprietary blend of palladium, alpha-lipoic acid, vitamins B1, B2 and B12, the amino acids formyl-methionine and acetyl cysteine, and trace amounts of molybdenum, rhodium, and ruthenium.

I have the most experience of any practitioner in the world in the use of this product, and I was the second doctor to give it to patients intravenously. I have also taught other doctors how to use it. It's not something that I give to all of our patients, but it's part of our toolbox. I use it mostly on my patients with brain cancer because it crosses the blood brain barrier, unlike many nutritional supplements. I also use it when patients aren't getting the response that I'd like from other therapies.

Near Infrared Sauna Therapy

God has provided us with many amazing ways to use light, heat, oxygen and other natural elements to overcome cancer. Another therapy we utilize that involves the use of light is the near infrared sauna. Near infrared represents physiologically relevant wavelengths of light that resonate with the body's natural energy, which means that the body recognizes it as familiar and non-threatening.

Like far infrared sauna therapy, which is the type of sauna therapy most people are familiar with for detoxifying and relaxing the body, near infrared light sauna also detoxifies the body but has a number of other benefits. Among these, it:

- Reduces the body's pathogenic load, by killing infection-causing bacteria and viruses.
- Helps to eliminate cancer-causing chemical toxins such as heavy metals, via the perspiration process.
- Reduces the body's radioactive "load" that patients may carry as a result of prior radiotherapy treatments and imaging studies.
- May relieve pain and improve blood flow.
- Stimulates the immune system and reduces inflammation.

Another benefit of near infrared therapy is that it can be used as a type of Photodynamic Therapy, which can help to eliminate cancer cells when used along with SP-Activate or another photosensitizer.

We recommend that our patients do infrared sauna therapy three-four times per week. You may want to purchase an infrared sauna for use at home. For information on where to purchase affordable and safe infrared saunas, check our book website, hopeforcancerbook.com.

Near Infrared Lamps

Focused near infrared lamp therapy, which uses the same type of technology as near infrared saunas, is another valuable supportive therapy that we employ.

Near infrared lamps aid in detoxification, reduce inflammation and pain, and promote deep tissue healing. Like near infrared saunas, they can also be used as a type of Photodynamic Therapy when used in conjunction with a photosensitizer like SP-Activate, and potentially aid in destroying cancer cells.

You don't need to go to a cancer clinic to benefit from infrared sauna or infrared lamp therapy. You can purchase your own sauna or infrared lamp online or at a variety of retailers.

SUMMARY OF NON-TOXIC CANCER THERAPIES

Table 4.2.

Non-Toxic Cancer Therapies	What It Is	How It Works	Benefits
Sono-Photo Dynamic Therapy	Uses a variety of light and sound therapies along with a photosensitizer to destroy tumors.	Light and sound therapies activate photosensitizers in cancer cells, which release oxygen radicals that are toxic to cancer.	Causes apoptosis, stops angiogenesis, stimulates the immune system.
Helixor (Mistletoe)	Plant extracts of mistletoe.	Compounds in mistletoe destroy cancer and support the immune system.	Suppresses tumors, stops angiogenesis, causes apoptosis, stimulates immune system, mitigates symptoms.
Amygdalin/Vitamin B-17/Laetrile	Natural substance found in apricot pits and other fruit seeds.	Selectively releases cyanide inside of cancer cells, which is lethal to them.	Destroys cancer cells, has analgesic and pain relieving properties.
Vitamin C	Vitamin that has both antioxidant and pro-oxidant benefits.	At low doses, it stimulates the immune system and scavenges free radicals. At higher doses it causes lethal hydrogen peroxide to form inside of cancer cells.	Strongly supports the immune system and connective tissue, scavenges free radicals, and directly kills cancer stem cells.
Hyperthermia	The application of heat locally and systemically, via hyperthermia chambers and devices placed over the tumor area.	Heat is directly applied to tumors to destroy them. Heat applied systemically kills cancer and induces a fever, which stimulates the immune system.	Causes apoptosis, stops angiogenesis, stimulates the immune system, kills cancer-causing pathogens.
Hyperbaric Oxygen	High-pressure oxygen therapy is administered in a chamber.	Oxygen penetrates deeply into tumors that thrive in a hypoxic environment.	Destroys cancer cells while supporting healthy ones. Heals the body, reduces inflammation.

continued on page 134

Non-Toxic Cancer Therapies	What It Is	How It Works	Benefits
Poly-MVA	Supplemental nutritional formula.	Provides energy to the body, facilitates proper cellular metabolism and repairs DNA.	Supports the overall health of the body, indirectly destroys cancer cells.
Near Infrared Light Therapy (Lamp and Near Infrared Sauna)	Light therapy that uses infrared wavelengths applied both locally and systemically.	Infrared heat and light reduces inflammation, kills pathogens and cancer cells, and supports healing.	Reduces pain and inflammation, while also helping to destabilize cancer cells.

Final Thoughts

Our experience and research has demonstrated that all our treatments, when done together, are extraordinarily beneficial for a majority of our patients. All are safe, non-toxic, powerful, and heal the body while also destroying cancer cells—which is how cancer treatment should be.

If you can't come to our treatment centers, you can still take advantage of the benefits of some of these therapies by doing them at home or with the help of your local doctor. We encourage you to call or email us at Hope4Cancer to learn more about this program!

SUMMARY

- Some of the most powerful and beneficial cancer treatments come from plants and other elements that God created in nature, such as light, water, oxygen and sound.
- Every therapy that we use at Hope4Cancer is non-toxic, natural and safe for the body, yet has powerful cytotoxic effects.
- Sono-Photo Dynamic Therapy (SPDT) is one of our signature treatments; it uses sound and light along with a photosensitizer, to help eliminate cancer cells.

KEY PRINCIPLE #1 | EFFECTIVE INTEGRATIVE CANCER THERAPIES

- Vitamin C supports immune function at lower dosages; at higher levels it eliminates cancer cells by creating hydrogen peroxide within tumors, which destroys them.
- Amygdalin, or Laetrile/Vitamin B-17, a natural compound that's found inside the seeds of apricots and some other fruits, releases cyanide within cancer cells, while leaving healthy cells unharmed.
- Hyperthermia uses heat to disable cancer through a variety of mechanisms. Whole-body hyperthermia stimulates immune function by inducing a fever, while also heating up tumors and destroying their vasculature and other cellular components. Local hyperthermia focuses on applying heat directly to the tumor.
- Ozone therapy oxygenates the body while also killing microbes and cancer cells via its oxidative properties. Oxygen supports the body's healing processes, yet is toxic to cancer cells.
- Helixor, an aqueous solution of mistletoe extract, supports immune function and has powerful cytotoxic effects upon cancer.
- Poly-MVA is a nutritional supplement that supports energy production, DNA repair and the normalization of metabolic processes.
- Near infrared sauna supports detoxification and creates a fever-like effect in the body, which stimulates the immune system.

QUESTIONS FOR FURTHER REFLECTION

1. What are some of the principal benefits of Sono-Photo Dynamic Therapy?
2. How does hyperthermia heal the body in patients with cancer?
3. Why does low dose Vitamin C have different effects upon the body than high dose Vitamin C?
4. Why does the cyanide in amygdalin affect cancer cells, but not normal ones?
5. How does ozone support the body, in addition to directly killing cancer cells?
6. Why must multiple therapies be combined for optimal effect?

5

Tools That Empower Your Immune System

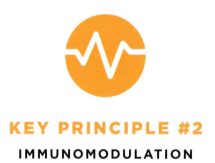

KEY PRINCIPLE #2
IMMUNOMODULATION

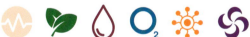

Contrary to popular belief, no medical treatment can heal you from cancer. Rather, it's your God-given immune system that does! Consider this: you can do all of the cancer treatments in the world, but none will work unless you have a strong, functioning immune system.

Our immune system is complex and intelligent, yet when faced with cancer, it often needs help to recognize where the cancer is and how to eliminate it. For this reason, the second aspect of our 7 Key Principles approach involves supporting and empowering the amazing immune system that God has given us to protect and heal us from disease.

The immune therapies that we use at Hope4Cancer do several wonderful things: they help the patient's body to more readily identify the cancer and adapt to its ever-changing survival mechanisms; and they enable cytotoxic—or cancer-killing—treatments to work better. Each therapy addresses the immune system in a unique way, and when the therapies are taken together, they have a powerful, synergistic effect upon the body.

We have designed all of the following immune therapies to enhance the function of both the innate and adaptive immune systems, and to be non-toxic and free of side effects. The innate immune system, also called the non-specific immune system, is your body's short- or quick-acting system; the "first responder" to infections and cancer cells. The cancer cells that form in all of us daily before we get active cancer are kept in check by the innate immune system.

Physical barriers, such as the skin and mucous membranes in the sinuses and gastrointestinal tract, are integral components of the innate immune system. They provide a first line of defense against pathogens like bacteria, fungi, parasites and viruses, so they don't gain a foothold inside us in the first place.

Some of the major functions of the innate immune system include recruiting immune cells, such as chemical mediators like cytokines, to the site of infection and activating what's called the "complement cascade." The complement cascade helps the body to identify bacteria, and promotes the clearance of dead cells and antigen-antibody complexes from it.

Antigen-antibody complexes are formed when the body sends proteins also known as Immunoglobins (Ig) to remove antigens, which are foreign proteins produced by cancer cells and pathogens. The antibodies bind with the antigens, forming antigen-antibody complexes that are then digested by macrophages and phagocytes, which are immune cells that "engulf" cancer cells so they can be eliminated by the body.

The innate immune system is also involved in identifying and removing damaged cellular debris from the organs, tissues and lymphatic system. When there is inflammation, the innate immune system responds

KEY PRINCIPLE #2 | TOOLS THAT EMPOWER YOUR IMMUNE SYSTEM

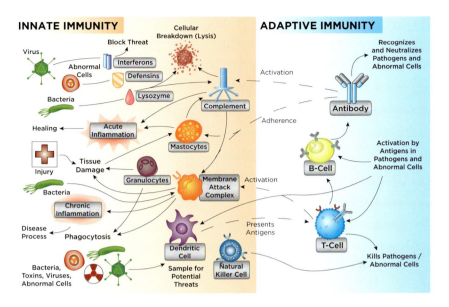

Figure 14. The immune system is a highly differentiated system of cells, each playing a unique role in the maintenance of the body's homeostasis—or steady environment. The innate immune system is designed to respond to perceived attacks (both internal and external), while the adaptive immune system learns from these attacks to launch a long-term immune response and preserve memory of the aggressor.

---

by sending out a variety of immune cells, such as macrophages, dendritic cells, natural killer (NK) cells, neutrophils, mastocytes, and Kuppfer cells (the latter of which come from the liver).

The innate immune system, in turn, triggers the body's adaptive system. This is also known as the long-term immune system, because it has a memory of sorts and can remember the body's initial exposure to a pathogen or cancer, which then leads to an enhanced response to any subsequent infections caused by that same pathogen and/or cancer.

Lymphocytes, which are white blood cells that look for harmful antigens, or foreign proteins in the blood, are a major component of the adaptive immune system. B- and T-cells are two types of lymphocytes that target antigens produced by cancer cells.

Your body uses both your innate and adaptive immune systems, and all of these immune cells and mechanisms to fight cancer. In addition, it's not just good enough to have an optimal immune system that is able to eliminate the cancer; your immune system must also be able to recognize the cancer in the first place.

This is because cancer cells can cloak or shield themselves from your immune system and effectively hide from it. It is possible for your immune system to be strong and yet unable to recognize the cancer. Therefore, **any immune therapies you do must not only strengthen and stimulate your immune system, but also help it to recognize the cancer.**

As part of strengthening a patient's immune system, we work on healing and balancing their gut and microbiome (or the community of microbes in their gut) because research shows that about 70% of the immune system is in the gut.[1] For instance, there's an area in the gut called Peyer's patches, where many immune cells are made.

If the intestinal flora isn't healthy, or the microbiome is imbalanced, then the Peyer's patches don't get enough nutrition to build up an adequate immune defense and protect you. In the chapter on nutrition, we share with you some ideas for healing your gut.

The remaining 30% of your immune system is spread throughout your body; in your lymphatic system and bloodstream, as well as in your mucous membranes such as the sinus cavities.

In addition, recent research has shown that your brain has an immune system. So when people get full brain radiation, it really negatively impacts their immune system. Both chemotherapy and radiation, in fact, suppress the immune system—the one thing that you most need to fight cancer (which is another reason I prefer not to prescribe them).

Interestingly, many of our cancer patients have said to me, "I was never sick a day in my life until I got cancer!" Which means that their immune system was probably never really challenged until they got cancer.

I equate the phenomenon of an immune system that's never been challenged to a soldier who has been to boot camp, but never into battle. Think about it: when the going gets tough, do you want a soldier fresh out of boot camp to protect you, or someone who has done three tours of duty in Afghanistan or another war-torn area? That's right, you want the one who has been in battle!

Similarly, you want your immune system to be challenged once in a while by a cold or virus. Patients who were rarely sick before they got

Key Principle #2 | Tools That Empower Your Immune System

> For many years, I was a vegetarian. However, a few years ago, I started eating fish and chicken again, because I felt like my body needed some animal protein, although I still do not eat red meat.
>
> Well, in late 2017, on a trip to Nashville, Tennessee, I was invited to eat at the best steakhouse in the city with a few friends. So I went, and decided that since I was at the best steakhouse in Nashville, I would break my beef fast and order a nice steak—now, this was after having not eaten any beef in years!
>
> Perhaps not surprisingly, after I finished eating, I got the chills, and started to feel really cold and nauseous inside, like I was going to pass out. It was a very scary feeling, so I got anxious.
>
> I said to myself, *Tony, calm down.*
>
> I drank a lot of water (maybe two glasses), took deep breaths, and tried to relax. Fortunately, after a while, the symptoms went away.
>
> Reflecting upon the event, I realized that because I hadn't eaten red meat in years, my immune system hadn't recognized the foreign proteins, and probably "kicked in" an antigen-antibody reaction to them, and this is what caused the symptoms.
>
> One of the main reasons we don't recommend animal protein to our patients, especially in the acute phases of cancer, is because the body mounts an antibody-antigen response against animal protein every time we consume it. Animal protein is foreign to the body—and we want our patients' immune systems to rest and not have to deal with the burden of the foreign proteins.
>
> In addition, the body uses up to 33% of its energy to digest food, especially animal protein, and we want the immune system to have as much energy as possible to heal the body from cancer.
>
> *~ Dr. Jimenez*

cancer are at somewhat of a disadvantage, because their immune systems haven't been "trained" to respond to disease.

For this reason, I welcome patients getting colds and flus because I think having to battle a virus, bacteria or infection now and then helps activate your immune system. In essence, these "training sessions" make it ready and "on call" to fight cancer. It's good for your body to have an alarm system that gets triggered once in a while!

Finally, cancer suppresses the immune system, but so can many other things, including an unhealthy lifestyle, negative thoughts, and environmental toxins. This is why we strengthen and support a patient's immune system not only with immune-specific therapies, but also with diet, detoxification and spirit-soul-body lifestyle strategies for healing. You will want to do the same.

In this chapter, I share with you some of the remarkable immune-enhancing therapies that we use to support our patients' immune systems. Like our cancer-killing treatments, these therapies all come from things that God has created in nature, and as such, are incredibly safe, effective and beneficial!

Sunivera Immunotherapy™

Sunivera Immunotherapy[2] is a protocol comprised of a number of powerful immune-modulating substances that function synergistically to strengthen the immune system.

Like all of our immune therapies, Sunivera modulates both the innate and adaptive immune systems, and is the combined result of 25 years of research expertise at leading Japanese- and U.S.-based research centers, as well as our clinical experience in natural cancer therapies.

One of Sunivera's main benefits is that it "turns on" the immune system's ability to recognize cancer and rebuilds the immune system from a variety of angles. It also enhances the effects of the other therapies that we do.

GcMAF, A Powerful Macrophage-Activating Substance

GcMAF stands for Gc Protein Derived Macrophage Activating Factor, which is a regulatory protein that supports the immune system. GcMAF is naturally present in your body, and is primarily responsible for activating macrophages, which are a type of immune cell that is involved in recognizing and killing cancer cells. Researchers suspect that GcMAF may also activate the immune system in other ways, although the ways in which it does this aren't yet clear.

GcMAF may be one of the most powerful anti-cancer proteins or substances that God has given us to heal from cancer as well as a variety of other chronic and degenerative conditions.

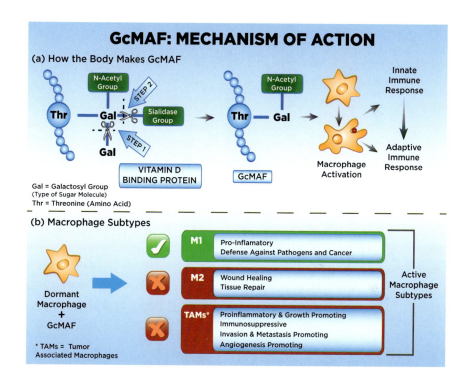

Figure 15. (a) Under normal conditions, the ubiquitous protein, Vitamin D Binding Protein (VDBP) is converted by the body to GcMAF which, in turn, results in the activation of macrophages, key innate immune system cells. Cancers and viruses have evolved ways to prevent this conversion, suppressing the body's innate immune response. External supply of GcMAF restores this response, and helps program the adaptive immune system for long-term response.

(b) Dormant macrophages are extremely flexible molecules that can be activated into a variety of sub-types, including ones that can be subverted by tumors to support their growth. These macrophages behave differently based on the way they are activated. GcMAF is known to stimulate the production of only M1-like macrophages that defend the body from pathogens and cancer.

Foremost in the Sunivera protocol, GcMAF is essential for increasing your immune system's ability to kill cancer cells, induce apoptosis, stop angiogenesis, and inhibit cancer cell proliferation and metastases.

GcMAF levels are typically low in people with compromised immune systems. Also, cancer cells produce an enzyme called alpha-N-acetyl-galactosaminidase or nagalase, which neutralizes your body's own production of GcMAF, so that your macrophages don't receive the signal to attack the cancer. When this happens, cancer can flourish in your body.

Studies have proven that GcMAF is effective against various types of cancer, including advanced and progressive cancers, especially breast, prostate, colorectal and lung cancers, and melanoma.

For instance, a study in *Anticancer Research* revealed that GcMAF inhibited breast cancer cell proliferation, or multiplication, in the lab, as well as halted metastases and angiogenesis.[3] And in a 2014 study on a 55-year-old woman with terminal breast cancer with metastases to the spine, GcMAF combined with Sonodynamic and hormonal therapy, eliminated the tumor and metastases, and with that, the woman's symptoms.[4]

Another study, published in 2016 in *Anticancer Research* showed that GcMAF, along with Sonodynamic Therapy, ozone and a type of frequency therapy called Tumor Treating Fields (TTF), stabilized the tumor of a 77-year-old man with stage 3B non-small cell lung cancer. The median survival time of those with non-small cell lung cancer using conventional medicine is about 8 months, whereas this man's tumor had not enlarged for 15 months following the therapy. He experienced improvement in his symptoms, as well.[5]

For your body to adequately utilize GcMAF, your Vitamin D levels need to be within an optimal range, which for someone with cancer is between 80-120 mg/dl. In people with lowered levels of Vitamin D, Vitamin D supplementation and/or larger doses of GcMAF may be required.

Next Generation Injectable and Oral GcMAF

Researchers at the University of Tokushima and Saisei-Mirai immunotherapy centers in Japan have recently developed a patented process to create the world's most advanced injectable form of GcMAF, which is 15 times more potent than the first-generation product. After treating over 1,000 patients at Saisei-Mirai, the researchers have concluded that it is safe and effective against a variety of cancers.[2]

Colostrum MAF, an oral version of GcMAF, also has anti-cancer benefits. Both the injectable and oral forms of GcMAF cross the blood-brain barrier, which means they can get into the brain and help eliminate any cancer there, unlike some other treatments.

GcMAF is easy to administer, and generally doesn't cause side effects, unlike other conventional immune therapies, which can over-stimulate a cancer patient's immune system. GcMAF also doesn't introduce genetically altered immune system cells to the body, making it safer than many other immune therapies.

In contrast, newly developed conventional immunotherapies that include immune checkpoint inhibitors that target the PD1, PD-L1 and CTLA-4 proteins, deliver a high degree of toxicity to the body, which means they can have adverse effects upon normal cells.[6] These treatments are also very specific to patients who express these proteins in sufficient quantity and often need to be co-administered with chemotherapy.

Another easy way to reap some of the benefits from it is to make it from kefir. Yes, you can actually create your own GcMAF! GcMAF kefir is not as potent as the pure, injectable form, but it is likely to have some immune-supportive benefits.

If you have an advanced, progressing cancer, however, you'll want to work with an integrative doctor who can administer the injectable form for you. While not available in the USA, GcMAF can easily be brought back from cancer clinics in Mexico, Asia and Europe.

Bee Propolis

The second component of Sunivera is bee propolis, also known as "bee putty" or "bee glue." Bees produce propolis from the resin they collect from trees and shrubs, which they then combine with beeswax, pollen and secretions from their salivary glands. They use it to repair their hives, and to protect themselves from predatory microbes and diseases. Propolis also maintains the temperature and health of the hive.

Bee propolis is also incredibly healing to the human body. Research has shown it to contain a variety of compounds that modulate the immune system, reduce inflammation and provide antioxidant benefits[7]. In addition, studies have shown it to be quite toxic to cancer cells.

A review published in 2014 in the *Asian Pacific Journal of Biomedicine* summarizes its effects. The researchers state: "Bee product peptides induce apoptosis (or programmed cancer cell death) in vitro in several transformed (cancer) human cell lines, including those derived from renal, lung, liver, prostate, bladder and lymphoid cancers." They also note that some bee products, including propolis, stop tumor cell growth and metastasis.[7]

Isn't it remarkable that God created bees to produce such amazing healing properties? We have found it to be helpful for our patients, as well.

Other Supporting Supplements and Nutrients

The Sunivera Immunotherapy protocol also incorporates several other supplements designed to fortify the immune system through targeted nutrition, detoxification, lymphatic drainage, and enzymatic and probiotic replacement. These products include: Solray-D Liposomal Spray, Flora Syntropy, Hepatagest, Vita LF Powder, and Lapacho Intrinsic. Chapter 7 describes these supplements in greater detail.

Oncolytic Virotherapy[8]

Did you know that not all viruses are bad, and that some can actually be used to treat cancer?

One of the more recent advances in cancer therapy is oncolytic virotherapy which involves the use of viruses to target and kill cancer cells. Viruses that are known to target cancer cells are injected into the patient. Most of the time, the viruses are genetically engineered to minimize their capacity to cause disease, which requires us to be cautious because of the unknown potential side effects from this modification. Once the virus is in the patient's body, it selectively targets cancer cells and modulates the immune system.

The history of cancer virotherapy actually goes back to the early 1900s, when cancer patients who were vaccinated with viruses were found to have unexpected improvements in their condition. In the 1940s, scientists discovered that cancer cells showed increased sensitivity to viruses.

It was found that viruses could proliferate, or replicate selectively, in animal tumors.

This selective targeting of cancer cells is also known as oncotropism. In some cases, this behavior was accompanied by oncolysis, or a breakdown of the cancer cell. From these discoveries, researchers learned that viruses could be used as anti-cancer therapies, at least theoretically.

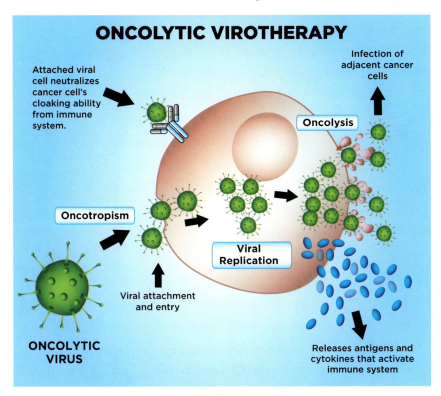

Figure 16. Mechanism of action of oncolytic virotherapy.

In subsequent years, more experiments were done. Unfortunately, doctors found that while some viral therapies were able to destroy cancer, they also infected the patients with what were sometimes dangerous viruses! That is why it is important to focus on viruses that are natural predators of cancer cells, and yet can naturally co-exist within the human ecosystem without causing harm to the host.

After the virus is injected into the patient, it selectively seeks out and infects the cancer cells, including those found in both localized and systemic tumors. In an ideal scenario, the virus would not cause infection and leave healthy cells and surrounding tissues unharmed.

Once the virus attacks the cancer cells, it either breaks them down, in a process known as lysis, or indirectly targets them by stimulating the immune system to go after them, much like a normal antiviral response. That a virus can elicit an immune response in the body shouldn't come as a surprise, since our bodies do this every day to fight off a number of potential infections.

When you get cancer, however, your immune system may fail to stop the growth of the tumor. Initially, it was believed that cancer cells lacked the appropriate cell surface receptors needed to communicate an immune response. Now, scientists believe that it is not just a lack of receptors that is the issue, but the cancer cell's ability to avoid the immune system altogether.

Oncolytic virotherapy "retunes" or modulates the surface receptors of tumor cells, thereby making them vulnerable again to cell-disrupting immune mechanisms. Even in cases where the cancer is insensitive to the anti-cancer effects of the virotherapy, the virus can still modulate the immune response, so that the cells become vulnerable once again to the body's defense mechanism. Oncolytic virotherapy, metaphorically speaking, lifts the invisible cloak off the cancer cells so that they can no longer hide from the immune system.

Recent research has shown that oncolytic virotherapy can enhance the effects of other immunotherapies as well.

While no studies have proven that oncolytic virotherapy also targets microbes, clinical evidence points to its benefits against infections such as Epstein-Barr and hepatitis, among others. But enough studies have not yet been done to know for sure for which infections it might be most effective.

In recent years, the pharmaceutical industry has joined the oncolytic virotherapy bandwagon and developed their own viral therapies. Their approach generally involves taking disease-causing viruses and genetically altering them so they aren't virulent or dangerous to the body.

Yet, introduction of these live viruses is the equivalent of introducing a new species into the body which is capable of altering our cells at a genetic level, with unknown, potentially dangerous consequences.

AARSOTA Bio-immunotherapy

Autologous Antigen Receptor Specific Oncogenic Target Acquisition (AARSOTA) is a vaccine-like bio-immunotherapy that I developed, which boosts the immune system's natural cancer-fighting abilities by using the cancer's antigens against itself. Antigens are proteins that are produced by cancer cells, and are characteristic of the tumor(s) from which they originate.

These antigens, or cancer proteins, show up in the patient's blood and urine, and have been used as tumor markers to identify and track how the cancer is progressing or regressing. For example, the markers CA 15-3 and CA 27.29 indicate breast cancer; CA 125, ovarian cancer; and CA 19-9, gastrointestinal or pancreatic cancers. When we measure these tumor markers in blood, we are really measuring proteins (or antigens) from the cancer cells. In addition, we can collect them from the urine to create a vaccine against the cancer.

A study conducted at University of California Los Angeles (UCLA) and Veterans Administration (VA) Medical Center demonstrated that the urine of 86-100% of patients in different cancer type groups positively tested for tumor-associated antigens. In contrast, only 7% of healthy donors tested positive, demonstrating the potential of using urine as a source for tumor-associated antigens.[9]

For the AARSOTA process, we first extract the antigenic proteins from the patient's urine, or other bodily fluids such as pleural fluid and ascites. From these, we create a therapeutic vaccine that's tailored to the specific tumor(s) in the patient's body. The antigen concentrate is then delivered back into the patient via an intramuscular injection at discrete intervals, which has the effect of building up his or her antigen-antibody response.

Once the antigens are reintroduced back into the patient's body, his or her own antibodies recognize them and form what's called an "antigen-antibody complex." This complex basically gives the antibodies, which help to fight the cancer, important immunological information, so that the immune system can mount a more specific and targeted response against the cancer.

The specific immune benefits of AARSOTA include:

- Upregulating the immune system's T and B lymphocyte population—which are part of the adaptive system.
- Increasing the cytotoxic effects of natural killer (NK) cells.
- Shifting the cell's cycle and taking cancer cells out of the "cellular synthesis" phase, and bringing them into a "resting" phase; basically, stopping their rapid turnover rate.
- Upregulating apoptosis, or programmed cancer cell death.

Because the AARSOTA vaccine is created using the patient's own antigens—hence the name "autologous," which means "your own"—there is no risk of side effects from the vaccine.

That said, the success of AARSOTA is somewhat dependent upon the quantity of antigens that are released into the urine. The greatest advantage of the therapy is that the antigens are naturally specific to the patient's cancer, and as such, are highly targeted and precise. Yet its biggest drawback is that we can't yet predict how strong the antigenic concentrate will be for each patient, and whether it will elicit a strong enough immune response for them.

This is partly why we combine AARSOTA with other immune therapies such as Sono-Photo Dynamic Therapy. Unlike some of the other immune therapies that we give our patients, however, we don't give AARSOTA to everyone (although there are no specific criteria for determining which patients should or should not receive it).

To prescribe AARSOTA, I rely greatly on my God-given physician's intuition. I usually find it more beneficial for people who have more aggressive cancers, because such people tend to have more antigens in their urine. In those cases, we can create potentially stronger therapies for them.

The beauty of the therapy is that it allows us to keep up with the cancer's adaptive mechanisms, because each subsequent treatment accounts

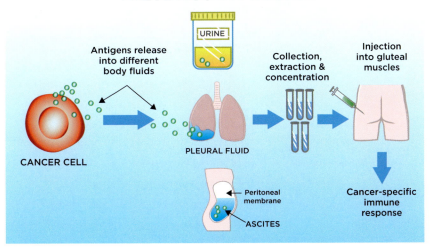

Figure 17. Cancer cells and pathogens carry unique proteins known as antigens, which the immune system uses to recognize their presence. These antigens are often found in the bloodstream and other body fluids. AARSOTA relies on extracting these cancer antigens from the body fluids, concentrating them, and then re-injecting them into the body to elicit an immune response that is specific to the cancer cell or pathogen.

---

for any mutations that may have occurred in the cancer. As you know by now, cancer cells mutate and change their characteristics periodically to bypass and evade the immune system.

Therefore, by giving patients weekly injections for five weeks, and then again every two-three months after that, we are continually presenting new antigen-antibody complexes to the patient's immune system, which enables us to keep effectively targeting the cancer in its evolving environment.

We are the only clinic in the world I am aware of that does this type of therapy. And like all our immune therapies, it works on both branches of the immune system. It triggers both the T and B lymphocytes, which are a part of the adaptive immune system, while the antigen-antibody complexes created by the vaccine are mostly a part of the innate immune system.

Immune Power Plus

Garden Food Plan's Immune Power Plus is a highly beneficial immune supplement that we give our patients as part of their home treatment program. I developed this supplement years ago while studying the nutritional needs of deeply immune-compromised HIV patients in South Africa.

Through my studies, I ended up discovering some key micronutrients, macronutrients and herbs, which I found really helped to reactivate the HIV patients' immune systems. In turn, this greatly improved and prolonged their quality of life, even the lives of those who were extremely sick!

Even though I created this formula years ago, I also ended up using it on my cancer patients; like HIV and AIDS, cancer is also a disease in which the immune system is deeply compromised. Immune Power Plus restores the essential nutritional building blocks that the immune system needs to be strengthened and brought back to life.

Some of the main constituents and benefits of Immune Power Plus include:

1. **Restoring key micro and macronutrients** needed by the immune system to function properly, such as the minerals magnesium, selenium and zinc. Following is more information on each of these:

   Magnesium - The fourth most abundant mineral in the body, magnesium is needed for more than 300 biochemical reactions in the body. It helps to maintain proper muscle, nerve and heart function, and healthy blood sugar levels.

   Selenium - This is an essential trace mineral that works as an antioxidant by scavenging damaging free radicals from the body. It is also necessary for proper immune function.

   Zinc - This trace mineral is found in cells throughout the body and plays a crucial role in proper immune

Key Principle #2 | Tools That Empower Your Immune System

system function, as well as cell growth and division. It also helps to regulate the action of insulin in the body. In addition, research has shown that zinc decreases angiogenesis and may increase apoptosis.

2. **Beta-glucans** are important immune modulators that activate specific immune cells including T-cells, macrophages, antibodies, and natural killer (NK) cells so that they can better respond to the cancer. Beta glucans also reduce the growth rate of cancer cells while stimulating a stronger immune response to pathogenic microbes.
3. **Turkey tail** is a wild-growing mushroom that has been shown in clinical studies to improve cancer patients' immune status. Two components of the mushroom—specifically, polysaccharide-K (PSK) and polysaccharide-P (PSP)—have anti-cancer properties. They enhance the workings of a variety of immune system cells that the body needs to combat cancer, especially helper T-cells. The T-cells signal all of the other cells in the immune system about what to do and how to attack the cancer cells.
4. **Astragalus** is an adaptogenic herb that has been used in Oriental medicine for centuries to improve immune function, as well as to protect the body from stress and disease. Studies show that it may also have anti-cancer benefits.

All the ingredients in Immune Power Plus are potentiated and enhanced by one another. We studied the effects of Immune Power Plus on 50 patients with full-blown HIV-AIDS in South Africa, and found that all had significant improvements in their symptoms, longevity and quality of life. The improvements that these people experienced in their health were so amazing!

Now, we also give it to our patients and have found it to be incredibly helpful for them, as well.

Immune Imagery

Immune imagery involves utilizing guided imagery, meditation and other techniques to harness the power of the mind and emotions to heal the body. It is based on psychoneuroimmunology, or the study of the interaction between the mind and emotions, and the nervous and immune systems. It is a powerful therapy that profoundly affects healing.

Research has shown that the brain and immune system communicate through an intricate network of neurons. This is evidenced by the fact that people tend to get sick during periods of high stress: the negative emotions and thoughts they experience result in an overwhelmed and impaired immune system.

The good news is, one of the most powerful immune-boosting tools God has given you is your own mind! Later, I will share with you some ways you can harness the power of your emotions and thoughts to heal your soul and body. Here, I provide just one example so you can see that immune boosting therapies aren't just limited to medical treatments.

They also include tools that utilize the power of your God-given mind and God's Spirit within you, to direct and control your cellular behavior. You have been given great power to overcome any and every assault on your body!

Immune Imagery teaches you, among other things, how the right visualizations and thought processes can induce a positive biological response in your body, as well as how you can open up your mind to focus on more of the right thoughts.

The tools typically consist of professional guided imagery, deep relaxation exercises, and visualization techniques shared via audio or video, all of which help to establish a more beneficial mind-body connection. Visual tools illustrate how your body defends itself, so that you can visualize and activate your body's natural defenders. Relaxation techniques increase the efficiency of your immune cells and alleviate stress.

Videos that are a part of the Immune Imagery program show and teach you how to visualize your immune system as it attacks viruses, fungi, bacteria and cancer cells. Much research has shown that our patients' immune markers improve following Immune Imagery, as measured by blood tests that are drawn before and after they view the material.

Other Immune Therapies

In Chapter 4, I described the benefits of five more immune-supportive therapies that we use: Sono-Photo Dynamic Therapy, Vitamin C, Helixor, hyperthermia and ozone. All are powerful immune-boosting therapies that also have significant cancer-killing properties. Please refer to Chapter 4 to learn more about their benefits as cytotoxic agents.

Choosing an Immunotherapy Protocol for Patients

In my 25-plus years of clinical experience, Sono-Photo Dynamic Therapy has proven to be an important core therapy for our patients, in addition to three other immune therapies: Sunivera, Helixor and virotherapy. All of these therapies can be combined and used together at the same time, but we find that it isn't necessary for our patients to do all of them.

Finally, I just want to re-iterate that medical treatments aren't the only factors that impact your immune function! Other factors, such as laughter, social interaction, meditation, prayer, proper nutrition and exercise all affect the immune system. The impact of lifestyle, diet and these other factors upon your healing (among others) are sometimes unquantifiable, but plenty of research has shown that they can powerfully enhance immune function, and are no less important than any of the immune therapies I just shared with you.

If you'll recall, I mentioned in Chapter 1 that your human spirit is in charge of your soul and body. So, when you focus on strategies that strengthen your spirit, such as cultivating a relationship with God through prayer, they can enhance your immune system just as much as—if not more than—any other tool that we have in medicine.

I encourage you to keep this in mind as you read, as it will greatly empower you in your healing journey. And remember, even if you can't do every single treatment I share with you, you can strengthen your immune system in other ways.

Now, I am not saying that you should not do any medical treatments. I'm just saying there's a lot that you can do on your own, from the comfort of your home, to support your immune system—and these strategies often won't cost you anything but a bit of your time!

TOOLS THAT POWER THE IMMUNE SYSTEM

Table 5.1.

Immune Therapy	What It Is	How It Works	Benefits
Sunivera	A variety of immune-supportive substances such as GcMAF and propolis, combined in a protocol.	Modulates immune system and disables cancer in a variety of ways by delivering missing key components. Supports whole body healing.	Modulates both the innate and adaptive immune systems.
Oncolytic Virotherapy	Naturally occuring or genetically engineered virus which selectively targets cancer cells.	Virus is attracted to cancer cells through oncotropism; once in the cell, it causes it to break down (lysis). Also, makes cancer cells visible to immune surveillance system.	Directly destroys cancer cells while stimulating the immune system.
AARSOTA	Non-toxic therapy using patient's own cancer antigens.	Antigens are collected from urine, pleural fluid, or ascites and injected back in the body to elicit an immune response.	Boosts immune system by stimulating a response against the antigens.
Immune Power Plus	Supplement containing key nutrients and herbs.	Reactivates the immune system and provides essential building blocks to the body.	Gently modulates the immune system.
Immune Imagery	Utilizes guided imagery, meditation and other techniques.	Patient watches video imagery that stimulates mental pathways that affect the immune system.	Stimulates an immune response by using the power of the mind to influence the body.
Helixor (Mistletoe)	Plant extracts of mistletoe given via injection.	Compounds in mistletoe stimulate and modulate the immune system. Are also cytotoxic.	Suppresses tumors, stops angiogenesis, causes apoptosis, stimulates immune system, mitigates symptoms.
Sono-Photo Dynamic Therapy	A variety of sound and light therapies that kill cancer and stimulate the immune system when activated by a photosensitizer.	Light and sound therapies activate photosensitizers in cancer cells, which release reactive oxygen species that are toxic to cancer.	While toxic to cancer cells, also activates the innate and adaptive immune systems.

SUMMARY

- Your God-given immune system is the most important tool you have to overcome cancer, which is why supporting both your innate and adaptive systems with the right combination of immune therapies is vital for your success.
- Hope4Cancer's immune therapies modulate, stimulate and strengthen the immune system, in addition to helping it recognize the cancer.
- The Sunivera protocol consists of powerful immune modulating agents such as GcMAF and bee propolis. It "turns on" your immune system's ability to recognize cancer and re-builds it from a variety of angles.
- GcMAF stands for Gc Protein Derived Macrophage Activating Factor, and is a regulatory protein that activates macrophages, a type of immune cell involved in killing cancer cells.
- Oncolytic virotherapy involves injecting a virus into your body that selectively infects cancer cells, while leaving your healthy cells unharmed.
- Autologous Antigen Receptor Specific Oncogenic Target Acquisition Bio-immunotherapy, or AARSOTA, is a vaccine-like therapy that boosts your immune system's natural cancer-fighting abilities by using your cancer's own antigens against itself.
- Immune Power Plus, a supplement originally developed for HIV patients, consists of key micro and macronutrients and herbs that powerfully support the immune system.
- Immune Imagery involves utilizing guided imagery, meditation and other techniques to harness the power of your mind and emotions, to heal your body.

QUESTIONS FOR FURTHER REFLECTION

1. Describe the basic difference between the innate and adaptive immune systems, and how Hope4Cancer's immune therapies address both.
2. What does GcMAF do in your body, and why is it the most important component of Sunivera?
3. Describe some of the benefits of bee propolis.

4. How does oncolytic virotherapy work?
5. Why are mind-body therapies like immune imagery important in healing?

CHARLES' STORY

Charles was diagnosed with bladder cancer in 2007, at the age of 51. What was initially supposed to be a somewhat quick recovery became much more complicated and difficult over time, but Charles beat the odds and has enjoyed an unexpectedly good outcome. Here, he shares his story. He currently lives in Woodland, Georgia with his wife.

I was diagnosed with invasive bladder cancer in January 2007. I didn't know much about cancer at the time, but soon learned that when it comes to bladder cancer, the word "invasive" means the disease has gotten into the muscle wall of the bladder. When this happens, it can spread throughout the body

The doctors did scans, X-rays and other tests on me, and fortunately, told me that the cancer was confined to my bladder and had not metastasized. The "gold standard" treatment in conventional medicine at that time for invasive bladder cancer was to remove the bladder, prostate and surrounding lymph nodes. And because the cancer had apparently not metastasized, with this surgery I would have about a 90% chance of a cure and would not need chemotherapy.

I was interested in combining conventional with alternative treatment, but the mainstream doctors I asked didn't give me the information I requested. Yet, a 90% cure rate just by doing surgery and no chemotherapy sounded relatively good to me, so I went ahead and had the surgery in March 2007.

Everything went fine with the surgery, but afterward the surgeon came back to me and said that the cancer was also in my lymph nodes.

Remember, the initial test, scans and X-rays showed that the cancer had not metastasized. So with the new diagnosis, my chances of a cure had now dropped to somewhere around 40%, and my doctor told me that I was now going to need chemotherapy.

At this point, I didn't have an oncologist because no metastases had been previously detected. My doctor had initially told me that if I just did the surgery, that would be enough, and I would not need chemo.

So after the surgery, I met with an oncologist, and he said, "Let's do another scan."

I told him, "I have recently had a scan and don't need another one."

But again he insisted and said, "Let's do another scan."

In the meantime, he started me on chemotherapy.

The scan revealed more bad news. The oncologist said, "You have three tumors in your liver."

A biopsy confirmed that the bladder cancer had also metastasized to my liver. When I asked the oncologist if there was a chance of a cure, he said, "Not really." He stated that the average life expectancy of a person with bladder cancer with metastases to the liver was about nine months, although some people 'go' in four.

But then this doctor, who specialized in urological malignancies, added that he had never seen anyone with bladder cancer with metastases to the liver, live for more than twelve months.

So, in a very short period of time I went from having a diagnosis and a surgery that would have given me around a 90% chance of a cure, to a diagnosis and treatment (chemotherapy) that would give me about a 40% chance, to now, with the oncologist telling me I didn't have much of a chance to be cured.

I was devastated by the diagnosis.

I was facing death within a year.

I continued with chemotherapy, however, and did not get a response from it; but the tumors didn't grow, either. So I did another protocol that involved doing 50% of the initial chemotherapy treatments, and with that additional chemo, two of the smaller tumors became undetectable on a CAT scan, and the larger tumor shrank.

Then, the oncologist recommended liver surgery to remove the remaining tumor. So he connected me with a liver surgeon, and in the beginning of September 2007, I had liver surgery. The doctors removed the tumor, and for a while, I had a brief remission.

But in March 2008, another scan revealed that the cancer had returned to my liver, and the doctor told me that my prognosis was still the same—and that this cancer was ultimately going to "get me."

He told me I could do another liver surgery, but that I couldn't have any more chemo. I was fine with that, because quite frankly, I didn't want to do any more chemo. My body was still torn down from the effects of all the chemo I had already done, as well as from the disease.

For the first liver surgery, the surgeon had cut me open, removed the tumor, and then sewed me back up. The second surgery, however, was an ablation; meaning, it was a surgery, but it would not be as invasive. So I had a second liver surgery.

Around the same time as this second surgery I started to look harder into alternative treatments for cancer.

My wife helped me research, but she was really "holding down the fort"—working and taking care of me, and my then 11-year-old daughter, so she didn't have much free time. Fortunately, my brother and his wife offered to help me research alternative clinics.

We researched clinics everywhere; from New York to California, to the Bahamas and Mexico. After three weeks, I had almost settled on a place in the United States that I felt pretty good about. But one day, my sister-in-law, who had been sending and receiving emails to and from cancer clinics, received an email from a doctor in New York. He said that he could not help me, but recommended I give Hope4Cancer a call.

So I did, and I spoke to Marcy, Dr. Tony's wife. She was the patient coordinator there, and as I spoke with her, I felt like this was my last chance. I literally had pages of questions for her; about the types of therapies the treatment center offered, and so on.

Marcy thoroughly answered most of my questions and I then did a follow up interview with Dr. Tony, who answered all of the medical questions that she wasn't able to answer. After doing multiple interviews with them both, I decided to go to Hope4Cancer in May 2008.

Once I started treatment at Hope4Cancer, I did Sono-Photo Dynamic Therapy, along with localized and full body hyperthermia, and local laser and sauna therapy. In addition, I was given supplements to fight cancer and help my immune system.

I did Hope4Cancer's initial program at the clinic for two weeks, and then continued with a home program after that.

In the meantime, I kept my oncologist and urologist, because they were good doctors, and I resumed my scans in the summer after my second liver surgery and my stay at Hope4Cancer.

A few things had really helped to sell me on Hope4Cancer. First and foremost was their success at being able to remove cancer from the liver. The liver is a difficult place to get cancer out of. Because the body has an almost unlimited blood supply there, the tumor has easy access to nutrition from the blood.

When I was interviewing clinics, my first question to all the staff was whether their particular clinic had been successful at removing cancer from the liver. I don't remember a place other than Hope4Cancer that seemed confident about their ability to do this. The other places that I had talked to gave vague answers like, "Well, we'll try to do this or that (treatment) for you." But when I spoke with Marcy, she told me that their therapies were successful at removing cancer from the liver.

Another thing that was very encouraging about Hope4Cancer was their home treatment program. I would be able to continue with their main "bread and butter" treatments at home, just as I did at the clinic. That was very important to me. Many cancer clinics I had interviewed had what I considered to be a strong, aggressive in-patient program, but their follow up home programs seemed quite weak.

By then, I had already done everything that could be done in conventional medicine to get well. I had done all the chemo that I could do, and had all the possible surgeries. Yet, the prognosis was still grim—that the cancer was ultimately going to get me.

I wanted to do something to see if I could stop it.

My urologist had told me that one predictable thing about cancer is that it is unpredictable. My oncologist continued to do scans on me every few months, while I was doing the Hope4Cancer home program.

I started to feel better once I started treatments at Hope4Cancer. Every time I was about to have a scan, however, I was a nervous wreck. But once I got a year under my belt I realized that I had been alive for a year following my last recurrence of cancer. It hit home that I had reached a milestone in my healing.

My oncologist told me that once a person is in remission for three years, that's another huge milestone.

I had only been in remission for seven months following my liver surgery before the cancer came back. That's why it was a pretty big deal to me when I made it to that year mark without a recurrence!

Around three years later, my scans were still coming out clear. My oncologist started saying that the longer I went without a recurrence, the greater the chances that it would never come back.

He declared me to be cancer-free though, and I have been declared cancer-free ever since—12 years at the time of this writing.

My oncologist also told me that in all his years of practice, he had never seen anyone survive bladder cancer with metastases to the liver. And my urologist, who has had extensive training and experience with urological malignancies, told me that I was a miracle.

To this day, I continue with certain aspects of Hope4Cancer's home program, voluntarily. I do it as a maintenance program, to keep the cancer from coming back, and so that I will remain healthy.

Cancer affects everybody—everyone who loves and cares for you, whether family or friends. Both of my parents were still alive at the time of my diagnosis and treatment, as were my wife, daughter, son, and brother. They were all affected by what I went through, but their support and help were critical for me. Thankfully, I'm doing well today.

Now I feel good! I just got the results of an AMAS test, which is a blood test that can detect cancer before scans and X-rays, and the results came out normal.

My current bladder doesn't work like the one I was born with, but it's pretty cool and works well.

If you're battling cancer and have been given a prognosis like mine, I just want to encourage you to not let that be "it" for you. Keep on looking for better answers. I was encouraged by a friend not to accept my prognosis of death. I was encouraged by another friend not to give up. I took their advice.

There are other options besides conventional treatment, and there is always hope.

The stars lined up for me.

6

Nutrition Based on the Garden of Eden

KEY PRINCIPLE #3
PART 1: FULL SPECTRUM NUTRITION

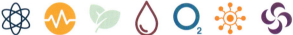

Behold, I have given you every plant yielding seed that is on the surface of the entire earth, and every tree which has fruit yielding seed; it shall be food for you.

GENESIS 1:29

When God put Adam and Eve in the Garden of Eden, he gave them some very clear, simple directions.

Wouldn't it have been nice to live there in the Garden, where the food was fresh and nutrient-rich, and you didn't have to think about what to eat, because God put it all right there in front of you?

Our early ancestors thrived on a nutritious plant-based diet that included an abundance of fruits and vegetables, and possibly other plant-based foods, like nuts and seeds. These foods gave them energy, vibrancy and perfect health.

Since the time of the Garden and Adam and Eve, however, we have been progressively consuming increasingly toxic foods that were not part of God's original plan, and have paid a price for it. In recent decades especially, we have been eating foods that are genetically modified, nutrient-depleted, and polluted by antibiotics, pesticides, plastics, herbicides, and hormones. We also consume unnatural "food-like substances"; or, foods that have been created by man, not God, which are foreign and actually disease-causing to our bodies, rather than life-giving!

What's more, we've created many "diets," including anti-cancer diets, which have sometimes confused us about what foods are best for our health or recovery. And at times, such diets led us to believe that we needed to follow a rigorous food regimen in order to get well.

But what if nutrition wasn't meant to be complicated? What if we were simply meant to eat foods similar to what God originally gave us in the Garden of Eden?

After all, if God created plant-based foods for the first humans, then why wouldn't those foods be healthful for us today, too?

Well, my experience with many cancer patients has shown me that they are! And while we can't go back to the Garden and a perfectly nutrient-rich food supply, we *can* find healthy foods that resemble what God gave us in the Garden. Foods that are healthful for people with cancer, because they are what God originally created for our benefit at the beginning of time.

The Bible also says that God has allowed us to consume meat, but this was *after* man disobeyed God's commandments and sin and disease entered the world (see Genesis 9:3). One could infer from this that we were originally created to be vegetarians.

However, because we live in a very different world than that of our first ancestors, meat is now permissible, and even necessary, in certain situations and societies (e.g., Inuit peoples, who only had access to a meat-based diet). But because meat was not part of God's original plan for humanity, we can infer that it is generally less healthful than plant-based food.

KEY PRINCIPLE #3 | NUTRITION BASED ON THE GARDEN OF EDEN

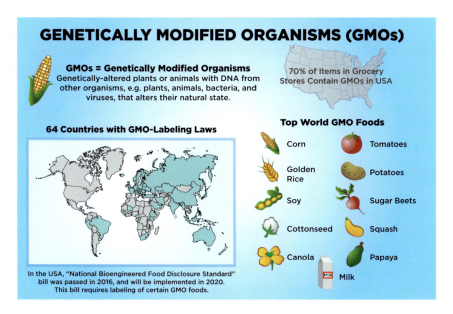

Figure 18. Products of the biotechnology revolution, genetically modified plants and animals bring unpredictable dangers to humans as consumers and, over the years, have been implicated in a number of diseases.

Don't let that discourage you, however, if you feel that your body needs some meat. We are unique and all have somewhat different nutritional requirements. I encourage you, though, to follow Garden-based eating as much as possible. I have found that this is the food plan upon which most cancer patients thrive best, and which I believe God created for our well-being.

Following are some Garden-based food guidelines, which I collectively refer to as the Garden Food Plan.® The foods in this plan will bring life, vibrancy and healing to your whole being. The plan is not meant to be difficult to follow, because God isn't complicated. I don't believe food is meant to be so, either. **So please don't allow food to be a source of stress and worry for you.** Stress can override any benefits that you may receive from following the Garden Food Plan, and we don't want that. Just do your best to follow the basic guidelines I share, without trying to be perfect.

The Garden Food Plan isn't meant to just keep you alive; it is supposed to be medicine for your body, as much as any cancer treatment.

Your body heals and repairs itself when it is given the proper raw materials, which come from healthy food, but can be further damaged and diseased if you consume the wrong foods.

In addition, no vitamin supplement, therapy or drug can heal you like food! Neither can any supplement take the place of food, and no manipulated or genetically modified food could possibly be better than how God originally created it. In fact, whenever man has tampered with the food supply, it has had negative consequences upon society's health.

For instance, genetically modified foods (GMOs) are difficult for the body to digest, and have been linked to a number of diseases, including autoimmune conditions and cancer. A study entitled "Genetically Engineered Crops, Glyphosate and the Deterioration of Health in the America," published in 2014 in *The Journal of Organic Systems* shows significant correlations between GMOs and 22 diseases.[1]

How important is organic food? A pivotal study conducted collaboratively at leading research centers in France (as part of the *NutriNet Santé Prospective Cohort Study*) was published in October 2018 in the *Journal of the American Medical Association (JAMA) Internal Medicine*. This study clearly showed that a higher frequency of organic food consumption was correlated to a significantly reduced cancer risk.[2] The authors also clarify that the role of pesticides for the risk of cancer "could not be doubted given the growing body of evidence linking cancer development to pesticide exposure."

What does this mean? It simply confirms what we have known all along: that your eating habits could potentially determine not only whether you get cancer in the first place, but also how effectively you can reduce your risk of tumor growth and metastasis if you have the disease.

We all have different levels of tolerance to toxins and GMO foods, but most of us can't consume an unlimited amount of harmful chemicals without repercussions. Nonetheless, you won't know how much better you will feel unless you try eating clean, organic food the way God created it!

So, if there's just one thing I want you to remember as you read this chapter, it's this: The cleaner and more natural your food is, and the more it resembles what our first ancestors ate in the Garden of Eden, the more likely it is to benefit you.

KEY PRINCIPLE #3 | NUTRITION BASED ON THE GARDEN OF EDEN

If you truly can't afford clean, organic food, I encourage you to ask God to bless your food and protect you from the effects of any contaminants in it. Jesus says of His followers in Mark 16:18, "If they . . . (Jesus' followers) drink anything deadly, it will not hurt them" (HCSB). This may apply to our food, too, although none of us live entirely unaffected by the environment. That's why I recommend eating clean, as much as possible, as you bless and thank God for your food in the process!

NATURAL FOOD

The man that feeds on nuts and grains
Crisp herbs and roots, sweet fruit and water,
Knows little of disease and pains
And of the many ills that bother.

His body well, his brain is clear.
His soul is full of every goodness.
He lives a life that knows no fear
Of Nature's roughs, revenge and rudeness.

His passions are in harmony
With spirit, soul and better senses.
In consequences Morality
Accuses him of no offenses.

Tobacco, coffee, meat and beer
And salt and pepper, wine and whiskey,
Are words that harshly grate his ear;
He knows their use is low and risky. [3]

~ Anonymous

The Benefits of the Garden Food Plan® for People with Cancer

Eating clean, Garden-based foods will do all of the following for you:

- Reduce the amount of cancer-causing toxins in your body
- Improve your gut health
- Help you maintain a healthy weight
- Avoid triggering cancer-causing genes and encourage the expression of cancer-suppressing genes
- Modulate your immune and endocrine systems
- Improve your detoxification pathways
- Reduce the demands on your body's enzymatic system
- Reduce inflammation
- Counteract muscle wasting

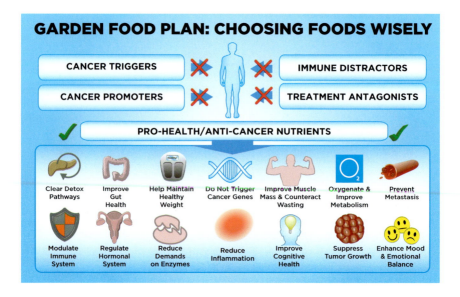

Figure 19. The Garden Food Plan is based on Hope4Cancer's nutritional philosophy that provides our patients a clear outline of what constitutes healthy eating.

This translates into a variety of symptomatic improvements such as greater energy, better digestion, along with less pain, brain fog, depression and other symptoms.

In addition, the Garden Food Plan improves muscle mass and strength in advanced cancer patients, and helps to rebuild their tissues.

The Five Categories of Food and How They Affect Your Health

Every food or drink can be broadly categorized into one of five different groups as they relate to cancer and your health:

1. Foods or food-like substances that directly cause cancer (Cancer Triggers). These include trans fatty acids from food-like substances such as margarine, french fries, potato chips and most processed foods. Such foods contain acrylamide, which is a cancer-causing substance that is formed when foods are cooked at high temperatures. High-temperature cooking also generates free radicals that can lead to cancer. These substances also include aspartame, a chemical that is found in artificial sweeteners such as Nutrasweet and Equal, and products such as Diet Coke; monosodium glutamate (MSG) and polyunsaturated oils such as corn oil.
2. Foods that feed and strengthen cancer cells and pathogenic microbes (Cancer Promoters). These include: refined sugar and flour products, soft drinks, and most dairy products.
3. Foods that directly interfere with cancer treatments (Treatment Antagonists). These include chlorinated and fluoridated water, alcohol and coffee.
4. Foods that occupy and distract your immune system from focusing on killing the cancer (Immune Distractors). These include beef, turkey and other animal proteins that are foreign to the body. They require extra energy to digest, and because the body recognizes them as foreign, they tax the immune system.

5. Foods that contain cancer-killing nutrients, stop the spread of cancer, or in some other way support your body and help it to heal from cancer (Pro-body + Anti-cancer nutrients).

These are Garden-based foods, and are what we will mostly be focusing on in this chapter.

Life Giving Garden-Based Foods

The Garden Food Plan includes lots of fresh, raw vegetables, fruits, nuts, seeds, healthy oils and sprouts. These provide your body with the highest quality sources of protein, fat, carbohydrates, fiber, vitamins and minerals that you can get, in forms that are readily digestible and assimilated. Most of our patients have followed this plan for a long time and found that it improves their symptoms and accelerates their healing.

Plant-based protein is superior to animal protein, especially for advanced cancer patients, for the following reasons:

- When consumed raw or lightly steamed, it contains more nutrients than cooked animal protein.
- It contains fewer environmental toxins and poisons than what's found in animal protein.
- It is present in foods that also contain a variety of other anti-cancer nutrients, such as antioxidants and phytochemicals.
- It is easily digested and assimilated by the body.
- It is of sufficiently high quality to meet all of your body's nutritional requirements.

I recommend consuming a wide variety of fruits and vegetables (unless you have an allergy to any specific varieties, a blood sugar regulation problem, or other health condition like diabetes. In other words, unless you have dietary restrictions that preclude you from eating higher glycemic fruits and vegetables, like bananas or potatoes).

KEY PRINCIPLE #3 | NUTRITION BASED ON THE GARDEN OF EDEN

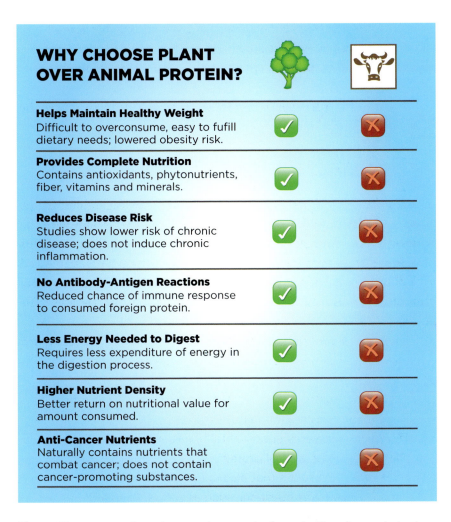

Figure 20. Reasons to favor plant protein over animal protein. Since the protein intake needs of each individual, especially cancer patients, may vary greatly from person to person, you are advised to consult a nutritionist prior to making large-scale changes to your nutritional protocol.

The basic key here is to choose foods that are as God created them; fresh and natural, and which come from one of four places: the ground, a plant, a tree or (perhaps) the sea, rather than a box, can or factory.

Anti-Inflammatory Super Foods

Foods that lower inflammation foster healing. While most fruits and vegetables are anti-inflammatory, some of my favorites for lowering inflammation include:

- All kinds of spices and herbs (e.g., curcumin, basil, rosemary, mint)
- Wild-caught, cold-water fish (if you need animal protein)
- Hot peppers
- Extra virgin, cold-pressed olive oil
- Leafy green vegetables (e.g., spinach, lettuce, chard, kale)
- Cruciferous vegetables (e.g., broccoli, cauliflower)
- Pumpkin, butternut squash, sweet potatoes, carrots
- Antioxidant berries (e.g., blueberries, raspberries, blackberries)
- Dark chocolate (one of my favorites!), with only natural sweeteners added, like Stevia

Super Foods that Affect Estrogen-Driven Cancers

Some cancers, like breast cancer, are affected by estrogens. Breast cancer is one of the most prevalent cancers, with 1 in 8 women in the United States now being diagnosed with it. Nearly three-quarters of all breast cancers are estrogen-receptor positive; meaning, certain estrogens and estrogen-like substances cause these cancers to develop, grow and metastasize.

Unfortunately, many environmental toxins act as estrogens in the body. These "fake" estrogens, called xenoestrogens, which come from pollutants such as polychlorinated biphenyls (PCBs), food additives, drugs and phthalates (chemicals from plastics) can enter the body and occupy estrogen receptor sites on cancer cells and cause them to multiply and grow.

Eliminating excess estrogen and xenoestrogens from toxic foods and the environment is therefore important for halting the growth of hormonally influenced cancers like those of the breast and prostate. Fortunately, I believe God knew before time began that we would one day be faced with an epidemic of cancer. That is why He provided us with foods such as those described in the following sections—the kinds that help our bodies eliminate cancer-causing toxins like xenoestrogens.

Cruciferous Vegetables

Cauliflower, broccoli, cabbage, Brussels sprouts, kale and Bok choy, among other cruciferous vegetables, have hormone-regulating compounds such as sulforaphane and indole-3 carbinols (I3Cs) that aid in liver detoxification. As part of this, they remove estrogen metabolites and clear excess estrogen from the body.

According to a review published in October 2016 in *Seminars in Cancer Biology*, many studies have reported that consuming cruciferous vegetables may reduce cancer risk.[4] The same review stated that Diindolylmethane (DIM), which is a compound that's produced in the gut, in combination with the medication Herceptin, induced apoptosis and caused cancer cell cycle arrest in some types of breast cancer cells.[4]

Allium Vegetables

Onions, scallions, garlic, chives, and leeks belong to a family of vegetables called "allium", which means "garlic" in Greek. These vegetables also have been found to have significant anti-cancer properties, so I encourage you to consume ample amounts as part of your daily food intake, both for cancer prevention and treatment.

A review of several studies, published in August 2016 in the journal *Nutrition*, concluded that garlic has potent anti-cancer effects, particularly upon the digestive system. The researchers state that garlic inhibits cancer by inducing apoptosis, and halting cancer cell proliferation, invasion and metastasis. Further, it regulates hormones and/or hormone receptors involved in breast and prostate cancers.[5]

Garlic also has potent immune system effects. Another review published in 2015 in the *Journal of Immunology Research* showed that garlic stimulates the production of macrophages, lymphocytes, natural killer (NK) cells, dendritic cells, and eosinophils, all of which play an important role in fighting cancer.[6]

Green Leafy Vegetables

Most green leafy vegetables have phytochemicals such as beta-carotene, indoles and luteins, which have antioxidant and anti-inflammatory properties. Enjoy a wide variety of green, leafy vegetables as part of your Garden Food Plan.

Other healthful vegetables, in addition to those I've already mentioned, include (but are not necessarily limited to) the following:

- Asparagus
- Artichoke
- Avocado (although this one is technically a fruit!)
- Bean sprouts
- Beets
- Carrots
- Celery
- Collard greens
- Cucumber
- Green beans
- Lettuce (all types)
- Mushrooms
- Mustard greens
- Parsley
- Peppers (all kinds)
- Radishes
- Seaweed
- Spinach
- Sprouts
- Squash
- Turnips
- Tomatoes
- Watercress
- Zucchini

In general, the darker or more vibrant in color are your vegetables, the more nutrients they will contain. So, consume as many of these as possible.

Flaxseed

Flaxseed is another super food that particularly benefits people with hormonally influenced cancers like breast cancer. It contains lignans, compounds that have a weak estrogenic effect upon the body. These weak estrogens occupy estrogen receptor sites on cancer cells so that the cancer-causing xenoestrogens can't occupy them. So in the end, lignans actually end up acting like relative anti-estrogens in the body, even though they have estrogenic properties. Basically, they prevent other, more harmful estrogens from causing the breast cancer to grow.

In addition, the lignans in flaxseed are an excellent source of omega-3 essential fatty acids and alpha-linoleic acid, both of which decrease inflammation. Alpha linoleic acid decreases cholesterol and blood sugar in diabetics, and has a multitude of other benefits.

Fruits

All kinds of fruits are permissible on the Garden Food Plan, unless you have Candida, a blood sugar regulation issue, an allergy or infection, or you know that your body doesn't respond well to specific fruits. In general, though, fruits are very healthful because they cleanse your body of contaminants, and contain free radical-quenching antioxidants, essential vitamins, minerals and fiber. Some also have anti-cancer properties.

For instance, citrus fruits like oranges, grapefruits, lemons and limes eliminate cancer-causing free radicals and boost immune function. They contain Vitamin C, as well as flavonoids and nobiletin, which help to stop angiogenesis. Some studies have found reduced incidences of certain cancers, including lung cancer and colorectal cancer, among people who consume large amounts of citrus on a regular basis.[7]

Berries are another anti-cancer super food, because they contain high amounts of antioxidants and flavonoids that protect healthy cells, quench free radicals and lower inflammation. A summary of the anti-cancer nutrients in berries include: ellagic acid, Vitamin C, Vitamin A and folate. The anti-cancer antioxidant benefits of many berries, including blueberries, raspberries, black berries, cranberries and strawberries is summarized in an article published in 2015 in the *International Journal of Molecular Sciences*.[8]

In addition to citrus fruits and berries, some other delicious fruits to enjoy include:

- Apples
- Apricots
- Bananas
- Cherries
- Clementines (Tangerines)
- Grapes
- Guavas
- Kiwis
- Mandarins
- Mangos
- Melons
- Nectarines
- Papayas
- Peaches
- Pears
- Pineapples
- Plums
- Pomegranates
- Watermelons

Nuts and Seeds

Nuts and seeds are wonderful anti-cancer foods as well, especially walnuts and almonds. Other nuts, such as Brazil nuts, pecans, pistachios and macadamias are also healthful, and provide an excellent source of nutrients, including protein, fat, vitamins, minerals, carotenoids, and phytosterols. The only nuts that I don't recommend are peanuts, as most have been found to contain mold.

When preparing nuts for consumption, it's best to soak them overnight to remove phytates, which are sticky antioxidant compounds found in most nuts and seeds that can affect your gut, and interfere with the digestion of certain minerals like iron, zinc and manganese. By soaking the nuts and seeds, you remove the phytates and make them more digestible and bioavailable.

Rice and Beans

Rice and beans were most likely not found in the Garden of Eden, so they aren't first on my list of recommended anti-cancer foods, but I have found that some people tolerate them well, and they are an excellent source of protein and carbohydrates which don't feed cancer. In fact, when taken together, rice and beans provide all of the essential amino acids your body requires for life. Further, many cultures worldwide have subsisted on them as dietary staples for centuries, which attests to their nutritional value.

That said, rice and beans should not take the place of fruits or vegetables as the primary source of nutrition in your Garden Food Plan. You should consume them only as an adjunct to fruits, vegetables, nuts, sprouts and seeds, which are meant to be the basis of the plan.

Basmati rice is perhaps the most nutritious rice, and I highly recommend it. Other non-gluten grains and legumes, such as quinoa, gluten-free oatmeal, lentils and all kinds of beans, are also healthful, as long as you do not have diabetes or any other blood sugar regulatory condition that could make consuming these foods a concern.

Healthy Oils and Fats

Plant-based oils that have not been adulterated or processed are also an integral component of the Garden Food Plan. I encourage you to consume them in abundance as they have a multitude of health benefits. For instance, your body uses fat as a source of energy, to build cell membranes, promote healthy cholesterol levels and strengthen your cardiovascular system. Fats also provide your body with a nutritious source of protein and carbohydrates.

Olive, flaxseed, avocado and coconut oils are especially healthful oils for people with cancer. Most other oils, especially those that have been processed, are not healthy. For example, most of what is labeled "vegetable oil" is heavily refined soybean oil, which is produced under high heat and pressure, using industrial solvents. Similarly, cottonseed, safflower, corn, and grape seed oils are unhealthy, because they are polyunsaturated fats, which are prone to oxidation and free radical production when exposed to heat and light. Avoid these types of oils.

Purchase olive and avocado oil in dark glass bottles whenever possible, as it can easily become rancid when stored in clear plastic bottles.

The Problem with Animal Protein

I prefer that people with cancer don't consume meat, especially red meat, during their initial phases of treatment, for two reasons. First, about 30% of your caloric expenditure or energy is spent on digesting food, and animal protein requires more energy to digest than plant-based proteins. Your immune system needs as much energy as it can get to fight cancer, especially if it is in an advanced stage. I've also found that a plant-based diet helps patients who are fatigued and anemic to feel better.

In addition, I don't recommend animal protein during the initial stages of treatment because animal proteins are foreign to your body, and your immune system will create an antigen-antibody response against them. That means that every time you have poultry, beef or another animal protein, you are taxing your immune system to some extent.

That said, I recognize that some of you may have other health challenges that require you to consume animal protein. We have found that to be true for some of our patients as well so don't panic if this is you. Your Garden Food Plan must be based on your unique biochemistry as much as upon the guidelines that I share here. We are all biochemically unique and no one food plan strictly fits everyone.

If you do decide to consume animal protein as part of your daily food intake, make sure it comes from animals that were humanely raised. Seafood must be wild-caught, and beef, chicken and other meats must be from pasture-raised, non-GMO fed animals. Meat should be free of any added antibiotics or hormones, which can cause systemic inflammation, dysbiosis and other gastrointestinal problems, hormonal imbalances and immune system disturbances.

Fish

Small wild-caught fish such as salmon (e.g., from Alaska), are healthier for you than farm-raised fish, which are fed a non-native diet of corn, soybeans and other unhealthful foods. Wild salmon contains ample amounts of brain-healthy, anti-inflammatory omega-3 fatty acids, and much less unhealthy saturated fat than farm-raised fish.

Pacific sardines are one of the best fish you can buy, because they contain less mercury and heavy metals than larger fish, which tend to accumulate greater amounts of these toxins over their lifetime.

Visit any gourmet or natural food store, and you'll find sardines in all manner of flavors, whether plain or marinated in garlic, tomatoes, or olive oil.

Herring are a third good choice of fish, as they also contain high amounts of omega-3 fatty acids, as well as Vitamin D, and are smaller, lower mercury-containing fish.

I don't recommend eating shellfish, as the Bible tells us that these fish are not clean. Deuteronomy 14:9-10 states: "Of all the creatures living in the water, you may eat any that has fins and scales. But anything that does not have fins and scales you may not eat; for you it is unclean."

Pasture-Raised Poultry and Eggs

Pasture-raised chicken and turkey that are fed non-GMO grains and insects (rather than GMO corn, soy and grains, which are the dietary staples of most US-raised chickens), and which are not given hormones or antibiotics, are the best choices of poultry.

Be sure to read labels: free-range chicken may not be the same as that which is pasture-raised. Free-range chickens may be fed a non-native diet, and are only required to roam outside of their pens for five minutes daily, and may therefore not be as healthful as truly pasture-raised chickens that have spent most of their lives outdoors. Some companies, like US Wellness Meats, sell pasture-raised chickens: www.USWellnessMeats.com.

The same guidelines apply to eggs. Choose eggs that come from pasture-raised chickens that were fed a native diet, raised in uncrowded living conditions, and allowed to roam outside of their pens for most of their lives. In addition, they should be antibiotic and hormone-free.

Beef, Lamb, Bison, Elk and Other Red Meats

I discourage people with cancer from eating red meat, because it is inflammatory to the body. If you do choose to eat red meat from cows, lambs or other animals, make sure that it comes from 100% grass-fed animals, and is raised without synthetic hormones, antibiotics and other harmful chemicals.

Avoid pork though, as pigs are unclean animals that eat unsavory things, which then end up in your body! In the Bible, God also discouraged His people from eating pork. Leviticus 11:7-8 says, ". . . and the pig, for though it divides the hoof, thus making a split hoof, it does not chew cud, it is unclean to you. 'You shall not eat of their flesh nor touch their carcasses; they are unclean to you." Pork is one of the least healthful meats there is, even if it is tasty!

Green Tea: An Anti-Cancer Super Food

Green tea contains a multitude of powerful anti-cancer nutrients. The polyphenols in green tea, known as flavanols or catechins, comprise 30-40% of the solids found in green tea leaves. They have been proven in many studies to have significant anticancer properties. Among these, they halt tumor growth, induce apoptosis, and stop angiogenesis and tumor cell invasiveness. They have even been known to kill cancer stem cells. In addition, they modulate the immune system and activate detoxification enzymes that may help guard against tumor development.

In one study, published in *Nutrients* in March 2017, a combination of ascorbic acid (Vitamin C), lysine, proline, green tea extract, and quercetin was found to significantly suppress ovarian tumor incidence and growth, and lung metastasis in mice with ovarian cancer.[9]

Another study, published on Oct. 31, 2012 in the *Journal of Clinical Nutrition*, found that women who consumed green tea on a regular basis had a lowered risk of developing digestive system cancers, especially those of the stomach, esophagus and colon.[10]

Finally, a review of multiple studies on green tea, published in *Molecules and Cells* in February 2018, revealed EGCG, a principal anti-cancer compound in green tea that has been found to kill cancer stem cells, to either shrink or completely eliminate skin tumors when administered intravenously.[11]

Choose only organic green tea that hasn't been irradiated and which is caffeine-free. While it isn't always easy to determine whether a food has been irradiated, certified organic foods are less likely to be so. You can also ask the green tea company that you buy tea from whether they have an irradiation-free policy.

Water

Did you know that you are mostly made up of water? That's right: your blood is 92% water; your brain is 75% water, and your muscles are 75% water. Proper hydration is therefore very important: adequate intake of clean water cleanses and nourishes your cells, increases your body's ability to remove metabolic waste, and improves your digestion.

In addition to drinking ample amounts of clean water, you also want to drink water that balances your pH. Your body's pH, which is a measure of your acid-alkaline balance, should be around 7.36, or in a slightly alkaline state, in order to maintain homeostasis, or balance. **Most cancers thrive when your body is in an acidic state, and your water, along with your food and state of mind, can powerfully influence your acid-alkaline balance.**

Most bottled water is acidic, so I generally don't recommend drinking bottled water, unless you know for sure that it is alkaline. Water that's bottled in plastic also contains phthalates, which are inflammatory xenoestrogens, so you'll want to avoid drinking water from plastic bottles, as well.

Instead, I highly recommend hydrogen water, a subject on which I have published several recent papers with my colleagues across organizations.[12] This is a type of water that is enhanced with hydrogen, or H_2 molecules. Hydrogen is a selective antioxidant that bonds with cancer causing "OH" free radical molecules inside of your body, thereby converting those harmful molecules in your cells into hydrating ones. This is because when you combine OH free radicals with H_2 molecules, you get water!

At this point, you might be thinking, "Wait a minute, doesn't OH plus H_2 equal H_3O, not H_2O? To explain this anomaly, Gerald Pollack, PhD, BSEE, a brilliant researcher from the University of Washington, proposed that water exists in our bodies in a fourth state of matter that is similar to a crystal structure. This structure gives it form, unlike the liquid state. The empirical formula for this "structured" water averages out to H_3O_2. Hydrogen water creates conditions that help the body's water attain this "structure," helping cells and organs function well while staying hydrated.

Hydrogen water is also extraordinarily beneficial because almost every biochemical reaction in your body requires hydrogen, and most of us don't have enough of it. For instance, research shows that hydrogen water increases telomere length. Telomeres are the part of your chromosome that has to do with longevity. What's more, as an antioxidant, hydrogen decreases inflammation and improves metabolism.

To get hydrogen water, I recommend purchasing a hydrogen machine, which attaches to your kitchen faucet, and dissolves hydrogen into the water via a process called electrolysis. Many companies make quality hydrogen machines that you can buy. The machine should include a multi-stage filter that removes chlorine, chloramines, fluoride, heavy metals, pesticides, pharmaceuticals, VOC's, bacteria, viruses, algae, fungus, and other pollutants from tap water. Having a water filter is important since most tap water contains these cancer-causing pollutants.

You can also adjust the pH of your tap water with the machine, and choose more alkaline water for drinking purposes, and more acidic water for disinfecting purposes.

Further, you may even be able to program energetic frequencies into the machines to create homeopathic remedies, so it functions not just as a water filter, but also as a remedy maker! (You can learn more about hydrogen water machines through our resource page in the back of the book.)

I highly recommend a hydrogen machine because it has many healing benefits, which are priceless. If you can't afford one, I recommend at least purchasing bottled water in glass bottles, and choosing water from a reputable company that has verified its water to be free of contaminants and which is at least slightly alkaline.

Some refrigerators come with a water filter built in. While such filters are definitely better than drinking water straight from the tap in most parts of the world, make sure to change the filter cartridge regularly.

Your ultimate goal is to drink lots of water—half your body weight in ounces per day (e.g., if you weigh 140 pounds or 64 kilograms, drink 70 ounces)—that is, in order of preference:

1. Hydrogenated by a hydrogen water machine
2. Glass-bottled water (i.e., such as a home delivery service)
3. Filtered water using a clean cartridge that removes the maximum amount of cancer-causing agents from your water

WHAT ABOUT COFFEE?

Coffee is a controversial beverage. Of late, researchers have discovered that roasting coffee beans releases acrylamide into the coffee, which is a toxic carcinogenic substance. So now in California, all coffee shops are required to put a warning label on their coffee!

I know a thermographer in Los Angeles, who, when he relocated to a new office a few miles away from his former one, noticed that his thermography machines were showing a greater temperature variance in his patients' breasts more than in his previous location, indicating a greater abnormality in the breasts.

He didn't understand this, because he was seeing the same demographic of patients as before, and his new office was only a short distance from his former one.

Then one day, he noticed that many of his patients were drinking coffee in the waiting room. The receptionist told him that many were going across the street to a coffee shop while they were waiting for their appointment!

He concluded that the patients' breast tissue was absorbing some toxic ingredient in the coffee and causing the thermography to "light up." Perhaps it was the acrylamide.

In any case, even though I am Colombian-born (where we love our coffee!) I neither drink nor recommend coffee, not only because of the toxic chemicals in it, but also because it is a stimulant that dehydrates the body, which advanced cancer patients should avoid. Stimulants put the body in sympathetic dominance, or "fight or flight" mode, which is not conducive to healing. In addition, many people with cancer have insomnia and gastrointestinal issues, and coffee can exacerbate these problems.

Finally, most coffee contains mold. If you drink coffee, at least try a brand like Bulletproof, which has apparently been tested to be mold-free.

Juicing

Juicing is a fantastic way to get the most out of your fruits and vegetables. When you juice, the nutrients in the fruits and vegetables are readily assimilated by your cells, and you receive highly concentrated amounts of nutrients that your body doesn't have to expend much energy to digest and utilize.

Juicing is also the best way to cleanse and purify your blood from any cancer-causing contaminants. Use a variety of fruits and vegetables for making your juices, and switch them up as much as possible. All fruits and veggies contain a variety of healing nutrients.

Some excellent foods to use for juicing include: carrots, wheatgrass, pears, apples, pineapples and berries; all green leafy vegetables, including beet and carrot tops, collard greens, escarole, kale, dark lettuce, parsley, spinach and Swiss chard. Organic blueberries and other berries like raspberries and strawberries are excellent. While fresh berries are best, frozen organic berries are also permissible.

Most fruits and vegetables support the body in a variety of ways: for instance, parsley supports the thyroid, kidneys and adrenal glands, and cucumber has a lot of potassium and helps to cleanse the liver, as do beets and dandelion greens. Carrots cleanse the bloodstream.

Very often patients will ask me for a list of the best fruits and vegetables that will give them an optimal balance of nutrients. Don't get too caught up in making the perfect choices but try to rotate the foods you use, at least every three-four months. God put a unique set of nutrients in every fruit and vegetable, so by switching things up, you'll be providing your body with a broad range of nutrients, which is beneficial for healing.

Finally, I recommend drinking 4-5 glasses of fresh organic juice daily, that's composed of 80% vegetables and 20% fruit. It is best to freshly prepare each serving of juice, as the enzymes degrade the longer the juice sits on the counter or in the fridge. However, if you find preparing juice to be too time or energy consuming, go ahead and prepare multiple servings for the day, but keep them cold and refrigerated. Doing this is better than not juicing at all!

Herbs and Spices

In biblical times, herbs and spices weren't just tasty condiments: they were used in religious ceremonies such as burials, and in beauty care. They are featured throughout both the Old and New Testaments, highlighting their importance as healing and ceremonial agents, as well as savory additions to food.

Incidentally, many herbs and spices mentioned in the Bible have anti-cancer properties. These include (but are not limited to): aloe (John 19:39), anise (Mathew 23:23), cinnamon (Exodus 30:23), black cumin (Isaiah 28:25), mint (Matthew 23:23), and frankincense (Matthew 2:11).

The anti-cancer properties of a few of these, as well as other spices are summarized in an article published in *Food Chemistry* in 2012.[13]

In the meantime, I encourage you to include ample amounts of herbs and spices in your Garden Food Plan, as they are important healing foods that can add zest and nutrition to your smoothies, veggies, and other foods.

Curcumin

Curcumin, a compound found in the popular spice turmeric, has anti-cancer and other healing properties that are so powerful and numerous that some treatment centers, including ours, administer it intravenously as a cytotoxic treatment.

Among its benefits, curcumin stops inflammation, scavenges free radicals that cause cellular damage, regulates gene expression, and down-regulates the expression of pro-inflammatory cytokines or chemicals such as IL-6, IL-8, IL-1, and TNF. In addition, curcumin is a photosensitive substance and we use it in PDT Plus Therapy.

In higher dosages, it causes apoptosis, halts metastases, reduces cancer cell proliferation, impedes vascular endothelial growth factor (VEGF) from which tumors create blood vessels, activates tumor suppressor genes and can even halt cancer stem cell growth! It also inhibits the synthesis of proteins that play a role in tumor formation and suppresses oncogenes, or tumor promoter genes, that drive cancer's growth. By keeping inflammation down, it also keeps healthy cells from becoming cancerous.

According to an article, "The Benefits of Curcumin in Cancer Treatment," published on Mercola.com on March 2, 2014, Dr. William LaValley, a top natural medicine cancer physician, states that of all the nutrients, curcumin has the most evidence-based research to support its use as a cancer treatment. Not only does it affect more than 700 genes, but it also affects more than 100 different pathways once it gets into the cell. [14,15,16,17]

Soy

Soy is a mixed blessing. Most soy in the United States is genetically modified and therefore not healthful. However, non-GMO fermented soy products such as tofu and tempeh have powerful anti-cancer benefits for some types of cancer.

For instance, soy contains isoflavones, which are phytoestrogens that modulate the body's estrogen levels in a similar manner to the cruciferous vegetables. So ironically, soy can be both mildly estrogenic and yet have anti-estrogenic properties.

Among the isoflavones contained in soy, genistein has been shown to reduce cancer risk and inhibit the growth of cancer cells, especially in breast, prostate, colon and skin cancers. For instance, a study published in *Nutrients* in January 2018, concluded that soy is significantly associated with a lower risk of prostate cancer.[18]

But again, if you include soy in your nutritional plan, I advocate consuming only fermented non-GMO soy products. Asia has a very low incidence of breast cancer, and many researchers believe that it's because the people there consume an abundance of soy in their diet.

Whey Protein

Many people believe that whey is a healthy protein source. But I've found that it causes allergies or sensitivities in some cancer patients because it contains a protein called beta-casein, which they don't tolerate well.

KEY PRINCIPLE #3 | NUTRITION BASED ON THE GARDEN OF EDEN

People with cancer are often protein-deficient and at times are concerned about getting enough protein in their diet. But you can actually get sufficient amounts of protein from just vegetables, fruits, nuts and seeds!

Albumin is the most important and abundant protein in the body, and we have found that our patients who have albumin levels of 4 or above (the normal range is 3.5-5.5 mg/dcl) generally have better prognoses. Having adequate albumin is important, so one of our nutritional goals is to optimize our patients' albumin. We do this by recommending that they consume plant-based albumin-containing foods, such as pears, peas, beans, apples, bananas, barley, coconut, figs and oranges. You'll want to do the same!

Another way to increase your albumin is to have a plant-based protein drink daily. In the next chapter, I share some healthy options for plant-based protein powders.

The Absolute No-No's: As Far from the Garden as You Could Be

I don't have many stringent requirements as far as foods that you must absolutely avoid during recovery. However, a few categories of food you'll want to completely stay away from include:

1. **Gluten-containing foods.** Gluten has been known to damage the gut and cause inflammation and allergic reactions in most people.
2. **Dairy products.** Many people have sensitivities and/or allergies to dairy-containing foods. Like meat, they are also composed of proteins that are foreign to the body.
3. **Processed and refined sugars.** These inflame the body and feed cancer cells.
4. **Extensively processed foods with artificial ingredients.** This includes most foods that come in a box or a can, which are not natural and have more than just a few ingredients on their labels.

Does Sugar Feed Cancer?

Perhaps you've heard it said that cancer loves sugar, and that sugar is the number one food-like substance you want to avoid at all costs. This is true if the sugar you are consuming is unnatural, processed, refined or created by man. These sugars, which are typically found in baked or processed foods—like donuts, cookies, cakes, cereals, pasta and even things like yogurt and granola bars—do feed cancer and inflame your body, so it's imperative to avoid them.

Processed and refined sugars are rapidly absorbed into your bloodstream and create a systemic stress response. They spike your insulin, cortisol and cholesterol levels, and your adrenals become stressed as they produce adrenalin to try to remove all that sugar.

Yet not all sugars are bad for you, and not all sugars feed cancer! In fact, God has given us foods that contain natural sugar, such as fruit, and the body typically responds to these foods differently than it does to foods that contain processed or refined sugars. Fruit, honey, molasses and sugarcane—which are all-natural sugars—don't create the same alarm response in the body as processed sugar.

You may still be thinking, "But if fruit, honey and molasses still contain natural sugars, why wouldn't those sugars feed cancer, just as synthetic or processed sugars?"

Based on my clinical experience and patient outcomes, I believe there's a very important difference between sugars created by God and those created by man, and it's this: the sugars found in nature, or in "real" food created by God, have a left-spin movement energetically, while processed or refined sugars have a right-spin movement. In other words, the molecules in healthy sugars spin to the left energetically, and only normal, healthy cells can absorb left-spin molecules. Processed and refined sugars, on the other hand, spin to the right, and are selectively absorbed by cancer cells.

The fact that cancer cells cannot absorb left-spin sugars; only right ones, is why foods like fruit, which contain left-spin sugars, do not cause inflammation or feed cancer cells.

Consider the famous cancer doctor Max Gerson, MD, who frequently recommended carrot juice as part of his juicing protocols for cancer patients. Well, carrot juice has a high amount of natural sugar, but carrots are composed of left-spin molecules, so Dr. Gerson knew that they boost the function of healthy cells, but don't feed cancerous ones.

Similarly, studies have found that eating a ripe banana a day decreases the incidence of colon cancer significantly.[19] This lends further evidence to the fact that healthy, non-cancer causing sugars are found in fruits.

Conversely, for PET scans, a contrast medium is used which is a right-spin sugar molecule called fludeoxyglucose, which is absorbed by cancer cells, but not healthy ones.

Allergies and Food Sensitivities

Whatever nutritional plan you choose, you'll want to avoid any foods within that plan that you are sensitive or allergic to, because these cause inflammations, which can worsen cancer.

Allergies are not the same as food sensitivities. Food allergies will tend to cause a readily identifiable and immediate response in your body, like a rash, and can often be quite severe. Allergic responses are not dependent upon the amount of food you eat, whereas food sensitivities usually are.

If you have sensitivity to a particular food, you might tolerate very small amounts of that food but react to a larger amount. You may also not immediately perceive the negative reaction in your body from that food, but the food in question is taxing your immune system every time you eat it. Sensitivities can cause a broad range of symptoms as well, including irritability, fatigue, rapid heart rate, and brain fog. Sometimes, the detrimental effects of a food may be delayed and you may not feel poorly until one, two or even three days after you eat it.

For this reason, you may want to consider doing food sensitivity and allergy testing to determine what foods compromise your immune system. For allergy testing, I recommend Meridian Valley Lab in the Seattle, Washington area, which is directed by integrative doctor and author, Jonathan Wright, MD. To learn more, see: www.MeridianValleyLab.com.

Food is supposed to give you energy and mental clarity, and help you fulfill your daily activities to the maximum extent possible. If you eat a food, and the contrary happens, then that food is something you need to avoid.

Bloating, gas or flatulence, fatigue, brain fog, listlessness, irritability, increased heart rate, sleepiness, or even feeling like you were run over by a truck following a meal, are all signs that you ate something your body didn't like. So, pay attention to how you feel after you eat, as well!

How You Eat Is as Important as What You Eat

Hippocrates, known as the "Father of Medicine," said that we are what we eat. Yet in today's world, we aren't just what we eat, but what we absorb and utilize, and what we eliminate. Many factors influence these things.

Throughout history, families worldwide have taken their meals together, and I believe that God intended for mealtimes to be times of sharing and communion, not just food consumption. But in our fast-paced world of many distractions, we have lost the tradition of eating relaxed meals with our loved ones in a harmonious environment.

Eating in a relaxed manner with friends or family is important because your body's ability to digest, assimilate and utilize the nutrition in your food is affected by your environment, how you eat, and the company you keep.

It goes without saying then, that you shouldn't eat while working on the computer, browsing the Internet on your cell phone or watching TV. Besides the fact that electronic devices emit energetic frequencies that are harmful to your body, multitasking while eating can compromise your digestion.

In addition, make sure that you thoroughly chew each bite of food; ideally, 15-20 times per bite. Most of us tend to shovel our food into our mouths, and this can cause it to be poorly absorbed by the gastrointestinal tract.

If you are in the habit of eating rapidly and not chewing your food thoroughly, one way to slow yourself down is to put your fork or utensil down on the table in between spoonfuls or forkfuls of food. That way, you give yourself a bit more time to chew your food, before going on to the next bite.

KEY PRINCIPLE #3 | NUTRITION BASED ON THE GARDEN OF EDEN

You also want to avoid drinking beverages 30 minutes to an hour before meal times, as well as during meals and for about an hour or two afterward, if you can. Drinking while you eat causes your stomach acids and enzymes to be diluted, so you don't digest your food as effectively.

When you eat also matters. Your biggest meal of the day should be lunch. I also advocate **having a green smoothie for breakfast, to start the day off right with a burst of nutrients.** It also helps remove any toxins that your body may have processed during the night. One of my favorite smoothies consists of a pea or rice-based plant protein, chia seed and a tablespoon of coconut oil.

Finally, your digestion is also affected by your attitude toward food and how you prepare and consume it, among other factors. For this reason, **I encourage you to prepare your meals with an attitude of love and gratitude toward God, who gave us food for our health, enjoyment and nourishment.** Also give thanks for your food and bless it before you eat it, as I believe that doing so can decrease any contaminants in it and increase its benefits to your body!

Additional Tips for Enhancing Digestion

Consider drinking a glass of warm water when you wake up, as this primes your digestive system for food. Thirty minutes later, eat breakfast.

I don't recommend drinking cold beverages during recovery as your body has to expend energy to heat up the drink before it can properly assimilate it. This wastes valuable energy that you need to heal!

When you sit down to eat a meal, eat your raw foods first. Raw foods contain lots of live enzymes that help your body to digest both the raw and any cooked foods in the meal. For instance, if you normally have fruit and poached eggs for breakfast, eat the fruit first. If you have a salad, rice and beans for dinner, eat the salad first.

In addition, you may want to take supplemental hydrochloric acid and pancreatic enzymes before your meals. Your body uses these to break down food, so if you have an insufficiency of hydrochloric acid and/or enzymes in your gut—as most people with cancer do—

you won't absorb or properly assimilate the nutrients in your food without some help. To aid in digestion, I recommend Physica Energetics' Symbiome, Hypo Zymase and CataZyme-7, in addition to our proprietary nutritional product, GFP Nutritional.

About 80% of our patients have dysbiosis, a condition in which there is an imbalance of microbes in the gut; more pathogenic ones and not enough healthy ones. When you don't have enough friendly flora and too many of the "bad" guys, food can rot or ferment in your gut, so aiding your digestion with supplements like hydrochloric acid and enzymes can be very helpful for prevention.

Chemotherapy, radiation and the stress of having a cancer diagnosis can also compromise digestion. Recently, at our treatment center in Tijuana, we saw two patients who had very serious digestive problems. After only a few days of taking hydrochloric acid right before their meals, however, they felt much better and had improved energy.

Food Preparation and Cookware

All cooked foods should be either baked, sautéed, steamed or slow-cooked preferably at low temperatures in a slow cooker. Food retains more of its nutrients when cooked in one of these four ways.

Avoid frying, grilling and overcooking foods, as this depletes them of nutrients and creates compounds in the food that are carcinogenic to your body. Similarly, avoid microwaving food, as evidence suggests that microwaves create radioactive substances in food and destroy its nutritional content.[20,21]

Using safe cookware is also important. I recommend using only glass, stainless steel or non-lead cookware such as Corningware for preparing, cooking and storing your food. Aluminum and plastic cookware, which are perhaps the most commonly used, causes toxic aluminum and plastic to leech into the food and then your body. Aluminum has been linked to all kinds of diseases, especially neurodegenerative diseases like Alzheimer's. Make sure also to store your food in glass, ceramic or Corningware.

Non-Food Nutritional Factors

Your body's nutritional status isn't just influenced by what you eat, but also by your life's activities. For instance, when you get adequate sunshine, you provide your body with the best source of Vitamin D that there is. When you exercise, you receive more life-giving oxygen to your cells so that they can better utilize the nutrition that you get from your food. And, when you get adequate rest and sleep, your body more effectively metabolizes your nutrients and synthesizes proteins for healing.

Taking supplements is also a crucial component of most of our cancer patients' nutritional plans. In recent decades, our soil has lost many vital nutrients, which translates into nutrient-deficient food. Even the best organic soil is not as nutrient-rich as in years past, so it's a good idea to take supplements to compensate for any deficiencies.

For instance, studies show that vegetables and fruits contain just 30-50% of the nutrients that they did just 50 years ago. An article published in *Scientific American* states, "A landmark study on the topic by Donald Davis and his team of researchers from the University of Texas (UT) at Austin's Department of Chemistry and Biochemistry was published in December 2004 in the *Journal of the American College of Nutrition*.

"They studied U.S. Department of Agriculture nutritional data from both 1950 and 1999 for 43 different vegetables and fruits, finding 'reliable declines' in the amount of protein, calcium, phosphorus, iron, riboflavin (Vitamin B2) and Vitamin C over the past half century. Davis and his colleagues chalk up this declining nutritional content to the preponderance of agricultural practices designed to improve traits (size, growth rate, pest resistance) other than nutrition."[22]

That said, **you are a food body first, not a supplement body.** So if you have a Ziploc bag of pills, tablets and capsules in one hand, and an apple in the other, know that the apple is likely to benefit you more than all of the supplements taken together. This is because God made food, not supplements, and science and medicine still haven't discovered all the nutrients in our food. We may only know about a fraction of them, which means that supplements can never make up for all of the nutritional benefits that food provides us.

Final Thoughts

The best anti-cancer food plan is based on consuming food as God created it in nature and in the Garden of Eden, with fresh veggies, fruits, nuts, seeds, oils and spices as the foundation. It avoids processed, artificial, and non-organic food products, especially those that have ingredients on their labels that you can't recognize or can't pronounce. As well, avoid dairy products, gluten-containing grains, animal proteins, and of course, processed and refined sugars. The Garden Food Plan should give you energy, vitality and an overall sense of well-being.

If you suspect that the foods you're eating aren't doing just that, you may want to consult your nutritionist, doctor or other practitioner. Have them conduct food allergy or other types of testing to help you identify what you most need.

By doing these things and following the guidelines outlined in this chapter, you should find yourself well positioned to overcome cancer, and experience a higher level of well-being than perhaps you ever have before—and not just during cancer treatment, but throughout the rest of your life!

**FOODS TO CONSUME AND AVOID
BASED ON THE GARDEN FOOD PLAN**   Table 6.1.

Garden Based Foods	Benefits	Foods to Avoid	Why?
All kinds of vegetables, especially allium (such as onion, garlic and leek) and cruciferous	Contain phytonutrients that have anti-cancer benefits, in addition to other healing nutrients, including fiber, vitamins and minerals.	Animal protein, especially red meat (Note: Limited amounts of fish, and pasture-raised poultry and eggs are acceptable if you have a health condition that requires you to consume animal protein).	Contains proteins that are foreign to the body and requires additional energy to digest. Red meat can be inflammatory.
All kinds of fruits, especially berries	Contain antioxidants, vitamins and other cancer-fighting nutrients.	Gluten-containing foods.	Damage the gut and cause systemic inflammation.

continued on page 197

Key Principle #3 | Nutrition Based on the Garden of Eden

Garden Based Foods	Benefits	Foods to Avoid	Why?
Seeds and nuts	Healthy source of protein and fat to heal the cells and provide energy to the body.	Dairy products.	Contain foreign proteins, and may cause allergies, sensitivities and inflammation.
Healthy oils (e.g., coconut and olive).	Healthy source of fat to heal the cells, reduce inflammation, provide energy and boost the metabolism.	Processed and refined sugars.	Feed cancer, damage the cells and cause inflammation.
Plant-based protein powder	Provides a healthful source of supplemental protein.	Other processed and refined foods.	Encourages cancer growth, causes inflammation and damages the cells.
Herbs and spices	Have anti-cancer properties and add taste to food.	Coffee.	Contains acrylamide, which is carcinogenic.
Beans and rice (preferably Basmati)	Healthful source of plant-based protein and carbohydrates.	Whey protein.	Causes allergies and sensitivities and contains foreign proteins.
Fermented soy	Has phytoestrogens that may have anti-cancer effects upon reproductive cancers.	GMO foods, and conventionally-raised meats and produce.	Contain antibiotics, hormones, pesticides and other harmful chemicals. Are DNA-damaging.
Hydrogen water	Hydrates the cells and provides hydrogen ions that are important for cellular function.	Any other food that causes an allergy or sensitivity.	Causes a systemic inflammatory response in the body.
Green tea	Has anti-cancer properties.	Alcohol and soda pop.	May feed cancer and cause systemic inflammation. Compromises liver function.

SUMMARY

- An anti-cancer food plan should resemble what God gave our first ancestors in the Garden of Eden, with plant-based foods such as fruits, vegetables, seeds and nuts as the foundation.
- The right foods will give you energy, vitality and well-being. They are medicine as well as fuel for your body.
- All healthy foods come directly from one of four places: the ground, a plant, a tree or the sea!
- Most of our food supply has been heavily contaminated by chemical pollutants and GMOs, which make us sick. Choose clean, organic food whenever possible.
- Avoid dairy, gluten, man-made sugars, and artificial, processed foods, most of which come in a box or a can.
- How you eat is as important as what you eat. Bless and prepare your food with gratitude, chew it thoroughly, and enjoy meals in the company of others.

QUESTIONS FOR FURTHER REFLECTION

1. How is the Garden Food Plan unique from other anti-cancer "diets" out there?
2. Why is plant-based protein healthier for you than animal protein?
3. What foods directly cause cancer or encourage its growth?
4. Why are fruit and other natural sugars such as honey acceptable on the Garden Food Plan?
5. Name some anti-cancer "super foods."
6. What behaviors and habits encourage healthy digestion?
7. should your food be cooked and stored, for optimal nutrition and to avoid contaminating it?

7

Supplements That Repair and Restore Your Body

KEY PRINCIPLE #3
PART 2: FULL SPECTRUM NUTRITION

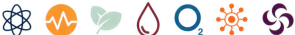

Please consult with your physician before taking any of the supplements recommended in this chapter, if you are currently receiving chemotherapy or radiation. While I believe that taking supplements during treatment is perfectly safe (and research shows that it actually improves recovery outcomes), controversy exists over whether patients who are receiving these treatments should take supplements, especially antioxidants. Some oncologists believe that antioxidants can reduce the efficacy of conventional treatments.

That said, according to a 2007 study review of the use of antioxidants during chemotherapy, published in the journal Cancer Treatment Reviews, *there is no evidence that antioxidant supplements interfere with the therapeutic effects of chemotherapy agents.[1] Despite this, a majority of oncologists remain opposed to their patients taking supplements during chemo or radiation therapy, so consult with your oncologist before taking any antioxidants.*

As you know by now, foods that most resemble what our first ancestors ate in the Garden of Eden are most optimal for cancer recovery. Yet today's fruits and vegetables are more nutrient deficient than those of our first ancestors. I mentioned in Chapter 6 that most fruits and vegetables contain anywhere from 30-50% of the nutrients that they did just 50 years ago. So, most of us need to take at least a few supplements to make up for what we may not be getting in our food.

Further, if you have cancer, your nutritional requirements are likely to be greater than average, because you have a process going on in your body that's taxing it. Similar to a marathon runner who needs more calories and nutrition than the average person to finish a race, your body is running a marathon to heal and so needs more of a nutritional "boost" to get to the finish line!

The Role of Supplements in Cancer Treatment

Supplemental nutrition is especially vital if you have had chemotherapy or radiation, since these treatments deplete your body of nutrients. For instance, chemotherapy and radiation affect your gut health by diminishing your appetite and causing nausea, vomiting and/or diarrhea, which compromises your nutrient absorption. For this reason, you will need to go a bit further than basic nutrition to optimize your nutritional status if you have received these treatments. At Hope4Cancer, 75% of our patients have metastatic cancers and about 70% have received chemo and/or radiation, so attention to nutrition is one of our foremost priorities for them.

The supplement plan we recommend to our patients is individualized, although we've found certain supplements to be foundational for

KEY PRINCIPLE #3 | SUPPLEMENTS THAT REPAIR AND RESTORE YOUR BODY

all people with cancer. These supplements support many aspects of healing encompassed in the 7 Key Principles of Cancer Therapy, and a few have already been mentioned in Chapters Four and Five, for their cytotoxic and immune-supportive benefits.

Therefore, these supplements not only compensate for any nutrients that your body may not be getting through food, but they also have powerful anti-cancer properties that have synergistic effects with other cancer treatments. A few are so strongly cytotoxic that they are really cancer treatments as much as nutritional supplements!

An effective, yet selective anti-cancer supplement protocol does all of the following:

- Modulates the neurological, endocrine and immune systems
- Restores intercellular and intracellular communication
- Detoxifies, cleanses and repairs the cells at a deep level
- Supports the organs, including the adrenal glands, thyroid, liver and gastrointestinal tract (stomach, small intestines and colon)
- Replenishes vitally needed nutrients so your whole body can function better

We focus on giving our patients targeted nutrients that we know are necessary for reversing disease, rather than trying to make up for every deficiency with dozens of different supplements. You can overwhelm your liver and GI tract by taking too many products, and complicate healing because your organs then have to process all of them.

Supplements That Restore Gut Health

Thermography testing has shown that 70% of all our cancer patients have gut dysbiosis, and/or fermentation and putrefaction. In dysbiosis, there is an excess of pathogenic microbes in the gut and not enough friendly ones. In fermentation, there is small bowel bacterial overgrowth in the stomach and small intestines (also called SIBO), which is caused by low stomach acid, immune system deficiency, malnutrition and other factors. Putrefaction is a condition in which undigested food simply stays in the gut and rots, rather than being digested by the body, and can also be caused by low stomach acid. It can cause bloating, digestive discomfort, chronic dehydration, or sometimes, no symptoms at all.

If you have dysbiosis, consider taking GI-supportive supplements to make sure your food and other supplements are actually getting to where they need to go, and that your body can break down, absorb and assimilate all of your nutrients. This includes, at the very minimum, hydrochloric acid, enzymes and a quality probiotic, which optimize the digestion and balance the flora, or beneficial bacteria in your gut.

I have found Physica Energetics' two products, Symbiome and Flora Syntropy, to be excellent gut-healing remedies. Symbiome delivers 50 billion CFU of ten probiotic strains in a unique symbiotic blend with pre and postbiotics in a nutrient-rich medium. Flora Syntropy delivers 50 million CFU of beneficial bacteria in a pre-probiotic formula. Together, these provide a complete array of pre-pro-postbiotics useful in applications ranging from constipation/diarrhea to irritable bowel syndrome (IBS), and for many chronic disease scenarios that involve a compromised gut.

In addition, hydrochloric acid (HCL) helps with the initial breakdown of food in your stomach, and enzymes further digest it as it passes through your small intestine and colon.

Protein Powder

Protein powders are a great way to ensure that you are getting enough healthy protein, in a form that is readily bioavailable to your body. I highly recommend plant-based protein powders, such as those that come from peas, which are much more effectively absorbed and assimilated than other types of protein. I discourage whey protein because people with cancer are often sensitive to it.

As I mentioned in Chapter 6, the most abundant protein in your body is albumin, which is synthesized in your liver. We have to emphasize albumin-containing foods in people with liver cancer or who have liver metastasis, because their albumin production is compromised. If this is you, a quality plant-based protein product can help to make up for any albumin or other protein deficiencies you may have.

The product I recommend for this purpose is GFP Nutritional. It provides a clean, rich source of protein and fiber derived from the pea plant, which also provides powerful immune support. With pea protein as the primary ingredient, GFP Nutritional delivers an assortment of essential and non-essential amino acids. This includes the all-important branched-chain amino acids, essential for rebuilding and strengthening muscles. The product is free from gluten, cholesterol and lactose, and can be used in both vegan and non-vegan diets.

Cytotoxic, Immune-Supportive and Detoxifying Supplements

Bee Propolis

If you'll recall from Chapter 5, bee propolis is a foundational supplement that contains compounds that modulate the immune system, reduce inflammation and quench DNA-damaging free radicals.[2] In addition, studies have shown it to be directly toxic to cancer cells.

One of the most well-studied compounds of propolis is caffeic acid phenethyl ester (CAPE). In a nutshell, CAPE destroys cancer cells, prevents angiogenesis and halts cancer cell replication.

Studies on cancer cells in vitro (i.e., cells that have been cultured in the lab) have been impressive. For instance, one study published in 2004 in the *Journal of Radiation Research* showed that CAPE eliminated 46% of lung cancer cells and reduced overall cancer growth by 60%. Three days after the treatment, 67% of all cancer cells were dead.[3]

Another study published in *Anticancer Drugs* in 2006 found that CAPE stopped colon cancer cells from multiplying and induced apoptosis in malignant cells without affecting healthy cells.[4] Similar effects have been found for breast, skin, gastric and pancreatic cancers, as well as for gliomas, a type of brain cancer.

Bee propolis is safe and has no side effects, even when it's consumed in higher amounts, so I recommend it to all of our patients with cancer.

Immune Power Plus

Like bee propolis, Garden Food Plan's Immune Power Plus has powerful anti-cancer ingredients. However, unlike propolis, which has significant cytotoxic, or cancer-killing effects, the benefits of this product are more strongly geared toward strengthening the immune system and restoring the essential nutritional building blocks the immune system needs to be revived.

In Chapter 5, I shared some of the main constituents and benefits of Immune Power Plus. These include restoring key micro and macronutrients that the immune system needs to function properly, such as the minerals magnesium, selenium and zinc. It also contains beta-glucans, which are immune modulators that activate T-cells, macrophages, antibodies, and natural killer (NK) cells, so they can better respond to the cancer.

Finally, Immune Power Plus contains turkey tail and astragalus. Turkey tail is a mushroom that has been shown to improve immune status, by enhancing the function of a variety of immune system cells, especially helper T-cells. Similarly, astragalus is an adaptogenic herb that improves immune function, and which protects the body from stress and disease.

All of the ingredients in Immune Power Plus function synergistically, potentiated and enhanced by one another. By enhancing your immune system, you can potentially decrease your risk of developing cancer. It is also very helpful for treating cancer, and for preventing any recurrences of disease.

If you are actively treating cancer, a standard dosage of Immune Power Plus is three capsules, three times daily. For maintenance, and to prevent disease recurrence, one capsule three times daily is adequate.

Vita LF Powder

Nature's nutrition comes in a variety of colors. It would only make sense that a complete nutritional supplement embodies all those colors. Vita LF Powder provides a naturally bioavailable product that delivers green, red, and blue colored nutrients from whole foods. The product is 100% organic, gluten-free, and non-GMO.

Lapacho Intrinsic

The immune system's function requires not only adequate nutrition, but also the fortification of key organs and overall health of the lymphatic system. Lapacho Intrinsic fortifies the spleen and supports lymphatic drainage, making it an important component of an immune support protocol.

Hepatagest

The liver is the hardest working organ in our body, constantly working to detoxify harmful chemicals (including heavy metals) and pathogens. Hepatagest is a synergistic combination of essential vitamins, minerals, amino acids, and botanicals designed to support the liver's detoxification pathways.

Energy Metabolism in Cancer

ATP, or adenosine-5-triphosphate is the energy currency of all cells. Cells require ATP, or energy to absorb nutrients, to react to changes in their surroundings, maintain their internal environment, and grow and replicate. ATP is especially important for cell division.

Healthy cells create energy via aerobic respiration, which occurs in the mitochondria, or energy powerhouse of the cell. This process involves breaking down glucose into a substance called pyruvate in the cytosol, transporting it to the mitochondria, and forming ATP in the presence of oxygen.

Cancer cells, on the other hand, use anaerobic respiration, which involves breaking down glucose into pyruvate in the cytosol, which is then directly converted into ATP and lactic acid. This process never reaches the mitochondria, and only generates 2 molecules of ATP. Thus, it is an inefficient way to create energy.

Cancer cells produce ATP at an accelerated rate. So, when we can slow or stop their production of ATP, we can trigger apoptosis and slow down cellular division, and angiogenesis.

Acetogenins are natural chemicals that inhibit energy (ATP) production in the cancer cells' mitochondria. As a result, they can slow down or stop the process of cancer cell division, so that the cells can't replicate.

What's more, angiogenesis, or tumor blood vessel formation, requires ATP, which means that acetogenins also stops new blood vessel formation.

GFP Nutritional is an excellent product that inhibits the energy production in cancer cells, while providing our healthy cells the necessary nutrition for improved metabolism.

Liposomal Vitamin C

Vitamin C plays a dual role in cancer recovery. As I mentioned in Chapter 4, Vitamin C has both cancer-killing properties and immune enhancing ones, depending on how it's used. At lower doses and when taken orally, Vitamin C stimulates the immune system and repairs the body, especially the connective tissue. At higher doses, and when it is taken intravenously, it kills cancer cells, including cancer stem cells.

A review published in *Nutrients* in November 2017 summarizes the immune-supportive benefits of Vitamin C. Among these, it:

- Is a potent antioxidant or free radical scavenger that helps to quench toxins that cause inflammation and cellular damage
- Is a co-factor for some gene regulating and other enzymes
- Supports both the innate and adaptive immune systems
- Strengthens connective tissue
- Accumulates in certain immune cells such as neutrophils, which play a vital role in fighting cancer
- Kills microbes, and cancer cells, especially at higher dosages[5]

I highly recommend doing intravenous Vitamin C treatments, in addition to taking a high quality, liposomal Vitamin C product. "Liposomal" means that the Vitamin C is encased in fatty membrane similar to a cell membrane, which makes it more bioavailable to your body.

Liposomal products are more expensive than regular supplements, but your body absorbs almost everything from liposomal supplements;

about 90%, compared to non-liposomal supplements, which have an absorption rate of about 70-75%, so that you don't need to take as much.

Physica Energetics makes quality liposomal Vitamin C products. Any product that you choose, like these, must be non-corn sourced and non-GMO and come from cassava, tapioca or beets. Most Vitamin C is made from corn and we have found that our patients' tumors grow aggressively when they take corn-derived Vitamin C, which is genetically modified, causes allergies, and damages the gut. For this reason, it is vital to choose a non-corn source of Vitamin C.

On that note, **all supplements that you take should be non-GMO, free of artificial ingredients and toxins.** Never take supplements that are potentially toxic due to their poor quality. So don't skimp and buy inexpensive products you know little about—they could literally do you more harm than good in the long run!

Instead, read the reviews for any products you are considering, which are often featured on product websites. Also, consult with a knowledgeable health care practitioner to find those supplement companies with a reputation for effectiveness.

To find your optimal Vitamin C dose, begin by taking 1,000 milligrams daily, and increase that by 500 or 1,000 milligrams per day until you get slightly loose stools. This is called the **"C-flush"** dose. Then, reduce that dose just slightly to get your ideal daily dose. You may also want to divide your daily amount into two doses, with one taken in the morning and the other in the evening, so that your body receives a continuous supply of Vitamin C.

Many integrative practitioners do IV Vitamin C treatments. If you aren't able to come to Hope4Cancer, I recommend researching a practitioner in your area who does.

Vitamin D

Vitamin D, which acts more like a hormone in the body than a vitamin, is a particularly powerful anti-cancer nutrient. **It positively affects more than two hundred genes in the body,**[6] **and research suggests that it can help to inhibit cancer cell's growth and replication cycle, stop new tumor blood vessel growth and even cause apoptosis.**

A medical research review on Vitamin D published in May 2017 in *Clinical Therapeutics* states that Vitamin D has particularly strong effects upon breast, prostate, and colorectal cancers, as well as melanoma.[7]

Studies also show that it reduces the risk of developing at least 17 different cancers, ranging from colon, breast, and prostate cancers to ovarian, esophageal, renal, and bladder cancers.[8] And, evidence suggests that it may improve treatment outcomes in people already diagnosed with cancer.

Current US RDA guidelines for Vitamin D supplementation are too low. Most sources recommend that your Vitamin D levels be 40-60 ng/ml daily, but for cancer prevention, you want your blood levels to be between 80-100 ng/ml. If you are actively treating cancer, the number should be closer to 140 ng/ml. I have never seen anyone with Vitamin D toxicity, so don't worry about these levels being too high. We've been led to believe that we need much less Vitamin D than we really do.

To get to 140 ng/ml daily, you might start off by taking 5,000-10,000 IU of Vitamin D daily, but you may need much more than that, depending on your current blood levels. I don't have cancer, and I sometimes take up to 10,000-20,000 IU per day. And if you're under a lot of stress and/or coming down with a cold, then you will need to take even more.

Our Sunivera Immunotherapy protocol includes Solray-D Liposomal Spray, a Vitamin D supplement I highly recommend. Required for the efficient functioning of GcMAF in Sunivera, this product delivers Vitamin D in its D3 form, and in combination with Vitamin K2. Vitamin K2 is essential as a co-supplement to Vitamin D3 to ensure proper absorption of calcium and prevent calcification of soft tissues. Most Vitamin D3-K2 supplements contain a synthetic version of Vitamin K2. However, Solray-D contains the natural form menaquinone-7, MK7, which is known to be 1,000-fold more effective than the synthetic version, MK-4.

Melatonin

Many people nowadays don't get enough sleep, yet seven-nine hours of quality sleep per night is important for recovery. Also, you'll want to **be asleep between 10 PM and 2 AM, because that's when your body detoxifies, repairs and regenerates itself.**

KEY PRINCIPLE #3 | SUPPLEMENTS THAT REPAIR AND RESTORE YOUR BODY

When you don't get enough sleep, your body is more inflamed and your insulin levels are higher. Sleep deprivation also causes your body to produce fewer natural killer (NK) cells, which are one of your principal defenses against cancer.

Melatonin is a hormone that your body naturally produces to help you sleep, but it can become depleted with aging and other factors, such as chronic disease. Fortunately, supplemental melatonin can make up for what your body may not be making on its own. It is a safe supplement that incidentally, also has anti-cancer effects at higher dosages.

For instance, a study published in the *Journal of Pineal Research* showed that melatonin reduced the risk of many cancers by up to 34%. From this, the lead researcher of the study concluded that melatonin has great potential as a cancer treatment.[9]

For sleep, lower doses of between 1-5 mg may be sufficient, but some people need more. For anti-cancer effects, 10-30 mg daily or higher may be used, but I don't recommend taking high doses as a cancer treatment except under the supervision of your doctor.

Many melatonin products work well. Physica Energetics makes a good liposomal melatonin product.

Curcumin

Curcumin is perhaps one of the most powerful anti-cancer phytochemicals that God has created. Thousands of studies demonstrate its anti-inflammatory and anti-cancer benefits. As I mentioned in Chapter 4, curcumin halts angiogenesis and tumor cell proliferation, prevents metastases, suppresses inflammation, stimulates your immune system, and quenches free radicals that cause cellular damage. These and other benefits are summarized in an article published April 2017 in the *Journal of Traditional and Complementary Medicine*.[10] In addition, curcumin is a photosensitizing agent that can be used in Photodynamic Therapy.

As we mentioned earlier, curcumin is found in the spice turmeric, but to benefit from its anti-cancer properties you'll want to take higher and more concentrated amounts, which you can get from curcumin supplements. Not all curcumin products are absorbed well when taken orally, though, so choose a product that has a reputation for effectiveness, and which contains ingredients that help your body absorb and assimilate it, such as bromelain and black pepper.

Curcumin products that I recommend include Physica Energetics' Bio-A Curcumin Phytosome. "Phytosome" indicates that the curcumin is bound to phosphatidylcholine, a fat that also helps to increase its absorption and assimilation.

Taking curcumin orally is a great way to reduce inflammation and quench cancer-causing free radicals that damage your DNA. For cancer treatment purposes, you'll want to take higher doses intravenously. Integrative doctors worldwide give curcumin intravenously, including ours.

Effective oral doses can vary widely. According to the European Food Safety Authority Panel, an acceptable daily curcumin dose is 3 mg/kg, or 1.4 mg per pound of body weight. In research studies, patients have been given anywhere from 0.5 grams (500 mg) to 7.5 grams (7,500 mg) of curcumin daily, divided into three or four doses. However, some people have taken oral doses of up to 12 grams without severe side effects.

Mild and temporary side effects can occur with curcumin. These include: gastrointestinal upset, diarrhea, bloating and nausea.

Supplements for Cellular Hydration

Dehydration is a common problem among cancer patients; therefore, **restoring cellular hydration is vital for recovery.** This is achieved not only by drinking enough water, but also ensuring that you have an optimal balance of macro minerals or electrolytes such as magnesium, potassium and sodium, which control the balance of water in and out of the cells.

Electrolyte balance is controlled by hormones from the adrenal glands and kidneys, so supporting these organs also can be helpful. Physica Energetics makes an excellent product called ReHydrate, which contains homeopathic dilutions of kidney and adrenal gland organs, as well as other ingredients that affect hydration and electrolyte balance.

In addition, we give our patients SpectraLyte, which is a broad spectrum, alkalizing trace mineral formulation that replenishes electrolytes. It is an excellent product for people whose electrolyte balance has become compromised by adrenal insufficiency, prolonged illness or digestive disturbances.

Green Tea Extract

In Chapter 6, I shared that green tea contains multiple polyphenols that have been shown in studies to have significant anti-cancer properties. Green tea extract halts tumor growth, induces apoptosis, and stops angiogenesis and tumor cell invasiveness. In addition, it modulates the immune system and activates detoxification enzymes that may help guard against tumor development.

While drinking green tea is a great way to receive anti-cancer polyphenols, I recommend taking a high-quality green tea extract to get concentrated amounts of EGCG and other polyphenols into your cells.

A number of companies make quality green tea extract products. Choose a reputable brand recommended by your doctor, though, as not all green tea products are created equal.

Cannabinoids

Cannabinoids come from cannabis, which is a plant family that includes many species, including hemp and marijuana. The plants within this family have been used medicinally for nearly 5,000 years, beginning with traditional Eastern medicine. Over the centuries, they have been used to treat a wide range of conditions, including cancer and symptoms caused by cancer treatments, including low appetite. In addition, they have anti-fungal, anti-inflammatory, and immune and nervous system modulating effects, among others.

Some cannabinoids have psychotropic, or mind-altering effects, while others don't. Tetrahydrocannabinol (THC) is the main compound that has mind-altering effects and is typically associated with marijuana.

Cannabidiol (CBD), on the other hand, is found in high amounts in hemp, and in lower amounts in marijuana. Pure CBD from hemp has zero psychotropic effects and it is this compound that I recommend for all cancer patients, for its multitude of benefits and ease of access. Unlike THC-containing products, which are only available via prescription in some countries and certain areas of the United States, you can get pure hemp-derived CBD everywhere.

CBD is safe, non-toxic and has powerful antioxidant and anti-inflammatory properties. It can alleviate insomnia, anxiety and pain, and relaxes the body.

Even more amazing, it has cancer-killing effects: it induces apoptosis; halts tumor invasion and metastases; and reduces angiogenesis and stops cancer cell proliferation.[11] A review published in June 2015 in the *Journal of Immune Pharmacology* states that in animal studies, CBD has been shown to inhibit the progression of many types of cancer, including glioblastoma, breast, lung, prostate and colon cancers.[11]

In general, though, experiments conducted by many research institutions have shown both THC and CBD to have profound effects upon many cancers, including seven of the most aggressive cancers (i.e., lung, ovarian, kidney and colon cancers; leukemia, melanoma, and triple-negative breast cancer).[12] Other cancers not mentioned in this list also respond to cannabis.

When CBD is used as a cytotoxic treatment, higher doses are required than when it is used as a sleep aid, pain reliever, relaxant, or to reduce other symptoms. I don't recommend self-treating with CBD to manage cancer; however, for symptomatic relief, I highly recommend over-the-counter CBD products such as ointments, extracts and capsules.

To my patients, I recommend the Garden Food Plan endorsed suite of CBD products. For more information, visit this book's website: hopeforcancerbook.com.

Bach Flowers

I am a fan of Bach flowers, which are liquid homeopathic remedies that can help patients process difficult emotions, many of which are the core cause of their cancer—its development, progression and metastases. These remedies are a helpful adjunct to other emotional healing tools, such as having a close relationship with God, which is paramount for emotional and spiritual health.

Bach flower remedies harmonize discordant or negative emotional energies within the body by introducing opposite frequencies to cancel out the discordant ones. Everything, including our emotions, contains

KEY PRINCIPLE #3 | SUPPLEMENTS THAT REPAIR AND RESTORE YOUR BODY

a measurable energetic frequency, so Bach remedies can assist with replacing negative frequencies with positive ones.

Homeopathic Drainage Formulas

Homeopathic drainage formulas are helpful for eliminating toxins generated by dying cancer cells and the environment. Drainage remedies do just what they sound like: they help to "drain" toxins out of the kidneys, lymphatic system and liver.

They are gentle and effective, and I highly recommend them, especially if you find that you are feeling toxic as a result of your treatments. There are many effective drainage remedy products. I prefer those by Physica Energetics.

Some of the drainage remedies by Physica Energetics that are beneficial for lymph drainage include:

- **Lymph 1 Acute,** which is for subtle inflammation and minor problems in the lymphatic system.
- **Lymph 2 Matrix,** which penetrates deeper into the extracellular matrix.
- **Lymph 3 Chronic,** which goes deep into the body and is most appropriate for people who have chronic, longstanding inflammation, and whose systems are rigid and not responding well to anti-cancer therapies.

In addition, I recommend Physica Energetics' Drainage Milieu for detoxification of the extracellular matrix, and a product called Burdock Intrinsic, which cleanses and supports the blood, lymphatic system, liver and spleen. However, I don't recommend taking all of these products at the same time, but rather, one at a time, in layers. You will want to work with a doctor at Hope4Cancer or with your own doctor to determine the regimen that's best for you.

Bio-Identical Hormone Replacement and Support

Your body's endocrine, or hormonal system, functions in concert with your immune and neurological systems. This means that if one system

HORMONES: ORIGINS AND FUNCTIONS

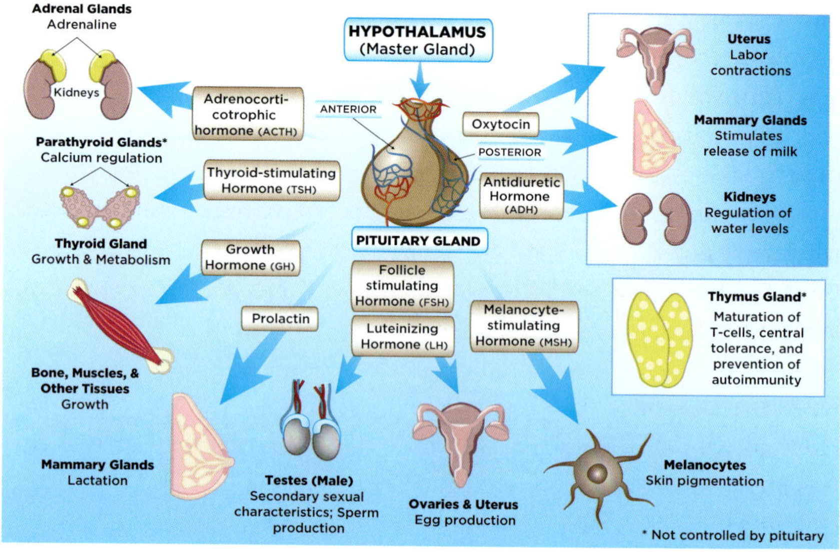

Figure 21. The endocrine system consists of a series of glands dispersed across the body that release biochemicals that we know as "hormones." These hormones have a profound influence on the functioning of every system of the body from metabolism, nervous system response, sexual development, etc. These hormones are not only individual messengers, but they often interact together as well. The cancer terrain is often characterized by hormonal imbalance that can trigger the growth of cancer, e.g., breast, ovarian, and uterine cancers are associated with estrogen and progesterone. In addition, cancers can affect the endocrine glands themselves, leading to hormonal imbalances that throw the body into functional chaos. That is why rebalancing the endocrine system is an essential step in a cancer therapeutic protocol.

is out of balance, the others will be, too. Proper hormonal balance is essential for recovery from cancer, so this is another area that you may need to address as part of your healing process.

That said, I don't recommend that you randomly take supplemental hormones, because hormone balancing isn't a do-it-yourself endeavor. You can easily cause more problems than you solve by taking supplements and hormones your doctor hasn't recommended, or which aren't based on lab test results. No hormone-balancing supplement or supplemental hormone is beneficial for all cancer patients so don't take something just because you read about it on the Internet.

However, I encourage you to ask your doctor whether you should do hormone testing, as hormonal imbalances can often be corrected by taking supplemental bio-identical hormones. These powerfully support the body and can be a critical piece of the healing puzzle for many people. I recommend doing a hormone test at a reputable lab such as Meridian Valley Labs. Jonathan Wright, MD, is the medical director of this lab, and was the first practitioner to develop and introduce the use of supplemental bio-identical hormones in integrative medicine.

Meridian Valley Labs also has an expert staff of naturopathic doctors who are well-trained in hormone balancing and who can prescribe compounded hormone and hormone-supportive products based on your lab results. To learn more see: MeridianValleyLab.com.

Nutritional Testing

How do you know if you have any specific nutritional deficiencies? It is often a good idea to do nutritional testing to find out whether you have any specific deficiencies that require additional supplementation. Two good laboratories to evaluate your nutritional status are Spectracell (SpectraCell.com) and Genova Diagnostics' NutrEval FMV (GDX.net).

SUPPLEMENTS THAT REPAIR AND RESTORE THE BODY — Table 7.1.

Supplement	Purpose and Benefits
GI-supportive nutrients: HCL, enzymes and probiotics	To optimize digestion, assimilation and uptake of nutrients, and balance healthy bacteria in the gut.
Pea and rice-based protein powder	Provides a healthy source of plant-based protein to the body.
Propolis	Modulates the immune system, reduces inflammation, and is cytotoxic.
Immune Power Plus	Strengthens and modulates the immune system.
Liposomal Vitamin C	Has both cancer-killing and immune-enhancing properties. Repairs the body, especially adrenals and connective tissue; is an antioxidant.
Liposomal Vitamin D	Has anti-cancer properties, supports immune function and affects more than 200 genes.

continued on page 216

Supplement	Purpose and Benefits
Melatonin	Aids in sleep and has cytotoxic effects at higher dosages.
Curcumin	Halts angiogenesis and tumor cell proliferation, suppresses inflammation, and stimulates the immune system.
CBD	Alleviates insomnia, pain, anxiety and other symptoms; has cytotoxic and anti-inflammatory properties.
Green tea extract	Induces apoptosis, halts tumor growth and angiogenesis. Modulates the immune system.
Supplements for Cellular Hydration	Hydrate and balance electrolytes in the cell.
Drainage remedies for organ support	Help remove toxins from the organs of elimination.

SUMMARY

- The right supplements will provide vital nutrients to your body, have healing and cytotoxic properties, and enable you to recover more effectively from cancer.
- Hydrochloric acid, enzymes and a quality probiotic optimize the digestion, assimilation and uptake of all your nutrients, and balance the flora in your gut.
- Protein powders from peas and other vegetable sources are a great way to ensure that you are getting enough protein in a form that is readily bioavailable to your body.
- Bee propolis contains compounds that modulate your immune system and reduce inflammation.[2] It is also toxic to cancer cells.

KEY PRINCIPLE #3 | SUPPLEMENTS THAT REPAIR AND RESTORE YOUR BODY

- Vitamin C has both cancer-killing and immune-enhancing properties, depending on how it's used. Choose non-corn-based liposomal Vitamin C supplements.
- Vitamin D affects more than 200 genes in your body,[6] and has powerful anti-cancer properties. Your Vitamin D level should be around 140 ng/ml if you are overcoming cancer.
- Melatonin is a great sleep aid and has anti-cancer effects at higher dosages.
- Curcumin is one of the most powerful natural cytotoxic compounds. Thousands of studies demonstrate its anti-inflammatory and anti-cancer benefits.
- Green tea extract has been shown in many studies to have significant anti-cancer properties. ECGC is one of its principal cytotoxic compounds.
- CBD is a compound found in cannabis and hemp that relieves pain, relaxes your body and mind, relieves insomnia, is not psychotropic, and has anti-cancer properties.

QUESTIONS FOR FURTHER REFLECTION

1. Describe three reasons why supplements are important in healing from cancer.
2. Why does the quality and type of Vitamin C you take matter?
3. What are drainage remedies and how do they assist your body with detoxification?
4. Which supplements have cytotoxic, or cancer-killing benefits, in addition to nutritional ones?
5. How do Bach flower remedies release harmful emotions?
6. Which supplements have anti-inflammatory properties?

JUAN'S STORY

Juan was diagnosed with stage IV kidney cancer in 2012, when he was 37, and underwent years of chemotherapy while also receiving natural treatments at Hope4Cancer, the latter of which greatly aided in his recovery. He lives in Temecula, California, with his wife and two sons.

I was diagnosed with cancer in my right kidney in 2012. A week or two after my diagnosis, I had a partial nephrectomy, or part of my kidney surgically removed. The doctors told me that I was cured, and to go live my life.

Fast forward to 2015. I began to have symptoms that resembled those I first had when I was first diagnosed, so I went to the doctor, who ran some tests on me and told me that I had kidney cancer—again!

At the time, I thought, *This can't be, I just had kidney cancer.* But it had come back.

So I had another surgery, this time a radical nephrectomy, and my entire kidney was removed. But I felt that removing the kidney wasn't all there was to this; something was really wrong.

Well, I soon learned that the cancer had metastasized and was now a stage IV disease that wasn't just in my kidneys, but also my lymphatic system.

When I asked my doctor what it meant to have a stage IV cancer, he responded, "This means that the cancer is now deadly."

I was in shock. The doctor put me on an oral chemotherapy drug called Afinitor two months following my surgery, and I went to see an oncologist in the meantime. From that point on, it was as if the doctors just kept giving me one bad news report after another.

One oncologist told me I could expect to live about 12 months, because I was young (as if that was good news!).

My wife decided that we needed a second opinion. So we went to the City of Hope cancer treatment center in Duarte, California, which is one of the top-ranked cancer centers in the United States.

In the meantime, we spent 12 hours a day researching treatment alternatives online. I have family in Tijuana, Mexico and they had told me there were many alternative cancer centers there. So after doing some research, I personally visited what I believed were the top five clinics in Tijuana, including Hope4Cancer.

In the end, we decided on Hope4Cancer Treatment Centers, because it was the most complete, offering the widest variety of treatments. Observing the other patients there also convinced me that it was the best place to be. They all seemed optimistic and healthy, and were running around doing all kinds of therapies, like IV Vitamin C, laetrile, ozone, sauna, Sono-Photodynamic Therapy, and so on. They were really well-informed about the treatments, and when I asked them why they chose the treatment center, they were able to tell me exactly why. So I thought, *Wow, this place is it!*

The atmosphere at Hope4Cancer was different than what I'd experienced at the conventional cancer clinics, where everyone felt sorry for you. Here, people were optimistic and actually believed that there was something they could do about their cancer, besides just wither away and die.

Another thing I liked about Hope4Cancer was that there was a really mixed crowd there. I saw people my age, older people, and even children. This really attracted me to the center.

My attitude changed after finding Hope4Cancer. I thought, *Well, this is it, give it your best shot, and give it all that you can.* Prior to that, I had been really down, and had believed that my life was ending. I had opened up a trust, did a will and stopped working. The doctors had already talked to me about hospice.

So about a month after my second surgery, I enrolled at Hope4Cancer and received treatment at the center for three weeks. Over the past few years, I have visited the center two more times. In between visits, I have continued to do Sonodynamic Therapy and some of the other treatments that Dr. Tony recommended, at home.

The same year I also visited another center to get a famous tonic called Hoxsey, along with some supplements, which I took at home, along with my other treatments.

At first, I had a large number of tumors in my lymph nodes. When I had surgery, the doctors removed some of them, but there were so many that they couldn't remove them all. So I did Sono treatment at home over the areas where the largest nodules, or tumors were: in my neck, chest and abdomen.

When I first went to Hope4Cancer, I brought my CT scans and tests that I had done in the US along with me. When Dr. Tony advised me about the dangers of CT scans, I asked my oncologist at City of Hope, where I was doing chemo, if I could instead do MRIs to assess my progress.

The oncologist was non-approving of my approach, and instead gave me a 15-minute lecture. He chided me about all these so-called "alternative" cancer doctors out there who are predatory and take advantage of patients. He stated that conventional medicine was proven and had a track record for treating cancer.

When I pointed out to him the dismal outcomes of conventional medicine for cancer, and how there hasn't really been any improvement in treatment outcomes over the years, he seemed to waffle and said, "Well, cancer evolves and changes..."

To which I responded, "Really? So cancer has been changing over the past 50-60 years and doctors can't keep track of it?" Medicine has made progress in developing treatments for other diseases, but not cancer. Imagine!

But my former doctor, who was an intern working under an oncologist, told me the same thing. She said that I shouldn't risk my life on alternative medicine—even though they had only given me 12 months to live, anyway!

I started to do chemotherapy two months following my first visit to Hope4Cancer, and decided to work with an oncologist anyway. Now I think it was more out of fear that I chose to do chemo in the first place.

In the meantime, my oncologist would assess my progress with MRIs and CT scans, and although I would fight with him about doing CTs, due to the dangers of the radiation I continued to do them.

Throughout 2015, there was no change in my lymph nodules. My oncologist was actually excited about this, saying, "Look, the tumors haven't grown. You could live a couple of years!"

Throughout most of 2016, the cancer remained the same; not shrinking but not growing either, although in late 2016 it finally started shrinking! I was still doing chemotherapy, alongside Dr. Tony's and the Hoxsey protocol. I was also taking frankincense, which I had discovered has many anti-cancer benefits.

Then, in about the middle of 2017, my test report stated, "No known nodules (or tumors)". The report didn't necessarily mean I was in remission, since the CT scan can't detect individual microscopic cancer cells, but it meant that my treatments were working!

Another test that I did later in 2017 showed the same results, so I began to cut my chemo pills in half. I guess it was a risky move at the time, but I didn't like the effects of the chemotherapy. It made me lethargic and tired, gave me cold sores, caused my nails to be fragile, and my hair to fall out. My oncologist said that it affects people differently.

In January 2018, after receiving chemotherapy for two and a half years, I stopped. I had seen firsthand the effects of long-term chemo on my mother, who also had cancer. During the five years she underwent chemotherapy, she seemed to age 15 years. Her speech became slurred and I could tell her brain was deteriorating from the effects of it. The chemo really took a toll on her body—especially her brain and bones.

My mother's life has not been the same since doing chemo. She was once a leader—a businesswoman and immigrant who had raised her children and was very independent—who became like a fragile little girl, dependent on others. She used to socialize and dance, and now she gets tired a lot, has to take naps, and is in bed often.

Chemotherapy changed her life, and I decided I didn't want to end up living like that. I have a wife and two children, and I didn't want to spend the rest of my days weak and in bed.

I'd rather pass away healthy than end up in the same kind of situation that she was in, so that's why I stopped taking chemotherapy. And in hindsight, I actually think I probably could have stopped chemo years ago. As I mentioned, I think I did chemo out of fear, not because I thought it was working.

Because I did more than just one cancer treatment, it's hard to say which ones have really helped the most; but I don't feel like I necessarily needed the chemotherapy.

At the time of this writing I have been off chemotherapy for almost a year, and my scans remain clear. I still consult with Dr. Tony from time to time, and he is always so generous with his time, which is amazing because so many people demand his time. He now wants me to do a blood test to determine how many cancer cells might be left in my bloodstream, so I still need to do that.

In the meantime, I continue to follow a healthy diet that is rich in organic vegetables and fruits, and low in meat. All our food is organic and non-GMO. Whenever I do eat meat, which isn't often, it's grass-fed. I also have wild-caught fish, and organic, pasture-raised chicken. I eat nothing canned; all my food is as fresh and natural as can be.

I feel great now. Whenever I talk to other people who have cancer, they will say to me, "I would never guess that you have cancer"—because I am doing so well. In fact, all that I went through now feels surreal, like a dream, as if I never even had cancer. I'm active, working, spending time with my kids, and doing lots of other things.

Cancer does give you a different perspective about life, though. You discover that you aren't going to live forever, but I'm grateful for that perspective. Everyone knows that they are going to die someday, but they often think that it's not now. Many people are in denial about death, I think, which isn't healthy.

My family and I have asked ourselves, though, how we can live today to make our tomorrow better. As part of that, we've made some changes in our lifestyle. We now take more chances. We used to travel once a year, if that; now we travel three times a year. We focus more on our children. I put my work second, not first anymore. So this really has been a very positive experience overall.

You know, when you get cancer, suddenly everybody around you gives you advice. Everyone becomes a guru, including your doctors. If you're battling cancer, I encourage you to take everything with a grain of salt, take a step back and evaluate your options. Get educated and do your research. Just because somebody tells you to do a treatment, doesn't mean that treatment is right for you. Only *you* know what's best for you.

If you believe you're going down a rabbit hole, then that will be true. But it doesn't have to be that way. You don't have to believe everything your doctor tells you. While your loved ones may mean well, cancer is a personal thing and you have to do what works for you.

Also, you tend to experience a lot of emotions when you have cancer, especially hopelessness. I think a lot of people go through what I call a "black hole" or a kind of depression when they first get diagnosed. I know that I did.

I would get really angry. I remember going to meet people for a barbecue or other event and they would say things to me like, "I know what you are going through. I broke my leg. . . " And it would make me so angry, because I'd think, *You have no idea what I am going through.*

It's important to work through these kinds of things. So if you need to cry, or take some time to be alone and process things—that's fine. Just take some time for yourself, whether a day or week, and then say, "Okay, what am I going to do about this?" And decide to get over the hopelessness bump. If you don't, you'll tend to believe the worst and focus on all the bad things that are happening to you. It can be difficult to come out of the depression, but you can do it!

My wife helped me to get over the hopelessness bump by telling me things like, "You're spending too much time in the dark," and encouraging me to get out and about. She would say, "Come on, let's go for a walk, or go shopping." She would put on music and let light into the house—things like that. I think my children played some part in helping me to get out of a dark place, too, but my wife was really pushy about it (in a good way!).

I made a deal with her. When she said, "We are going to do anything and everything that we can (treatment-wise) until something happens," —I agreed. We spent hours online every day, researching options. We spent a lot of time and money on supplements, pills, and blood tests, and eventually found treatments that worked. Now, my scans are clear and I am doing much better than my oncologists all expected!

Whereas I initially didn't know whether I'd live more than a year, as my doctors had told me, after some time, my perspective changed and I began to think, *Okay, maybe I'm going to make it after all.*

Now, I know that I will. If you have cancer, simply do your best and trust God to take care of the rest, and He will!

8

Detoxify to Heal and Live Long

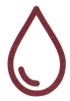

KEY PRINCIPLE #4
DETOXIFICATION

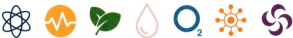

Our environment has changed dramatically from that which God originally created. We have polluted our air, soil, food and water with synthetic chemicals, electromagnetic radiation and other toxins, which have in turn polluted our cells. Every day, our planet becomes more toxic, as thousands of new chemical and electromagnetic pollutants are introduced into the environment; the ozone layer is being destroyed, and agricultural biotechnology companies continue to genetically modify foods, and then poison that food with things like antibiotics, hormones and pesticides.

Environmental toxins have even affected our telomeres, which are segments of DNA that are located at the end of our chromosomes and which protect the chromosome from deterioration. Scientists frequently compare them to the plastic tips of shoelaces (or aglets), that keep the laces together.

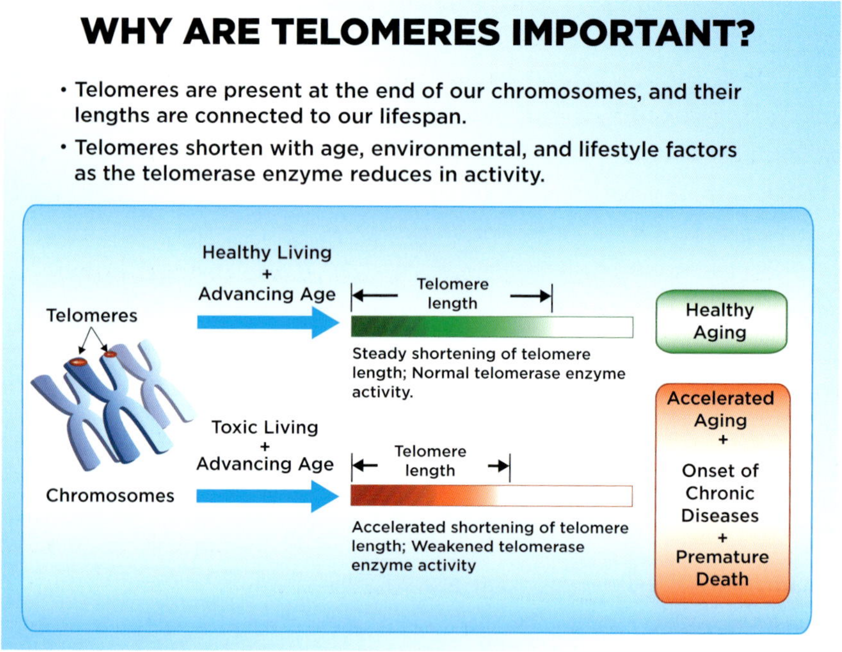
WHY ARE TELOMERES IMPORTANT?
• Telomeres are present at the end of our chromosomes, and their lengths are connected to our lifespan.
• Telomeres shorten with age, environmental, and lifestyle factors as the telomerase enzyme reduces in activity.
Telomeres
Chromosomes
Healthy Living + Advancing Age
Telomere length
Steady shortening of telomere length; Normal telomerase enzyme activity.
Healthy Aging
Toxic Living + Advancing Age
Telomere length
Accelerated shortening of telomere length; Weakened telomerase enzyme activity
Accelerated Aging + Onset of Chronic Diseases + Premature Death

Figure 22. How often do we find ourselves thinking about the ever-shortening small structures at the end of our chromosomes (telomeres) and how that affects our longevity? We don't. However, telomere shortening is the equivalent of a ticking time bomb, a process we may not want to accelerate, but that we unintentionally do through our lifestyles and environmental exposure. This infographic shows why minimizing toxin intake is essential to living a long and healthy life.

According to Drs. Elizabeth Blackburn and Elissa Epel, in their 2018 book, *The Telomere Effect,* we are born with 10,000 base pairs of DNA in our telomeres, but by the time we are 65, we only have about 4500 left![1] And just as the plastic sheath at the end of the shoelace eventually gets old and disintegrates, so our telomeres start to unravel as we age and with that, our DNA. This process is accelerated by toxic exposures.

In *The Telomere Effect,* the authors reference a Harvard study wherein people who had envisioned their telomeres lengthening, or repairing themselves on a daily basis, lived about 7.5 years longer than average![1] Our minds are very powerful.

At the same time, though, we need to do our best to live according to the natural laws God originally created for our well-being—especially when we are recovering from an illness like cancer.

One of the ways we can maintain the health of our telomeres and cells is by detoxifying our bodies from environmental pollutants, as well as from the toxins generated by cancer cells and the byproducts of our metabolism. Detoxification is imperative for recovery from cancer or any other chronic illness. In Chapter 2, I shared some types of toxins that have been linked to cancer. Here, I will share how you can remove these toxins from your body, so you can heal fully and faster.

All detoxification starts with toxin avoidance. You can do all of the therapies in the world but if you continually expose yourself to toxins from the environment, you will simply be putting back into your body whatever you are taking out of it. So you want to first make healthy lifestyle choices to keep your interior as clean as possible.

Detoxification is especially vital for late-stage cancer patients who have undergone chemotherapy and radiation, because these therapies create toxicity in the cells, and in turn affect the health and integrity of the cells. As I mentioned earlier, in a study involving 365 of our patients, we discovered that 92% had stage IV cancers along with recurrent and metastatic disease that traditional treatment had failed to adequately treat. Therefore, detoxification is a focal point of our 7 Key Principles approach for such patients.

After this, because the basic unit of life is the cell, detoxification and healing must start at the cellular level. When you detoxify your cells, your tissues and organs will function better, and your body's systems will self-regulate more optimally. It all starts with detoxifying at the cellular level, though.

In addition, detoxifying any negative emotions fosters cellular health. It has often been said that **a negative thought can kill you faster than a bad germ,** so I encourage you to also practice replacing any toxic thoughts with positive, life-giving ones. I share some tips for doing this in Chapter 13.

The Body's Five Means of Detoxification

Our body has many detoxification pathways that eliminate toxins through five main channels that include:

1. Our **breath**, when you exhale carbon dioxide.
2. Our **skin**, which is your largest organ. Perspiration is one of the most effective ways to cleanse and detoxify your body.
3. Our **urine**. to flush out toxins through your kidneys and bladder, for which it's vital to consume sufficient amounts of clean, filtered water.
4. Our **bowel** movements.
5. Our **thoughts** (emotional detox is vital).

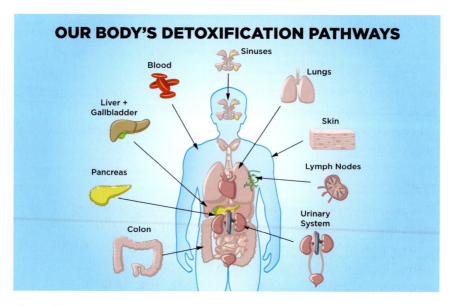

Figure 23. Our body is equipped with several pathways to remove toxins that engage a variety of organs and body fluids. Eventually, these pathways collect and eliminate toxins through urine, bowel movements, sweat and breath. Also important is our ability to detox emotionally through our thoughts (not pictured here). Maintaining the integrity of our detoxification pathways is vital to the healing process.

Here, I will share with you some simple detoxification therapies that make use of all your body's eliminatory channels. Your goal here is to remove any and all obstacles to optimal health. You can do most of these therapies on your own at home; although for a few, you will need the guidance or assistance of a healthcare practitioner.

At-Home Detoxification Therapies

Juicing

Juicing is an excellent way to detoxify your body, in addition to being the best way to infuse your cells with a multitude of nutrients. There's no better way to cleanse your blood, lymphatic system, kidneys, liver and gallbladder than with juice!

You can use all kinds of vegetables and fruits for your juices; however, I recommend that 80% of your juice be made from fresh organic vegetables, and 20% from fruit. Fruit gives juice a delicious flavor and both fruits and vegetables provide your body with an abundance of cancer-fighting antioxidants, phytochemicals and nutrients.

Refer to Chapter 6 for ideas on healthy veggies to include in your juices, and tips on how to prepare your juices. I recommend drinking at least two-three eight-ounce glasses of juice daily. For optimal detoxification benefits, you may want to dedicate one day per week to consuming only juices.

Coffee Enema

One great way to eliminate toxins from your liver, gallbladder and lower colon quickly and inexpensively is with a coffee enema. At one time, coffee enemas were recommended in the Merck Manual, which is considered by the medical community to be the bible of medicine. This was even before laxatives or medications existed to help detoxify the colon!

When you take coffee as an enema, it won't give you caffeine "jitters" like when you drink it. This is because it is absorbed preferentially into your body's hepatic system and so doesn't enter your bloodstream and spike your cortisol and adrenaline hormones, and over-energize you. I recommend doing one to two coffee enemas per day if you are actively treating cancer, and one enema three times weekly for health maintenance.

Some benefits of coffee enemas, in addition to removing toxins, include improved energy, mood and cognitive function. Enemas can even help to alleviate pain and headaches. This is because the health of your gastrointestinal tract and liver directly impact the rest of your body, especially your brain (gut-brain connection).

Doing a coffee enema is simple, painless and even relaxing. Enema kits can be purchased online and instructions for doing an enema can be found in the online resources section of this book's website, hopeforcancerbook.com.

Near Infrared Sauna

Your skin is your body's largest detoxification organ, and sweating with a sauna or other type of heat therapy has long been recognized in medical traditions worldwide as a valuable way to cleanse the body of many toxins. While there are several types of sauna therapy, many years of working with cancer patients has convinced me that near infrared saunas are the most beneficial type for eliminating toxins such as heavy metals, plastics, drug residues, acidic wastes and other chemicals from the body.

In addition, near infrared sauna therapy increases the circulation, oxygenates the tissues, stimulates the immune system, reduces systemic pain and inflammation, and even helps to remove plaque from the arterial walls. It is also very relaxing.

I prefer using near infrared light for sauna therapy because its energy is more physiological or aligned to the body than far infrared or other types of light, and it therefore resonates better with human cells. Near infrared light saunas also have very low electromagnetic fields (EMFs), which should be an important consideration when looking for a sauna.

I recommend doing sauna therapy three-four times per week, for 15-30 minutes each time. Drink a glass of water before and after a sauna treatment, to make sure you are well hydrated. I recommend adding minerals and sea salt to the water.

If you have a concurrent health condition, especially heart disease or high blood pressure, and/or you are on blood thinners, ask your doctor before doing sauna therapy, as it can be contraindicated in some people with these conditions. Some contraindications are absolute, however, while others are relative.

Practices for Proper Bowel Health

Many of us develop poor bowel habits as we go through life. Consider this: when we are babies, we eat, then immediately go to the bathroom afterward. Yet, by the time we get to kindergarten or first grade, many of us are a bit afraid or shy in school, so we begin to learn to "hold it in."

Then, when we get to grade school and start looking at girls or guys, we don't think about going to the bathroom. Or, our teachers may not allow us to leave class to go, which further encourages the habit of "holding it in."

After that, we go to high school and it's another level of learning, activities and busyness, so we continue to avoid going to the bathroom regularly. By the time we get a job or go to college, we think that having a bowel movement once every three-four days is normal!

Ideally, though, we should all have at least one, two or three bowel movements daily. If you aren't going to the bathroom daily, the toxins from your stools are getting reabsorbed back into your body, rather than being eliminated.

Sometimes, disease and medications make it difficult to have regular bowel movements. If you aren't going to the bathroom at least once daily, there are a few simple ways to correct this. First, take some magnesium, or increase your current dose of magnesium. Many people are magnesium deficient, even if their blood tests show that their levels are normal, because blood levels of magnesium don't always correlate with cellular levels.

If you believe you are receiving sufficient amounts of magnesium but are still deficient at a cellular level, consider taking a small amount of boron; perhaps 3 mg or so, which significantly helps with magnesium absorption.

In addition, drink plenty of clean, high-quality water throughout the day; approximately half of your body weight, calculated in pounds and ounces. So for instance, if you weigh 170 pounds, you'll want to drink 85 ounces of water, or about 10.5 8-ounce glasses daily. In addition, consider taking supplemental fiber, if the fiber in your fruits and veggies isn't sufficient to keep you regular. Exercise is another simple way to stimulate the bowels.

Interestingly, in my clinical and personal experience, I have found that bee propolis is also excellent for keeping some people regular, and propolis also has powerful anti-cancer properties.

Tools for Draining the Lymphatic System

Your lymphatic system is part of your body's circulatory and immune systems, and comprises a complex network of lymphatic vessels that carry a clear fluid called lymph directionally toward your heart. The system is also made up of nodes, glands and organs, which include the thymus, tonsils, bone marrow, spleen and what are called Peyer's patches in the gut. Approximately 1.5- 2 liters of lymph fluid circulates throughout your body daily. And overall, you have 6-10 liters of lymph in your body, compared to just 4.7-5 liters of blood! So in terms of quantity, you have nearly double the amount of lymph as blood.

Your lymphatic system has a number of different functions. Its primary function is to create immune cells called lymphocytes. The lymph nodes are full of white blood cells and act as vessels to filter out foreign matter. When your body fights off infection, your white blood cell count increases dramatically to ward off the infection, and the white blood cells collect in the lymph nodes.

Another function of your lymphatic system is to transport disease-fighting cells to the cancer cells, and to carry away dead germs and toxins from healthy cells, for elimination by your body.

Unlike your blood circulatory system, the fluids of which are moved along by the pumping of your heart, your lymphatic system doesn't have an organ to keep the lymphatic fluid moving along. So by comparison, lymph fluid moves quite slowly throughout your body, making it easy for it to become stagnant.

Stagnant, toxic lymph flow in turn produces thickened, cloudy, dirty lymph. When this happens, immune cells and toxins can get stuck in the fluid. As a result, they don't get to where they need to go, which then compromises your immune function. This in turn encourages degeneration of both the cells and organs, and contributes to tumor and cancer formation.

People who have received chemotherapy are even more prone to stagnant lymph, as are those who are sedentary or who can't move much due to illness.

Stimulating the flow of lymph fluid is important for ensuring that your immune cells get to their destination, which is the cancer cells, and that your healthy cells can effectively "take out the trash."

Lymph fluid is stimulated by movement, especially exercise. One great way to get your lymph moving is with a vibrating platform. For this, you stand on a platform, simply press a button and allow the device to vibrate your whole body for a few minutes. This has the effect of stimulating the flow of lymph fluid throughout your body. VIBE is one device that we use and recommend to our patients.

Another great way to stimulate lymph flow is with a Chi machine.

For this, you lie on your back on the floor, and then place your ankles in a cradle that sits atop a small device. The device then moves your lower body side to side in a fishlike movement while you relax.

The movement causes the muscles surrounding your lymph vessels to contract, which then stimulates the movement of lymph fluid.

A third way to stimulate the movement of lymph fluid is by bouncing up and down on a rebounder, or mini-trampoline. Start with five minutes of rebounding daily and work up to fifteen. This is also an excellent exercise for the body.

If you are in a wheelchair or too weak to move much, try lightly bouncing your legs on a rebounder from a seated position in an adjacent chair. Or, if you can't walk or stand, ask a friend or family member to move your arms or legs, or flex your legs and feet to get your circulation going. Movement is the most effective way to detoxify your body, so just do whatever you can to get some movement into your limbs!

Finally, I recommend taking lymphatic drainage remedies, which help to stimulate the flow and movement of lymph. Physica Energetics makes three great drainage remedies, which I discussed in Chapter 7. Please refer to that chapter for more information on those remedies, and consult with your doctor to find out which remedy you need, especially if you have an advanced cancer.

It is vital that your lymph fluid be flowing properly before you do any other type of detoxification. Otherwise, all the toxins from your body will just get stuck in your lymphatic system. So, I encourage you to make lymph drainage treatments a priority!

Liver and Gallbladder Cleanse

A liver and gallbladder cleanse is another powerful way to detoxify these organs, which can become overloaded and poisoned from processing environmental toxins and chemotherapeutic drugs.

Most cleanses focus on removing gallstones, which build up in the liver and gallbladder and over time, compromise their function. These stones are made up of cholesterol, bilirubin and other components of bile, and can be as small as a grain of sand or as large as a golf ball.

Liver and gallbladder cleanses can be somewhat taxing on the body, so it's best to do them under physician supervision and only if you aren't very weak. Nonetheless, cleanses are a powerful and effective way to improve the health of your liver and gallbladder, and with that, the rest of your body.

You can do them as often as every few weeks, or as your health allows. Some people become tired for a day or two following a liver cleanse, so it's a good idea not to do them more frequently than twice monthly. However, I recommend doing them periodically until you no longer expel stones.

There are many liver and gallbladder cleansing recipes out there, but most use similar ingredients and follow a similar procedure. For this cleanse you will need:

- 4 quarts or liters of fresh, organic apple juice
- 4 tablespoons of aluminum-free Epsom salts
- 1/2 cup of extra virgin olive oil
- 1 big, organic grapefruit, or 3 lemons
- A 1-2 quart or liter glass jar or pitcher

KEY PRINCIPLE #4 | DETOXIFY TO HEAL AND LIVE LONG

STEPS TO A GALLBLADDER CLEANSE

1. For four-five days prior to the cleanse drink as much apple juice as you can; ideally, a liter (or quart) or two. During the last two days, drink 8 ounces of apple juice every two-three hours. This will help to ensure that the cleanse is successful. Throughout the duration of the cleanse also make sure that you are following the Garden Food Plan.
2. On the sixth day, eat a light, fat-free breakfast. Then, do not eat any foods or consume any liquids for the remainder of the day.
3. At 2:00 PM on the same day, mix four tablespoons of Epsom salts with three cups of water in a jar or pitcher. Put the jar or pitcher in the refrigerator.
4. At 6:00 PM, drink 3/4 cup of the mixture.
5. At 8:00 PM, drink another 3/4 cup of the mixture.
6. At 9:45 PM, pour 1/2 cup of extra virgin olive oil into a large glass. Then, squeeze an entire grapefruit into the glass, removing the pulp with a fork. Mix the olive oil and grapefruit oil together with a spoon.
7. At 10:00 PM, drink the olive oil-grapefruit mixture. Try to ingest it relatively quickly; within a few minutes or so.
8. Lie down in your bed immediately, on your right side, for approximately 20 minutes. Remain in bed and go to sleep if you can, until morning. It is very important not to get up once you take the olive oil-grapefruit mixture. However, after 20 minutes, you can move around in bed a little, or use the bathroom if need be. Just don't get up and move around a lot.
9. The following morning, go to the bathroom. You should find that your stools are watery and contain green and/or brown stones. There may also be brownish debris and cholesterol crystals that have not yet become stones. You may continue to expel stones throughout the day, so you'll want to stay home all day.
10. After you get up, drink a third dose of the Epsom salts solution that you prepared the day before.
11. Two hours later, drink the remainder of the Epsom salts solution.
12. Wait two more hours before eating anything, and when you do eat, have some fruit. Later in the day, you can have other solid foods.

Castor Oil Packs

The castor seed plant and the oil from which it is made have been used for centuries to treat a variety of conditions, especially digestive disorders. Today, they are used as antimicrobial agents, anti-inflammatories and analgesics, as well as immune system and lymphatic stimulants. Centuries ago, the castor plant was referred to as "Palma Christi" because the leaves were said to resemble the hand of Christ. This association likely came from people's reverence for the plant's healing abilities.

Castor oil's main medicinal compound is ricinoleic acid, which is a unique triglyceride that can be used topically to treat skin conditions, as well as to remove toxins from the liver. We recommend that our patients take it for detoxifying their liver and gallbladder, in the form of a castor oil pack. It is a simple, gentle way to cleanse these organs of toxins.

To make a castor oil pack, simply spread a light layer of organic castor oil (which you can purchase at most health food stores), over a piece of cotton cloth large enough to cover the upper right quadrant of your abdomen. Your liver is located here, below the bottom of your ribcage, on the right side (but you won't necessarily be able to feel it).

Once the cloth is saturated, place it over your upper right abdomen, then place a large piece of plastic or a plastic bag atop the cloth. Finally, set a hot water bottle with hot (but not boiling) water atop the plastic bag. Heat the area for anywhere from 30-60 minutes.

The oil and heat appear to work by increasing blood circulation to the area and then drawing toxins out of the liver. They also improve the flow of lymph fluid, and speed the removal of toxins via the lymphatic system.

You will want to use a castor oil pack while lying down on a sofa, recliner or bed, so that the pack stays firmly put over your abdomen. Make sure to clean your skin when you are finished. You can reuse the oily cloth multiple times, and store it in wax paper for future use.

I recommend doing castor oil packs as often as you can, even daily, for maximum benefit.

Therapeutic Breathing

We in the West tend to underestimate the benefits of therapeutic breathing, but Eastern cultures have recognized it for centuries. **When you** practice therapeutic breathing, you more effectively uptake oxygen into your cells, and thereby improving their function, especially nutrient uptake and waste disposal.

Therapeutic breathing starts with inhaling through your nose, holding it for a number of seconds, then exhaling forcefully. Throughout the day and at night when you sleep, you should also aim to breathe through your nose. Don't take deep breaths, or breathe through your mouth, as this actually decreases the amount of oxygen your body receives. Here's why:

According to Patrick McKeown, author of *The Oxygen Advantage*, "Hemoglobin (a blood protein) releases oxygen into the cells, only in the presence of carbon dioxide. When we take deep breaths, carbon dioxide is washed from the lungs, blood, tissues and cells, and this actually causes hemoglobin to hold on to oxygen, resulting in reduced oxygen release and therefore reduced oxygen delivery to tissues and organs!"

He goes on to say that, "As counterintuitive as it may seem, the urge to take bigger, deeper breaths when we are tired does not provide our cells with more oxygen, but less."

McKeown advocates breathing through your nose, and avoiding taking deep breaths, especially through your mouth. When you breathe therapeutically, you temporarily increase carbon dioxide in your cells, which over time, actually increases your cellular tolerance to carbon dioxide and improves your oxygenation levels.[2] McKeown overcame his own asthma through the practice of therapeutic breathing, and has helped Olympic athletes improve their performance by teaching them to do the same.

I was raised in New Jersey, but as a child, I would often go to Colombia for vacation, to visit my grandparents. While at their house, I would sometimes peek out my bedroom window in the early morning to observe my grandfather, who would be out in the backyard doing breathing exercises, while he lifted his arms up to the sky. I'd watch him and think, *Why is he doing that?* Now I realize that he simply knew one of the secrets to optimal health: therapeutic breathing.

Heavy Metal Removal

Most of us have significant amounts of heavy metals in our bodies as a result of being exposed to them in the environment, through a variety of sources. They tend to congregate in areas of the body where other toxins and microbes are found. For example, metals have often been found inside molds and parasites, so it can be important to synchronize any antimicrobial therapies you do with heavy metal detoxification.

Heavy metals are important to remove from your body because they compromise your immune system, so I recommend taking one or more heavy metal binders on a regular basis, to mop up these toxins.

One gentle and safe way to do heavy metal detoxification is with EDTA (Ethylene Diamine Tetra Acetic acid) suppositories. These have been shown in studies to remove a variety of heavy metals, including mercury, lead, cadmium and uranium,[3] the latter two of which have been shown to be difficult to remove with other binders. You can order EDTA suppositories online; one reputable brand is by Detoxamin.

I recommend taking one suppository rectally, three times per week. One month of suppository therapy provides the same benefit as doing 10 intravenous chelation therapies, and the beauty of it is that you can do it from home.

If you take EDTA, you should also take a multi-mineral formula at the same time, so that you don't get mineral depleted, since EDTA also removes beneficial minerals from the body. SpectraLyte is an excellent product from Physica Energetics that can replenish lost electrolytes.

Other heavy metal binders include: DMSA, DMPS, Vitamin C, chlorella, zeolite and brown kelp, the latter of which is a species of algae.

The strongest and perhaps most effective of all these binders are DMSA, DMPS and EDTA. They should only be used under physician supervision, as they are powerful and can cause redistribution of metals into other areas of the body if they are used improperly or in the wrong doses.

Chlorella, Vitamin C, zeolite and brown kelp are weaker heavy metal binders and so may be a better choice for people who are sensitive or weak and cannot tolerate stronger binders.

Finally, cilantro and cilantro tinctures are powerful chelators that mobilize metals from the cells, and which can cross the blood-brain barrier. However, cilantro doesn't bind with metals, it only pulls them out of the cells, so it should always be paired with a binding agent such as DMSA.

Again though, it is imperative to work with a doctor who understands heavy metal chelation, to find out what binders your body most needs, and in what dosages. Before taking any type of heavy metal binder, you'll also want to make sure that your pathways of elimination are working well, so that any metals that you mobilize from the cells make it safely out of your body.

If you have stagnant lymph, a sluggish liver or impaired kidneys, for example, you may not be able to effectively eliminate toxins, including metals. When this happens, the metals can get redistributed throughout your body, rather than removed. So make sure to support your eliminatory organs and pathways before, during and after doing heavy metal detoxification.

Dental Detoxification

Dental toxins are a foremost cause or contributing factor to many chronic, degenerative diseases, including cancer. Therefore, eliminating any dental toxins with the help of a competent biological/holistic dentist is essential for healing. As part of our program at Hope4Cancer, we refer all of our patients to a biological dentist for a thorough evaluation and consultation.

Eminent cardiologist Thomas E. Levy, MD, JD, states that dental infections are the primary cause of most cancers and are chronically neglected, resulting in relapses and secondary cancers down the road. In his recent book, *Hidden Epidemic*, he discusses results from **3D cone beam imaging studies that have shown that 10-20% of all adult teeth are chronically abscessed, even though they may be asymptomatic.** He emphasizes that the treatment of all diseases, including cancer, not only require that existing damage be "repaired," but also that ongoing sources of endogenous toxins, such as dental infections present in cavitations, dental implants, root-canaled teeth, gums, tonsils and sinuses, be simultaneously addressed.[4]

There are four aspects of dental detoxification:

1. **Remove toxic amalgam fillings.** Dental amalgams are composed of heavy metals such as mercury, aluminum and tin.

If you have amalgams, whenever you chew your food, metal particles can dislodge from these fillings and enter your bloodstream, where they resettle in your brain and other parts of your body and poison them. Cancer has been strongly linked to oxidative stress and DNA damage caused by heavy metal toxicity.[5]

If you have amalgam fillings, I encourage you to replace them with a healthier composite material. Amalgams must be carefully removed using special procedures, so that the metals don't get re-distributed into other areas of your body. Skilled biological dentists understand how to do this. To find one in your area, see the International Academy of Oral Medicine and Toxicology (IAOMT): https://iaomt.org/for-patients/search/ or the International Academy of Biological Dentistry and Medicine (IABDM): https://iabdm.org/location/.

2. **Remove root-canaled teeth.** Research shows that most root-canaled teeth are infected.[6] This is because a root-canaled tooth is a dead tooth, which means that it doesn't have adequate vascular circulation to cleanse the area, making it a haven for sub-acute infections. These infections may not cause you pain or inflammation, but they are silently affecting your immune system every second of every day.

   A researcher named Dr. Robert Jones found an extremely high correlation between root canals and breast cancer. In a five-year study on 300 patients with breast cancer, he reported that 93% had undergone root canals, and that in the majority of cases, their tumors were on the same side of their body as the root-canaled tooth.

   The preferred way to remove toxins caused by root canals is to extract the root-canaled tooth and ensure that any infection is thoroughly cleaned out. At times, surgical debridement, or the removal of necrotic or dead tissue, is also necessary. Natural agents such as herbs, ozone, essential oils, and Photodynamic Therapy using lasers, all

Key Principle #4 | Detoxify to Heal and Live Long

work well for cleansing infected root canals. It is imperative to work with a skilled biological dentist who specializes in root canal extractions and in removing deeply embedded infections.

Following the root-canal tooth and infection removal, you may choose to have an artificial tooth implanted. A biological dentist should do this procedure, using biocompatible materials. Implants are not always feasible, but at times are necessary and/or helpful for maintaining proper teeth and jawbone alignment.

3. **Remove dental cavitations.** Cavitations are hollowed out areas in the jawbone that have become infected. They often occur where teeth have been extracted, especially wisdom teeth. Like root-canaled teeth, cavitations often become a haven for microbes, and must be surgically opened up and thoroughly cleansed.

    Several treatment agents and methods can be used to cleanse cavitations, including photobiomodulation or laser light therapy, platelet-rich plasma, ozone, and insulin—among others. Again, it is vital to work with a biological dentist who specializes in the removal of cavitation infections. These infections are important to address because they don't just stay in your mouth, but become systemic, and affect all of the organs and systems that lie along the meridians, or energy pathways, of the infected teeth.

    For instance, if you have a molar on the top left side of your mouth that's infected, and which connects to your breast via an energy meridian, the infection in that molar could contribute to disease in the breast or in any other tissues, glands or organs that are along the same energetic pathway.

    Studies confirm that infected teeth can cause or contribute to cancer. For example, one study published in the *Journal of Cancer* found that extracted molar teeth seemed to predict cancer risk in a group of otherwise healthy 30-40 year olds.

4. **Treat periodontal disease.** Over half of all Americans have some degree of periodontal disease, which is principally caused by infections and inflammation of the gums and bone that surround and support the teeth. In the early stages, periodontal disease is called gingivitis, and during this stage, the gums become swollen and red, and may bleed, especially when flossing. In the later stages, the disease is called periodontitis.

    It's not normal for your gums to bleed when you floss, but practicing good dental hygiene, including regularly visiting a biological dentist and flossing your teeth daily, can go a long way toward preventing periodontal disease and keeping your immune system strong.

Creating a Healthy Living Environment

You can detoxify your body but if your home is filled with toxic chemicals and electromagnetic pollutants, you will constantly be re-exposing yourself to toxins and putting back into your body what you are taking out. Unfortunately, most homes are filled with harmful chemical toxins, which come from household cleaning, building and personal care products, as well as from carpeting and furniture. Many of these chemicals have been linked to cancer.

Floor Treatments and Home Furnishings

Carpet contains cancer-causing chemicals such as formaldehyde, which has been shown to be one of the most carcinogenic indoor toxins.[7] So wherever possible, use non-toxic carpeting from companies such as Nature's Carpet. Or, remove the carpeting from your home, especially if it is newer, as new carpet off-gasses more formaldehyde and other toxic chemicals. Hardwood, linoleum and ceramic tile are better choices of flooring. Avoid toxic floor adhesives as well, such as glues, dyes, stains, grouts, sealers, and finishes that contain toxic chemicals.

The same goes for your home furnishings. For example, many companies now make mattresses and bedding from materials like bamboo, natural latex, organic cotton and wool that haven't been treated with toxic chemicals. Avoid conventional mattresses and bedding, which may be made from things like petroleum-based polyester and polyurethane foam, and are treated with toxic flame-retardant chemicals that have been linked to cancer.

Mold

Mold is a common household toxin that can make some people really sick. Most homes contain some mold, and while not everyone gets sick from mold and the toxins it produces, called mycotoxins, some people do. Mold expert Ritchie Shoemaker, MD, has found that **25% of the population has a genetic inability to detoxify mold, and it is these people who become sick from it and the toxins it produces.**[8] Mold is increasingly found to be a strong contributing factor to chronic, degenerative diseases of all kinds, including cancer.

According to a study review published on February 6, 2017 in *Oncology Reports*, many mycotoxins can cause major changes to the human genome, and trigger the development of cancer. Some mycotoxins that have been linked to cancer include: Aflatoxin B, Citrinin, Fumonisins, Patulin, Trichothecene and Zearalenone.[9]

Mold can be difficult to detect in your home environment because you can't always see or smell it; it hides behind walls, and some molds don't leave a musty smell. A musty smell or history of water leaks in the home can indicate mold, however, so it's worthwhile to do an at-home mold test called the ERMI, or Environmental Relative Moldiness Index. This test detects more than 36 species of mold via a simple dust sample. The ERMI can provide you with a basic analysis of potential mold in your home. For more information, see: Myco-metrics.com.

You can also do a urine mycotoxin (or mold toxin) test to determine whether mold toxins are contributing to the toxic load in your body, and even the cancer. The Great Plains Laboratory, Inc. and Real Time Labs both do mycotoxin testing. For more information see: RealTimeLabs.com and GreatPlainsLaboratory.com.

It is beyond the scope of this book to discuss mold treatment and remediation, but to learn more, I encourage you to read Ritchie Shoemaker's book, *Surviving Mold: Life in the Era of Dangerous Buildings* or

Dr. Neil Nathan's book, *Mold & Mycotoxins: Current Evaluation and Treatment 2016*.

Household Cleaning and Personal Care Products

Most commercial brands of personal care and household cleaning products, including things like soap, shampoo, deodorant, lotion and toothpaste, laundry and dish detergent, floor, carpet and household cleaners—all contain chemical toxins that have been linked to cancer.

Common toxic chemicals found in household cleaning products include phthalates, perchloroethylene, 2-butoxyethanol, sodium hydroxide, ammonia, chlorine and triclosan, among many others.

Studies confirm that these chemicals can cause cancer. For instance, a study published in *Environmental Health* in 2010 states that household cleaning products may contribute to breast cancer because many contain endocrine-disrupting chemicals or mammary gland carcinogens.[10]

Similarly, most commercial personal care products, such as deodorant, soap, shampoo, body lotion and cosmetics, contain chemicals that have been linked to cancer. These include, but are not limited to: parabens, mineral oils, petrolatum, propylene glycol, sodium lauryl (or laureth) sulfate, FD&C color pigments, aluminum and artificial fragrances.

For instance, a 2013 study published in the *Journal of Inorganic Biochemistry* suggested that high concentrations of aluminum in the breast caused by aluminum-containing antiperspirants, cause oxidative damage to the cells and inflammation, which can lead to cancer.[11]

Avoid aluminum-containing antiperspirants, and instead choose natural deodorants made from herbs and essential oils. This is also important because antiperspirants block your sweat glands, and sweating is one of your body's natural mechanisms for detoxifying. God gave you a sweating mechanism through your armpits for a reason: its purpose is to eliminate cancer-causing toxins!

In addition, avoid fluoride-containing toothpaste, as fluoride has been linked to cancer, as well as to thyroid dysfunction, which in itself has been linked to certain cancers. For example, a study published in a 2012 journal found that patients with osteosarcoma, a rare malignant bone tumor, had higher amounts of fluoride in their drinking water.[12] Fluoride has been linked to other cancers, as well.

Most cosmetics also contain cancer-causing toxins, so it's important to choose your cosmetic brands wisely. **Everything you put onto your skin is absorbed into your bloodstream the same as if you had eaten it.** So if you can't eat it, then don't put it on your skin!

Safe, non-toxic personal care products are made from ingredients that God created in nature; things like coconut, almond and olive oils—which are also natural fats that promote cellular health. They also work great for cleaning your body, and keeping your skin and hair healthy and lubricated.

It's not always easy to tell whether a product contains harmful chemical ingredients. Rather than try to memorize every potentially toxic ingredient out there, consult the Environmental Working Group (EWG) website, which contains a database where you can look up many thousands of household and personal care products, including cosmetics, and find safe ones are recommended by EWG. For more information, see: EWG.org.

In addition, you can download an App on your smart phone called Think Dirty, where you can check the safety of over 68,300 personal care and household products, using your phone. For more information, see: ThinkDirtyApp.com.

Most health food stores sell non-toxic household and personal care products, although some of these products also contain harmful chemicals (read ingredient labels carefully).

Seventh Generation is a well-known company that makes safe household cleaning products (SeventhGeneration.com), as well as My Green Fills (MyGreenFills.com).

I particularly like MyGreenFills.com because the company encourages consumers to recycle its jugs. They send you envelopes of detergent that you can use to refill the same jug, over and over. You just add water to the detergent and jug. This not only cuts down on waste, but you also don't have to lug around a heavy bottle of laundry detergent every time you shop. The detergent is also very high quality, and is made with essential oils and other natural ingredients.

Light and Electromagnetic Field Toxicity

Man-made electromagnetic fields (EMFs) are a potent, yet invisible toxin that we are all exposed to daily, through sources such as Wi-Fi, smart meters, cordless and cellular phones, power lines, appliances, and computers—among others. All of our cells are made up of energy and vibrate within a specific frequency range. When they are exposed to outside sources of electromagnetic energy, it can affect their functioning, for better or worse.

Research shows that too much exposure to the wrong electromagnetic fields causes the cells to vibrate and more rapidly divide and mutate. Some experts, such as the late Robert Becker MD, an orthopedic surgeon and electromagnetic field expert, have believed that electromagnetic pollution is one of the most dangerous toxins to which we are exposed.[13]

Thousands of studies have linked electromagnetic fields to cancer and other diseases. For example, one meta-analysis of multiple studies published in March 2016 in *Environment International* reported that low frequency electromagnetic fields (from things such as power lines) are associated with increased cancer risk.[14]

A database of over 2,000 studies and other publications that demonstrate the effects of EMFs, including increased cancer risk, can be found at EMF-Portal: EMF-portal.org. The publications have been written by scientists, including biologists, physicists, engineers, epidemiologists, physicians, etc., and have been published in peer-reviewed scientific journals to validate their credibility.

Here are a few simple and easy things that you can do to reduce your exposure to EMFs in your environment:

- Turn off your Wi-Fi and cell phone at night
- Use a hardwired Internet connection, rather than Wi-Fi
- Use a landline instead of a cordless phone
- Minimize cell phone usage
- Unplug your appliances whenever you aren't using them, especially those near your bed (if you don't turn off your circuit breakers at night)

In addition, if you know that you are sensitive to electromagnetic fields, as many people are nowadays, consider purchasing Graham-Stetzer filters, which plug into the wall outlets of your home and block EMFs that enter your home through the wall wiring and your smart meter.

Many companies also sell EMF stickers and other gadgets that you can put on your phone or computer to help block or modulate the effects of electromagnetic fields from these devices. Some are more effective than others. I have found GAIA products to be very helpful, although many companies make EMF-protection products. For more information, see: GAIA.com.

If you find that you aren't sleeping well, you may also want to purchase a metallic-lined mesh canopy, sometimes called a Faraday cage, to drape over a canopy bed and which you then sleep beneath at night. Faraday cages block frequencies from sources such as Wi-Fi, cell phones and microwave towers. They don't protect you from electrical or magnetic fields emitted by power lines and appliances, but they can dramatically improve your sleep and protect you from many sources of radio frequencies (RF) and other fields.

To learn more about Faraday cages, Graham Stetzer filters and other EMF-protection devices, see: LessEMFs.com and StetzerElectric.com.

Grounding

God created the earth to contain electrons that have powerful healing effects upon the body. Whenever you contact your feet or another part of your body to the earth, the electrons from the earth pass into your body and balance its energy. This is one reason why some people feel better when they walk on a beach, or sit or lie on the ground or grass. We were made to connect to the earth! So ground yourself to the earth, whenever possible.

If you can't get outside to ground, some companies, such as the Earthing Institute, sell grounding products, including mats, bed sheets, body straps, and other gadgets that you can use to ground yourself indoors. These products are attached to a cord and plug, which you insert into the grounding plug of your wall outlets. When you contact some part of your body with the product, you indirectly receive electrons from the earth, which are conducted through the grounding outlet. To learn more about grounding products, see: EarthingInstitute.net.

Light Toxicity

Some light bulbs emit radiation and energetic frequencies that disrupt the body's natural bioelectric energy field. Not all lights are toxic, but most commonly used light bulbs, especially compact and other fluorescent light bulbs, are harmful. Even light-emitting diodes (LEDs) are not healthy for your body, but they are better than fluorescent bulbs.

The most life-giving light is of course, sunlight, which is very healing to your body! Indoors, use incandescent light bulbs, which may be the least toxic of all bulbs. These are more difficult to find in stores, but you can still get them at places like 1000bulbs.com and at larger hardware stores like Lowes and Home Depot if you live in North America.

It's also generally a good idea to not stand or sit within a couple of feet of any indoor light source.

Final Thoughts

By detoxifying your body, you will greatly facilitate your recovery from cancer, help to prevent any recurrences of disease, and increase your chances of living a longer, healthier life. When you do therapies that make use of all of your detoxification organs, including your liver and gallbladder, skin, kidneys, lymphatic system and lungs, you maximize your body's ability to detoxify, while not putting undue stress on any one particular system or organ.

You are a system and your whole system is only as good as the sum of all of its parts. By having those parts work together collectively, you will be better equipped to eliminate toxins and heal—faster and more completely!

DETOXIFY TO HEAL AND LIVE LONG

Table 8.1.

Detoxification Therapy or Tool	Purpose and Benefit
Dental remediation (Consists of removing amalgams, infected root canals and cavitations, and treating periodontal disease)	To eliminate cancer causing infections and heavy metal toxins. To support the overall health of the body.

continued on page 249

KEY PRINCIPLE #4 | DETOXIFY TO HEAL AND LIVE LONG

Detoxification Therapy or Tool	Purpose and Benefit
Juicing	To cleanse the blood, organs and lymphatic system.
Coffee enema	To cleanse the liver, gallbladder and lower colon.
Near infrared sauna	To remove heavy metals, plastics, and other toxins from the cells. To stimulate circulation, reduce pain and induce relaxation.
Lymphatic drainage (using a vibrating platform, rebounder, Chi machine, or drainage remedies)	Stimulates the flow of lymph, which carries disease-fighting immune cells to cancer cells, and moves toxins from healthy cells for elimination by the body.
Breathing exercises	To eliminate carbon dioxide and bring life-giving oxygen to the cells.
Heavy metal toxin binders	To remove cancer-causing and immune-suppressive heavy metals.
Home Detoxification (Consists of removing all cancer-causing personal care and household products, as well as toxic furnishings and building materials, from your home)	To create a clean anti-cancer living environment that fosters health.

SUMMARY

- Our environment has changed dramatically from that which God originally created. We have polluted our air, soil, food and water with synthetic chemicals, electromagnetic radiation and other toxins, which have then polluted our cells.
- Juicing is an excellent way to detoxify, in addition to being the best way to infuse your body with a multitude of nutrients.

- Near infrared sauna therapy is the best way to remove toxins via the sweat. It also provides other benefits, including improved circulation, pain relief and relaxation.
- Coffee enemas stimulate the liver and gallbladder to release toxins, and also cleanse the lower colon.
- Standing on a vibrating platform, rebounding, and using a Chi machine are a few ways to stimulate the lymphatic system, which carries disease-fighting cells to cancer cells and removes toxins from healthy cells.
- Dental toxins seriously compromise health. You must remove any root-canaled teeth, infected cavitations and metal amalgams in order to have the best chance of healing from cancer.
- Replace all of your toxic personal care and household cleaning products with those made from all-natural ingredients.
- Detoxify your home by reducing electromagnetic pollution, removing mold, and replacing any furnishings and building materials that have been treated with toxic chemicals.

QUESTIONS FOR FURTHER REFLECTION

1. What are the five ways that our bodies eliminate toxins?
2. What are some of the benefits of stimulating the lymphatic system?
3. What are the four types of dental toxins that have been linked to cancer?
4. How often should you do a coffee enema if you are actively treating cancer?
5. Name the two main benefits of juicing.
6. What are some benefits of infrared sauna therapy, in addition to toxin removal?
7. How often should you do each of the detoxification therapies?

9

Oxygen: The Foundation for a Vibrant Life

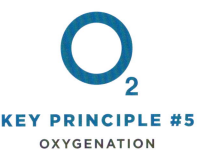

KEY PRINCIPLE #5

OXYGENATION

Have you ever considered how important oxygen is to your survival? You can live without sleep and water for a few days, and food for up to 40 days, but you can survive for only a few minutes without oxygen! It's an essential element that God has created for your survival, and every mitochondria, cell, tissue and organ in your body functions and thrives only in the presence of adequate oxygen.

The cells maintain a stable level of oxygen in part due to the chemical processes of aerobic metabolism associated with breathing. The red blood cells, specifically the hemoglobin, gather oxygen in the lungs and distribute it to the rest of the body via respiration.

Unfortunately, environmental toxins, including chemicals and man-made electromagnetic fields, as well as stress and negative thoughts, unhealthy lifestyle habits and poor breathing, cause oxidative stress in our bodies. In turn, this diminishes the amount of oxygen that our cells receive. The overall effect is compromised cellular health and the encouraged development of diseases like cancer.

Oxygenation can dramatically help reverse the damage caused by oxidative stress, and is one of our 7 Key Principles for recovery. We have experienced its amazing benefits with thousands of patients, and here I share with you oxygen therapies that you can pursue at our treatment centers or at home. These therapies can help you to more easily overcome cancer, and also create a healthier environment in your body. As a result, you can decrease the likelihood of any cancer recurrences in the future.

Cancer Cells Thrive in an Oxygen-Poor Environment

Healthy cells thrive in oxygen-rich environments, while cancer cells prefer hypoxic, or oxygen-poor ones. Normal cells need oxygen to convert energy from nutrients into adenosine triphosphate (ATP), as well as to release waste products, while cancer cells metabolize nutrients and create energy by fermenting sugar in an anaerobic, or a low-oxygen environment in a process called glycolysis. This is an inferior form of energy production that's activated when cellular oxygen levels drop below 40%, and leads to an acidic environment that encourages cancer growth.

The late German physiologist, physician and Nobel Prize winner Otto Warburg stated that the prime cause of cancer points to oxygen deprivation: "Cancer, above all other diseases, has countless secondary causes. But, even for cancer, there is only one prime cause. The prime cause of cancer is the replacement of the respiration of oxygen (sugar oxidation) in normal body cells by the fermentation of sugar."[1,2]

He continues, "In every case, during cancer development, the oxygen respiration always falls, fermentation appears, and the highly differentiated cells are transformed into fermenting anaerobes, which have lost all their body functions and retain only the now-useless property of growth and replication. Thus, when respiration disappears, life does not disappear, but the meaning of life disappears, and what remains are growing machines that destroy the body in which they grow. It is indisputable that all cancer could be prevented if the respiration of body cells were kept intact."

Oxygen deprivation is only one of many factors that can trigger the conversion of healthy cells into cancerous ones, yet it is one of the most important.

How Oxygen Deprivation Encourages Cancer Growth

Hypoxia or oxygen deprivation accelerates anaerobic metabolism in cancer cells. The result is increased angiogenesis, or new tumor blood vessel formation, resistance to apoptosis, increased cancer cell division and reproduction, and metastases. Chemotherapy and radiation also become less effective, and the body's terrain becomes more acidic, which further encourages cancer cell growth. In short, hypoxia creates optimal conditions in which cancer can flourish.

A review published in November 2015 in the journal *Hypoxia* confirms this, stating that hypoxia, or low oxygen levels, affects both cancer cells and the tumor environment, and plays a pivotal role in cancer progression and metastases.[3] It encourages new tumor blood vessel growth, favors cancer cell metabolism and survival, and even contributes to cancer cell migration and treatment resistance.

Normal cells communicate with one another for their survival, and cancer cells and tumors do, as well. Further, research shows that hypoxia encourages intercellular communication among cancer cells, so they interact with each other to enhance or diminish the hypoxic effects. Oxygenation can help to stop this intercellular communication.

Symptoms and signs of oxygen deprivation include fatigue, weakness, low hemoglobin counts, clumped red blood cells, anemia and cancer cell growth. The good news is that increasing oxygen at the cellular level with a variety of oxygen therapies can help to reverse all of these symptoms, signs and processes. In addition, it can better enable the cells to remove toxins, bacteria, viruses and other pathogenic microbes.

Clinical Oxygen Therapies

Some oxygen therapies that we give our patients and I highly recommend (again, with the help of a qualified healthcare practitioner) include:

1. Hyperbaric oxygen therapy (HBOT)
2. Ozone: rectally and vaginally, and in combination with ultraviolet blood irradiation
3. Low-level laser light therapy (Photobiomodulation)

In Chapter 4, I shared with you the anti-cancer properties of each of these modalities. Here I share a bit more on their benefits as oxygenating agents.

Low-Level Laser Therapy (Photobiomodulation)

While the precise, destructive power of high-powered lasers has found applications in medicine (especially in precision surgery), it has also been found that non-destructive, low-level (energy) lasers have unique beneficial physiological effects—known as Photobiomodulation. As part of Photodynamic Therapy, these low-level lasers can be applied intravenously or topically to activate photosensitizers.

The PDT Plus watch, a topical low-level laser delivery device, combines the latest research findings in the fields of Photobiomodulation and Photodynamic Therapy. Its blue, red, green and yellow light diodes emit specific frequencies, each of which has unique healing properties.

The light frequencies are transported into the wrist veins and carried throughout the body, where they energize, oxygenate and heal the cells. Just as God has created rainbows with a broad spectrum of colors and light energies, now we can harness the energy of the different colors of light that are represented in the rainbow, to oxygenate and heal the body!

The watch irradiates defined acupuncture points on the wrist, and during this process, the laser penetrates the vessel walls with a variety of wavelengths. An article published in October 2015 in the *Magazine for Acupuncture and Auricular Medicine* states, "The tissue under the laser watch absorbs the energy of the laser in order to produce lipoprotein lipase. Subsequently, the microcirculation and the oxygen transportation capacity of the red blood cells are improved."[4]

The watch can be used as a standalone treatment to oxygenate and boost the function of normal cells, as well as a supportive cancer treatment when combined with photosensitizing substances like curcumin. Among its many benefits, it increases cellular oxygenation and detoxification, improves Vitamin D production, reduces inflammation, activates telomeres, and improves energy.

A summary of the unique healing properties of each light color follows, especially as they pertain to increasing cellular oxygenation:

- The **red light** binds to hemoglobin and improves oxygen uptake by about 20%. It decreases hypoxia in the tissues, and stimulates an enzyme involved in cellular respiration, or mitochondrial energy production.
- The **blue light** plays a role in energy production, enhances nitric oxide production, decreases inflammation, activates telomerase (which plays a role in longevity) and optimizes oxygen utilization in the tissues.
- The **yellow light** promotes serotonin and Vitamin D metabolism. As you know by now, Vitamins C and D are essential for proper immune function. Serotonin is our "happiness hormone" which is involved in numerous body processes.
- The **green light** also binds oxygen to hemoglobin and improves mitochondrial function.

I recommend wearing the watch daily for an hour or two, for optimal benefit.

Hyperbaric Oxygen Therapy (HBOT)

HBOT involves delivering oxygen to your body under high pressure. For HBOT, you enter a chamber where the pressure of oxygen is steadily increased until it reaches a preset level. Then, oxygen is dissolved into all of your cells, and is carried to areas of your body where the circulation is diminished.

The biggest benefit of HBOT is that it penetrates the cells to a greater degree than other oxygen therapies, as the high pressure involved in the therapy allows the oxygen to go deep into the organs and tissues. It also allows for the lungs to gather much more oxygen than would be possible if you were breathing pure oxygen at normal air pressure. It is one of the best and most efficient methods of transporting oxygen to cells throughout the body.

While most people receive their hyperbaric oxygen therapies at an integrative therapy clinic, it is possible to purchase an HBOT chamber for use at home. However, these can be costly and it is best to receive the treatment under a physician's supervision, whether at home or at a clinic. I recommend doing this therapy as often as you can.

Ozone

Ozone is another life-giving oxygen therapy that has a multitude of benefits that include: stimulating the immune system, killing cancer cells and microbes, oxidizing toxins, reducing inflammation, and normalizing hormone and enzyme production.

In addition, by oxygenating the cells, ozone does all of the following:

1. Removes via oxidation, xenoestrogens and other carcinogenic, or cancer-causing toxins.
2. Increases levels of immune-stimulating and cancer-fighting cytokines, or chemicals.
3. Increases levels of superoxide dismutase (SOD). SOD is an enzyme that is involved in the body's antioxidant defense system.
4. Optimizes white blood cell counts. White blood cells are immune cells that are involved in warding off cancer and pathogens.
5. Increases microcirculation to healthy cells.

Ozone also improves the function of healthy cells, especially the mitochondria, which are the cell's energy producing "furnaces." Thomas Seyfried, PhD, author of *Cancer as a Metabolic Disease*, provides evidence that cancer is caused by mitochondrial dysfunction,[5] and that healing the mitochondria can help the body overcome cancer.

By oxygenating healthy cells and improving their mitochondrial function, ozone enables them to better eliminate cancer-causing toxins and uptake vital nutrients.

Studies also show that ozone decreases hypoxia in tumors. For instance, in one study published in 2004 in *Evidence-Based Complementary Alternative Medicine,* 18 people with cancer who were treated with systemic ozone therapy on three alternate days over a week were found to have a significant decrease in hypoxia. The researchers concluded that the more poorly oxygenated tumors benefited the most from the decrease in hypoxic state.[6]

Many studies also substantiate ozone's cytotoxic effects. I shared a few examples of these in Chapter 4.

Methods of Ozone Administration

Ozone can be delivered to the body several ways. We give our patients rectal or vaginal insufflation treatments, as we believe that these are the safest and most beneficial ways to deliver ozone to the bloodstream.

In addition, we do cold plasma ozone therapy, which involves using a cold plasma ozone generator to deliver high concentrations of ozone directly to the skin. Cold plasma ozone is primarily used to treat external tumors of the breast and lymph nodes, as well as liver tumors, while rectal and vaginal insufflation can be beneficial for people with all types of cancers.

Refer to Chapter 4 for more information on how to do ozone therapy and where to purchase ozone generators for at-home use.

At-Home Oxygen Therapies

God has given us many simple ways to oxygenate our bodies, in addition to clinical therapies. Therapeutic breathing and exercise are perhaps the easiest and yet most powerful of these. Many of our cancer patients report that their mental state improves when they take the time to practice therapeutic breathing and exercise regularly.

Exercise

Walking in nature and fresh air is one of the best ways to oxygenate your body, and is a peaceful, life-giving way to experience God's creation and even connect with God. He created us to be active and live in the outdoors; our first ancestors lived in a Garden, and throughout history, people have spent most of their waking hours outdoors.

For example, we used to hunt, gather and fish for food, unlike today, when most of us work indoors and get our food at a supermarket. Consequently, most of us are relatively sedentary compared to our ancestors. We can get back to God's original design for our health by going outside to walk, garden, swim or do other outdoor activities, daily.

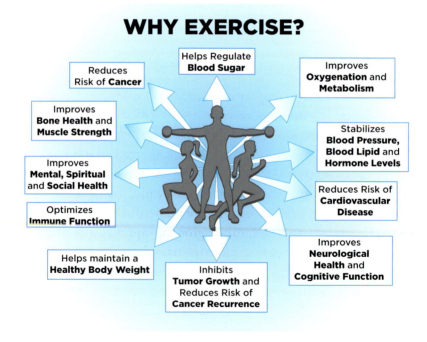

Figure 24. Daily exercise should be part of everyone's regimen to maintain a healthy body, sound mind, and uplifted spirit.

KEY PRINCIPLE #5 | OXYGEN

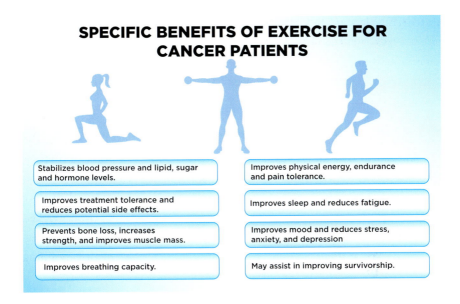

Figure 25. In addition to the general benefits, exercise has some very specific positives for cancer patients that help them traverse their treatment and recovery process with much greater success.

I recommend doing an outdoor activity that involves movement, at least five days a week, for 30-60 minutes at a time. If you are physically unable to do much, try moving your legs or arms around while sitting on a park bench, your front porch, or while wading in a pool. Even walking for 10 minutes daily, or practicing therapeutic breathing while sitting in a patio chair in your garden, can be profoundly beneficial.

The benefits of physical activity are numerous. For instance, exercise has been shown to inhibit tumor growth, improve cancer treatment efficacy, increase lifespan, and reduce the risk of cancer recurrence.[7] One study showed that people with breast and colon cancer who exercised regularly had half the relapse rate of those who didn't. And many studies show that women who exercise have anywhere from a 20-80% decreased risk of developing breast cancer than those who are sedentary.[8]

Studies also show that exercise improves immune function by stimulating the activity of some types of immune cells involved in fighting cancer; particularly, cytotoxic T-cells, natural killer (NK) cells, and macrophages.[9] The increased oxygen uptake created by exercise is likely a major reason for these improvements and outcomes.

Other benefits of exercise include: improved lymphatic movement, nutrient uptake and cellular detoxification; lowered insulin and inflammation; and improved mood and stress reduction.

Qigong and Yoga
Qigong (pronounced "*chee-gong*") and yoga are two great mind-body practices that I highly recommend for oxygenating your body. They combine therapeutic breathing and focused meditation with strengthening postural movements. You could do these practices outdoors, while grounding to the earth in your backyard, or at a park or beach.

While Qigong and yoga have some similarities, they are very different practices with unique philosophies. First, Qigong increases your body's "vital force" or energy, by combining mindfulness with gentle, flowing postural movements, and focused breathing.

Yoga also combines mindfulness with postures and intentional breathing, but its movements differ from those of Qigong in that they are more static, rather than fluid, and are held for longer periods of time. The movements involved in Qigong are slower and flow one into the other. Qigong is ideal for people of all fitness levels, as it requires less stamina and athletic ability than yoga.

While the practices of Qigong and yoga sometimes incorporate Eastern religion practices, I only recommend the breathing and exercise aspects (not the meditative or spiritual aspects) of these practices for health purposes.

Among their other benefits, which are due in part to increased oxygen uptake, Qigong and yoga increase your body's aerobic capacity, strength, mobility, endurance and immune function; promote relaxation, and help to dissipate anxiety and negative emotions.

Qigong is widely practiced in China, and one Chinese study revealed it to improve a wide variety of symptoms in more than 95% of patients with different diseases, including cancer.[10] In addition, a meta-analysis of 1,283 cancer patients found that Qigong dramatically improved the patients' sleep, energy, mood and even pain levels, when it was practiced for anywhere from 3-12 weeks.[11]

You can learn the basics of Qigong on your own, through DVDs that teach you the postures and techniques. Although, you may find it easier and more beneficial to take a Qigong class.

Similarly, many studies have confirmed the benefits of yoga for cancer patients. For instance, one meta-analysis of 138 clinical trials involving 10,660 cancer patients, the results of which were published in the *International Journal of Yoga* in 2018 revealed that yoga improved the overall physical and psychological symptoms, quality of life, and markers of immunity in most of the patients.[12]

Specifically, multiple studies have shown that yoga reduces stress, depression, and anxiety; changes the cellular milieu by altering genetic expression, and enhances cellular immunity. The authors conclude that it is very likely that yoga can prevent or halt tumor growth and even possibly help eliminate cancer. They cite a number of case studies in which yoga was shown to regress tumor growth.

Another beneficial resource is the book, *Yoga for Cancer: A Guide to Managing Side Effects, Boosting Immunity, and Improving Recovery for Cancer Survivors*, written by breast cancer survivor Tari Prinster. In this book, the author shows the benefits of yoga in reducing the side effects of radiation and chemotherapy. Prinster also addresses the unique needs of cancer patients, and teaches you how to create a safe home-yoga practice. She includes many yoga poses and 20 practice sequences in the book.

Like Qigong, you can learn basic yoga poses by following a DVD teaching, or you can take a class. If your fitness level is less than optimal, you might start out by doing just a few stretches or poses for a few minutes per day, and then gradually work up to 20-45 minutes, three to five times per week.

Before starting a yoga regimen, particularly, check with your physician about the type and intensity of yoga you should practice. Some yoga positions, for instance, can be quite difficult and strenuous, so take caution and be mindful of injury dangers. And if you take a beginning yoga class, you may want to inform the instructor beforehand of your cancer background. They might have helpful alternative poses and positions for you to practice in lieu of the more difficult ones. Ultimately, listen to your body and don't overdo it.

Therapeutic Breathing

As we discussed in Chapter 8, many in the West tend to underestimate or are simply unaware of the benefits of therapeutic breathing, but Eastern cultures have recognized its powerful healing potential for centuries. **When you breathe therapeutically, you increase your cellular oxygen levels, and in so doing, improve the functioning of your entire body.**

Many diseases have been linked to hypoxia, or oxygen deprivation, including cancer, heart disease, diabetes and chronic fatigue, among others. By improving oxygenation through therapeutic breathing, you can help to reverse cancer and any other chronic conditions that you may have.

As a brief refresher, therapeutic breathing starts with inhaling and exhaling through your nose, even at night while you sleep. Don't take deep breaths, or breathe through your mouth, as this actually decreases the oxygen to your cells, contrary to popular belief.

Hemoglobin releases oxygen into your cells only when carbon dioxide is present. Whenever you take a deep breath, you reduce the amount of carbon dioxide in your body, which causes hemoglobin to hold on to oxygen, rather than releasing it into the cells. This leads to less oxygen at a cellular level, rather than more, contrary to what most of us would think.

Patrick McKeown, author of *The Oxygen Advantage* overcame his own asthma through the practice of therapeutic breathing, and has helped Olympic athletes and many others to improve their performance by teaching them to do the same.

In *The Oxygen Advantage*, McKeown shows you how to nasal breathe through your diaphragm and abdomen, rather than your lungs, which is the most effective way to oxygenate. He then shares some exercises for improving your breathing. The first and easiest involves simply keeping your mouth closed while breathing throughout the day, and resisting the urge to take in deep breaths, or breathing through your mouth.

McKeown also teaches you how to put pressure on your abdomen and chest, to create resistance to breathing, and how to slow down and reduce your breathing movements, until you feel a tolerable hunger for air. By doing this simple exercise, you actually increase your body's capacity to utilize oxygen over time.

Once you have mastered the simpler exercises that McKeown recommends, he advocates progressing to more advanced ones, like practicing closed-mouth breathing while doing physical exercise.

Some people have found that sleeping with a piece of tape over their mouth is a successful way to encourage effective breathing at night, while their body is regenerating. This may be a beneficial practice, but consult your doctor before tying anything like this. In any case, regardless of how you choose to improve your breathing, know that therapeutic breathing at night is especially important for helping you to get deep, restful sleep and in turn, regenerate your cells.

To learn more about proper breathing techniques, I encourage you to read *The Oxygen Advantage*. McKeown's website also contains a list of practitioners that can coach you in therapeutic breathing: OxygenAdvantage.com.

Other Ways to Oxygenate

- Exercise with Oxygen Therapy (EWOT). This involves breathing higher levels of oxygen during exercise, using supplemental oxygen. For EWOT, you use an exercise bike, treadmill, stepper, elliptical machine or any other aerobic device, while breathing in oxygen through a generator and mask.
- EWOT has been shown to increase immunity, strength, and endurance and to reduce inflammation. Maxx O2 is a special type of equipment used to do EWOT and is purported to dramatically increase oxygen levels in the body. To learn more about Maxx O2 and EWOT, see: EWOT.com.
- Blowing up balloons. This increases your lung capacity and body's tolerance for carbon dioxide. If you'll recall, your body needs carbon dioxide to carry oxygen into the cells, so by increasing your carbon dioxide capacity, you increase the ability of hemoglobin to deliver oxygen into your cells.
- Breathing into a spirometer, which is an apparatus that's used to measure the volume of air inspired and expired by your lungs. Over time, as you practice doing this, your lung capacity will increase.

- Decreasing inflammation with the Garden Food Plan® and other inflammation-reducing treatments that we've described throughout this book. Inflammation causes free radicals and oxidative stress, which decreases oxygen capacity. So by reducing inflammation, you increase your cellular oxygen uptake.
- Buying more plants. The greener your home and workplace are, the cleaner your environment will be because plants oxygenate and clean the air. Drs. Elizabeth Blackburn and Elissa Epel, authors of the book, *The Telomere Effect: A Revolutionary Approach to Living Younger, Healthier, Longer* book recommend buying two plants per 100 square feet to keep the air filtered. Some good choices of houseplants include Peace Lily, Boston Fern and English Ivy. You may also want to get an aloe plant, which has been reported to help neutralize EMFs.
- Consuming more "live" plant-based foods, especially green ones. Foods that contain high levels of chlorophyll, like spirulina and chlorella, may be especially beneficial for helping to bring energy to your cells and oxygenate them.

Sleep Better to Oxygenate Better

Improper breathing at night causes oxygen deprivation, which can have tremendous repercussions upon your health. Many people suffer from sleep apnea, a condition in which you either have pauses in your breathing, or stop breathing for short periods throughout the night.

There are two types of sleep apnea: central and obstructive. In central sleep apnea, your nervous system fails to activate your breathing muscles. In obstructive sleep apnea, your airway collapses or is blocked during sleep. Both cause hypoxia, and have been linked to a multitude of health conditions, including cancer, heart disease, and many others.

If you awaken unrefreshed or tired in the morning, are sleepy during the day, feel like you are suffocating during sleep, or your spouse or partner tells you that you snore or stop breathing in your sleep, you may have apnea. Apnea is a common condition, yet can greatly affect your health.

Consider asking your healthcare practitioner to order a sleep study if you suspect you have it.

If you find that you do, the treatments for it are simple. If the apnea is mild, and depending on the cause, you may be able to mitigate it by sleeping on your side, rather than your back, by avoiding taking certain medications, and/or by losing weight (if you are overweight).

More commonly, however, apnea requires Continuous Positive Airway Pressure (CPAP) therapy, which involves wearing a mask over your nose and mouth at night, while a machine delivers a continuous flow of air into your airways.

It's important to determine the cause of apnea to know what type of treatments you may need. CPAP machines should only be used under a physician's supervision.

If you have apnea, CPAP can make a world of difference in your energy and well-being, by dramatically improving your oxygen levels.

OXYGEN: for a Vibrant Life

Table 9.1.

Oxygen Therapy	Benefits
Hyperbaric Oxygen (HBOT)	Brings oxygen deep into the cells and improves the functioning of normal cells while reducing tumor hypoxia. Is toxic to cancer cells.
Ozone	Improves the functioning of normal cells and is toxic to cancerous ones. Removes carcinogenic toxins, stimulates the immune system; increases superoxide dismutase and microcirculation.
PDT Plus watch (low-level laser therapy)	Energizes, oxygenates and heals cells. Increases cellular oxygen and detoxification; lowers inflammation and improves Vitamin D production.
Exercise	Improves immunity, increases lifespan, reduces cancer recurrence, promotes relaxation and happiness-inducing endorphins.
Qigong and Yoga	Improves the body's aerobic capacity, strength, mobility, endurance and immune function; promotes relaxation and peace.
Therapeutic Breathing	Increases breathing efficiency and oxygen uptake into the cells, making cellular processes more efficient.

SUMMARY

- Cancer cells thrive in a low oxygen environment. Angiogenesis, cancer cell division and replication, and metastases are all facilitated by hypoxia.
- Oxygen therapies disable cancer's survival mechanisms and improve the functioning of healthy cells.
- Clinical oxygen therapies include: hyperbaric oxygen (HBOT), ozone (O_3), laser light, and ultraviolet blood irradiation (UVBI).
- The most important at-home oxygenation therapies include exercise, therapeutic breathing, and consuming "live" foods.
- Qigong, walking and yoga are great mind-body practices that increase oxygen to the cells via therapeutic breathing and movement.

KEY PRINCIPLE #5 | OXYGEN

- Other ways to oxygenate the body at home include: having plants in your living environment, blowing into a balloon or spirometer, and treating sleep apnea (if applicable).

QUESTIONS FOR FURTHER REFLECTION

1. How does oxygen disable cancer cells?
2. What are some benefits of oxygenation upon normal cells?
3. Name three clinical oxygen therapies, and three that you can do at home.
4. Which therapy draws oxygen deepest into the tissues?
5. What types of exercise are best for oxygenating the cells?
6. Why is it important to breathe therapeutically?
7. What causes sleep apnea, and how is it treated?

ISABEL'S STORY

Fifteen year-old Isabel was diagnosed with ovarian cancer in May 2017—just weeks after her thirteen year-old sister, Jimena, passed away from the very same cancer. Isabel lives with her parents and 10-year-old sister, Hernanda, in Puebla, Mexico. Isabel's story is told here from her mother, Veronica's, perspective.

On May 11, 2017, Isabel awakened with a pain in her ovary. Her sister Jimena had had the same problem two years prior, and it had turned out to be ovarian cancer. Jimena had passed away within a year of her diagnosis. Just three weeks later, Isabel had awakened with the same pain, and we discovered that she too, had ovarian cancer. We were devastated.

We had taken Jimena to a hospital in Houston, Texas for treatment, where she received very aggressive chemotherapy. In the end, though, it was the treatments that had killed her, not the cancer.

Yet, when Isabel was diagnosed with the same cancer, we took her to the same clinic in Houston, where Jimena had been treated, because we knew the doctors there.

The doctors removed Isabel's ovarian tumor, but then wanted to give her chemotherapy and put her on the same exact treatment protocol as her sister. But because the chemotherapy not only hadn't worked for Jimena but had actually killed her, my husband and I decided we would not go that route again.

So we turned everything over to God, and began to research other options. Then I remembered that not long ago, I had spoken to a woman named Betty, who had overcome ovarian cancer at a treatment center called Hope4Cancer. Like Jimena, she first underwent conventional treatment, but the cancer returned. So the second time around, she decided to go to Hope4Cancer. And when she did that, she finally recovered.

So I contacted Hope4Cancer and set up an appointment for Isabel. In July 2016, we took her to the treatment center in Cancun, and did all of the treatments that Dr. Tony suggested.

In December 2017, Isabel had a checkup with her conventional oncologist in Houston; the same one who had insisted that she do aggressive chemotherapy treatment. However, the doctor now noticed that Isabel's scans were clear, and so encouraged us to continue doing treatment at Hope4Cancer. She told us that we had done the right thing for our daughter, and that the treatments were working!

She said, "Even though I don't know much about—or even agree with—this kind of approach, continue with it because it's working."

That was over a year ago, and since Isabel's last checkup on April 9, 2017, all of her tests and scans now show no cancer.

Of course, the doctors have told us that she needs to continue having checkups over the next five years, but the real danger has passed and her cancer is now in remission.

Isabel leads a normal life now. She's in good spirits, and is completely normal in every way. She attends school and social events, and has many friends. She agrees with the treatment approach that we pursued, and is convinced that the treatments she received at Hope4Cancer are what have made her well.

My husband and I are very thankful for Dr. Tony as well as God, because they led us to a treatment plan that wasn't invasive, dangerous or difficult for our daughter. And while it has been incredibly difficult to lose our other beloved daughter Jimena, we have faith that at least she is in Heaven with God.

If you are battling cancer, I encourage you to not lose hope or faith. God will hear you and show you the way. Research your options, and don't believe everything your doctors tell you; listen to your heart and intuition, as well.

Update: As of May 2021, based on her latest laboratory and imaging tests, Isabel remains clear of any evidence of cancer. While I know that nothing can take away the pain of Jimena's loss, we feel blessed to know that the trajectory of Isabel's story is heading in the right direction.

Veronica, Isabel's mom, wrote to me (I translate from Spanish): "Thanks to God, Isabel is doing very well. She is now 19 years old and is going to study fashion design at a university in Italy. This month she completes 4 years since the operation. God is very good!"

What else do we need to hear? Hope is real!

10

Parasites, Viruses, Fungi and Bacteria: Their Role in Cancer and How to Treat Them

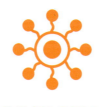

KEY PRINCIPLE #6
RESTORE THE MICROBIOME

At the beginning of time, in the Garden of Eden, there were no pathogenic, or disease-causing microbes in the world. But since sin entered the world, we have polluted our environment and are now exposed to increasingly greater numbers and types of pathogenic microbes, which cause acute and chronic infections. Many of these infections can contribute to or directly cause cancer. But because they don't always show up on tests or may cause few to no symptoms, conventional doctors don't often test or treat their patients for them.

Yet as you will soon discover, much medical evidence suggests that fungi, viruses, bacteria, parasites and lesser-known pathogens are linked to cancer. Further, all of us have pathogenic microbes in our bodies that may or may not be causing us problems. But if you have cancer, it's especially important to find out if you do, and if so, eliminate them.

Pathogenic microbes are ubiquitous in our environment: in the air, soil, food and water. We also get them via human-to-human contact and many other ways. These don't always cause us problems, but when our immune system becomes weakened by toxins like heavy metals (such as mercury and aluminum), an unhealthy lifestyle, overuse of antibiotics and other stressors, then the harmful bacteria, viruses, fungi and/or parasites can gain a foothold and start replicating and cause symptoms and disease.

For this reason, one of our 7 Key Principles is to treat any acute or chronic infections in our cancer patients. This is not just to eliminate the infections, but also so the dysfunction in the body created by the microbes—and which is contributing to the cancer—can be reversed. This also frees up the immune system so it can focus more of its resources upon the cancer.

The Role of Beneficial Microbes and How to Cultivate a Healthy Inner Terrain

Did you know that on average, we have 10 microbes for every normal cell in our bodies? This means that the average number of microbes in our bodies is about 372 trillion—or a whole lot of microbes! By quantity, we are composed of more microbes than normal human cells; however, by volume our normal cells make up a greater part of who we are.

Fortunately, many of the microbes that reside within us are non-disease causing and even an essential part of us. They exist predominantly in our gut, mucosal tissue and skin, but are also found elsewhere. They make up our microbiome, or the complex ecosystem of microbes in our

KEY PRINCIPLE #6 | PARASITES, VIRUSES, FUNGI AND BACTERIA

THE MICROBIAL MICROCOSM WITHIN US

THE MICROBIOME OUTNUMBERS US

372 Trillion
Symbiotic microbes in a human body

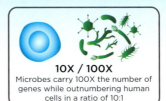
10X / 100X
Microbes carry 100X the number of genes while outnumbering human cells in a ratio of 10:1

THE MICROBIOME DIFFERENTIATES US

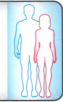
By Genomics
99%
Similar

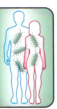
By Biodiversity
10%
Similar

SYNERGY WITH OUR MICROBIOME HELPS US FUNCTION

Human Cell-Microbiome Synergy

BUILDS IMMUNE SYSTEM
- Mucosal "firewall" restricts pathogen entry.
- Optimizes and "educates" the immune system.

REGULATES METABOLISM
- Unlocks our access to a wider array of nutrients.
- Aids enzymatic action.

VITAMINS AND MINERALS
- Helps acquire and produce key vitamins.
- Helps maintain mineral balance.

REGULATES OBESITY
- Obesity depletes the microbiome and is associated with many chronic diseases.

ANTI-INFLAMMATORY
- Regulates response to pro-inflammatory stimuli.

MICROBIOME-DEFICIENCY ASSOCIATED DISEASES

- Autism
- Anxiety & depression
- Diabetes
- Respiratory diseases
- Cancer
- Dental diseases
- Periodontal diseases
- Digestive tract diseases
- Cardiovascular diseases
- Malnutrition
- Skin conditions
- Autoimmune diseases

Figure 26. The role of the microbiome in our body.

body. When this system is healthy and in balance, our digestion and immune system work well, and we are able to easily eliminate pathogenic microbes, or at least keep them in check.

The friendly bacteria that reside in your gastrointestinal tract are also your body's first line of defense against any pathogenic organisms that enter your gut through your water or food, and play a major role in preventing infectious organisms from gaining a foothold in your body.

Yet when your microbiome becomes imbalanced by toxins and other stressors, these pathogenic microbes can begin to outnumber the beneficial ones, rendering you susceptible to disease.

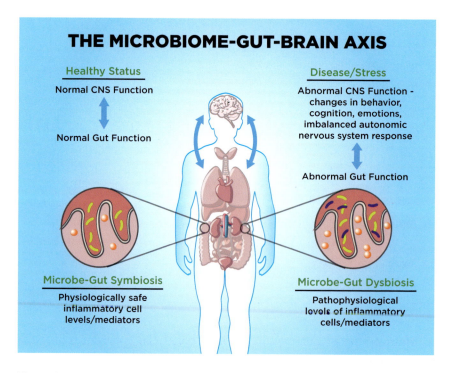

Figure 27. The microbiome, gut, and the brain work together to regulate many body processes; a deficient microbiome has the capacity to adversely affect the body's physiology in many ways, becoming the precursor to a variety of diseases. Most chronic diseases and conditions find their silent genesis in the progressive destabilization of the microbiome, which leads to imbalance in the immune system. A compromised microbiome affects the body's terrain in profound ways that can significantly promote the growth of cancer.

KEY PRINCIPLE #6 | PARASITES, VIRUSES, FUNGI AND BACTERIA

> ## YOUR HEALTHY TERRAIN
>
> Imagine what would happen if you dropped food scraps on your kitchen floor, ignored the mess, then went on vacation for a week? Chances are, you'd come back to find maggots, ants and other bugs crawling around everywhere! Where did these bugs come from? Well, they showed up because your kitchen's terrain changed, which then allowed them to come in and wreak havoc.
>
> Similarly, I have observed that in cancer patients, microbes are opportunistic and able to gain a foothold in the body only because they have an ideal environment in which they can grow and thrive. But when we build up our patients' immune system and clean up their terrain, the pathogenic microbes are no longer able to live in their bodies.
>
> Therefore, supporting your terrain is one of the most important things you can do to overcome infection, along with the appropriate antimicrobial treatments.
>
> Pathogenic microbes also thrive whenever you are in an unhealthy emotional state, so healing emotional trauma and learning to replace any unhealthy beliefs and thought patterns with healthy ones, is just as important as treating infections. In Chapters 12 and 13 I share with you how you can heal your emotions and choose life-giving thoughts.

Maintaining a healthy population of beneficial microbes is an essential first step toward eliminating infections and keeping any pathogenic microbes at bay. In Chapter 7, I shared with you tips for enhancing the health of your microbiome, which include taking gastrointestinal-supportive supplements, like hydrochloric acid, digestive enzymes and probiotics. This is the first step to disease prevention.

In addition, you can help to ward off pathogenic microbes by improving your inner terrain with the Garden Food Plan, detoxification therapies, and the other tools I share throughout this book. Microbes have many survival mechanisms; they want to live, too! They can be quite intelligent and will often mutate and hide from your immune system. Therefore, you need to go beyond treating them with antimicrobial agents and heal your terrain, as well. This will include supporting your microbiome and creating an environment in which the pathogens can't flourish.

Finally, targeted antimicrobial treatments are an important step to overcoming acute and chronic infections. In this chapter, I share with you some of the therapies that we use to treat infections in our patients. We address their cancers at the same time as their infections, because infections compromise their ability to overcome cancer. Pathogenic microbes create an inner terrain that favors cancer progression by weakening the immune system and unbalancing the body on multiple levels; for example, by compromising its ability to absorb nutrients.

How Pathogenic Microbes Cause or Contribute to Cancer

Pathogenic microbes create conditions in the body that favor cancer development, but some microbes also directly cause cancer. As I mentioned in Chapter 2, according to the American Cancer Society, 15-20% of all cancers are directly caused by infections. Microbes are suspected to cause cancer in one of the three following ways: [1]

- By directly affecting genes that control cellular growth and apoptosis
- By causing long-term inflammation and disturbances in the immune system, which over time leads to cancer
- By causing suppression of the immune system and those immune cells that protect the body from cancer

There are other theories about how pathogens cause cancer. Among these is that they produce toxins that disturb the cell cycle of normal cells. A disturbed cell cycle results in altered cellular growth and DNA that is similar to that caused by carcinogenic, or cancer-causing toxins.

Some researchers also believe that pathogenic microbes encourage a loss of cellular control by directly inducing or facilitating cellular mutations via the release of inflammatory cytokines, or chemicals that allow cancer to evade the immune system. Inflammation damages the DNA of healthy cells, induces cancer cell proliferation and halts apoptosis, all of which encourage cancer growth.

Pathogens also encourage cancer development by causing dysfunction in the endocrine and neurological systems, the microbiome, and other organs and systems of the body. The health of our microbiome is so important, because once pathogens affect our gut, they also affect our brain and in so doing, induce the brain to send wrong signals to our nervous, endocrine and immune systems. In turn, these systems send wrong signals to our cells, and cause us to be in sympathetic overdrive, or "fight or flight" mode, which is not conducive to healing.

These are just a few of the mechanisms by which pathogens may cause or contribute to cancer, but they are among the most important.

Cancer-Causing Pathogenic Microbes

The International Agency for Research on Cancer has compiled a list of cancer-causing infectious pathogens,[2,3] each of which has been linked in studies to the development of specific cancers. These pathogens and the cancers they can cause are as follows:

- **Epstein-Barr virus -** Cancers of the nasopharynx and stomach, among others
- **Kaposi/Sarcoma Herpes virus, (KSHV/HHV8) -** Kaposi sarcoma, lymphoma and multiple myeloma, among others
- **Human papilloma virus (HPV) -** Cancers of the cervix, anus, skin and aerodigestive tract, the latter of which includes the combined organs and tissues of the respiratory tract and the upper part of the digestive tract (including the lips, mouth and trachea)
- **Hepatitis B and C virus (HBV) -** Hepatocellular carcinoma
- **Human T-lymphotropic virus type 1 -** T-cell malignancies

- **Helicobacter pylori -** Gastric and esophageal cancers
- **Chlamydia trachomatis -** Cervical and ovarian cancers, ocular lymphoma
- **Salmonella typhii -** Gallbladder, hepatobiliary, pancreatic, lung and colorectal cancers
- **Streptococcus bovis -** Colon cancer
- **Chlamydia pneumoniae -** Lung cancer
- **HIV-1 virus -** Kaposi sarcoma, non-Hodgkin's and Hodgkin's lymphomas, cancers of the mouth and throat, and skin, cervical, lung, liver and anal cancers
- **Merkel Cell Polyomavirus -** Skin cancer
- **Simian virus 40 -** Mesothelioma, brain cancers, bone cancers, lymphomas

This list is not all-inclusive, and other pathogenic microbes are likely to play a role in cancer. The most common viruses I see in cancer patients are hepatitis, Epstein-Barr and human papilloma virus; among bacteria, *Helicobacter pylori* is common.

Ironically, many people with cancer acquire infections such as methicillin-resistant *Staphylococcus aureus*, (or MRSA), *Escherichia coli* and Klebsiella while receiving conventional cancer treatments in the hospital, and often die not from the cancer, but from these infections, instead.

While we don't know for sure how many people have infections as a contributing cause to their cancer, I suspect that a large percentage do, based on my experience with thousands of patients. For instance, years ago I had a patient who came to Hope4Cancer with an unspecified type of cancer. Her medical workup revealed that she had cytomegalovirus (CMV), Epstein-Barr virus and *Toxoplasma gondii*. When we treated her for all three infections, she had a dramatic recovery from both the infections and the cancer.

We treat all our patients empirically, based on the assumption that most have one or more sub-acute infections (even though they may not necessarily have symptoms). We also do tests whenever possible, and evaluate each patient according to their symptoms and clinical

KEY PRINCIPLE #6 | PARASITES, VIRUSES, FUNGI AND BACTERIA

history. That said, once microbes embed themselves deeply in the tissues, tests often can't detect them; so testing has its limitations, for this and other reasons.

Incidentally, many of our cancer-killing treatments are also effective for treating infections, so we can often "kill two birds with one stone" by doing a broad "sweep" and using the same tools that we use to treat cancer, to remove infections. This approach often enables us to remove the most harmful infections in our patients. So by treating cancer with natural therapies, you may also inadvertently end up eliminating pathogenic infections, or at least end up needing fewer medications to treat those infections!

Specific Pathogenic Microbes and Their Links to Cancer

Following I describe four main categories of pathogenic organisms, how they are linked to cancer, how you can find out whether you are infected with one or more of them, and finally—how you can eliminate them.

Parasites

As I mentioned in Chapter 2, the late Hulda Clark, PhD, was ahead of her time when she theorized that parasites were the underlying cause of a variety of diseases, including cancer. Parasites take advantage of a weakened immune system and further undermine it. The internationally renowned physician Dietrich Klinghardt, MD, PhD, also believes that parasites are a main cause of most chronic diseases.

Further, in medical researcher Connie Strasheim's doctor interview book, *New Paradigms in Lyme Disease Treatment: 10 Top Doctors Reveal Healing Strategies that Work*, Dr. Klinghardt contends that parasites are not only immunosuppressive, but also concentrate toxins, and harbor smaller organisms such as Lyme disease spirochetes, viruses, bacteria and toxins such as mold and heavy metals. Therefore, he believes that parasites should be treated first, before any smaller organisms, like bacteria or viruses, as you can't fully eliminate the smaller microbes until you eliminate the bigger ones.

Parasites suppress the immune system, and can even evade, or hide from it. For example, helminthic parasites (or worms) have been shown to do this, and are able to establish long-lasting chronic infections in the body. Many other parasites do the same. In addition, parasites form symbiotic relationships with cancer cells.

Further, the metabolism of cancer cells has been shown to resemble that of certain parasites such as helminths. What's more, some anti-parasitic medications, such as mebendazole and artemisinin that affect the metabolism of helminths also affect cancer cells.[4] For this reason, prescription and herbal anti-parasitic medications can sometimes have strong anti-cancer effects.

Studies have linked a few types of parasites to cancer, although much more research still needs to be done to evaluate the connection between most parasites and cancer. For instance, one study published in 2016 states that two types of parasites, Theileria and Cryptosporidium induce DNA mutations of healthy cells, while Plasmodium has been linked to lymphoma and what's called the "African lymphoma belt".[5]

Another study published in the *Nigerian Journal of Medicine* in 2013 states, "The most common parasites associated with human cancers are schistosomiasis, malaria and liver flukes (Clonorchis sinenses, Opistorchis viverrini)."[6]

A review of 1,266 studies on the relationship between cancer and parasites published in 2016 in the *International Journal of Cancer* expands on the 2013 findings, and states that all of the following parasites have been found in cancers or tumors: Echinococcus, Strongyloides, Fasciola, Heterakis, Platynosomum and Trichuris helminths.

Helminths (or worms) cause cancer by: inducing chronic inflammation; modulating immune function; re-programming the body's glucose metabolism; destabilizing genes; inhibiting tumor suppressor proteins, and triggering sustained cancer proliferation. In addition, they are believed to stimulate angiogenesis, to enable cancer cells to resist cell death, while also activating cancer invasion and metastasis.[7]

Treatments for parasites range from botanical remedies such as herbs and essential oils to pharmaceutical drugs, but the appropriate treatment depends upon the parasites present, because parasites vary greatly in their characteristics. For example, they can be tiny, unicellular organisms like protozoa, or they can be multicellular organisms like helminths, flukes, and roundworms.

According to parasite expert Omar Amin, PhD, owner of Parasitology Center, Inc., in an interview for the Alternative Cancer Research Institute, about 50% of all people in the United States probably have some parasitic infection.[8] Parasites are no longer just a Third World phenomenon as many of us have been led to believe, so it's worthwhile to get tested and treated for them!

Botanical remedies that are effective for treating parasites include, but are not limited to those for:

- **Protozoa (like *Giardia lamblia*):** myrrh, clove and oregano essential oils, *Phellodendron amurense*, *Andrographis paniculata*, garlic, wormwood, *Artemisia annua* and black walnut.
- **Helminthes (worms):** myrrh and clove essential oils, *Artemisia annua*, wormwood, stemona, black walnut hulls, peppermints, green tea.
- **Larger worms such as tapeworms:** *Mimosa pudica*, wormseed, garlic, oregano oil, olive leaf, clove oil, grapefruit seed extract.

Common pharmaceutical remedies for parasites include: ivermectin, albendazole, praziquantel and metronidazole. Again, the type of remedy you'll need if you find that you have a parasitic infection will depend on the parasites present and your individual biochemistry.

Two labs that do parasite testing are Dr. Omar Amin's Parasitology, Inc: ParasiteTesting.com, and Raphael d'Angelo, MD's ParaWellness Research: ParaWellnessResearch.com. If your test results indicate that you have parasites, I recommend consulting with your physician for an appropriate healing protocol, as treatment for these organisms can be complex.

Viruses

Many viruses have been linked to cancer. I listed some examples of these at the beginning of this chapter, although that list is not all-inclusive.

According to a study published in 2017 in *Cancer*, Human papillomavirus (HPV) causes greater than 5% of cancers worldwide, including all cervical cancers and an alarmingly increasing proportion of oropharyngeal cancers (OPCs).[9] **Cervical cancer remains the second most common cause of death from cancer in women worldwide, so treating HPV is essential if you have an active infection.**

Substantial evidence also indicates that a handful of viruses also play a role in breast cancer, including mouse mammary tumor virus (MMTV), bovine leukemia virus (BLV), human papilloma viruses (HPVs), and Epstein-Barr virus (EBV is also known as human herpes virus type 4).[10] HPV and EBV antibodies are common in a large percentage of the population, but that doesn't mean everyone with the antibodies has an active infection.

These are just a few examples. Like parasites, most of us have some latent or chronic viral infections that may be causing few to no symptoms, so it's worthwhile to get tested, or do a trial run of a treatment. Many of our anti-cancer treatments, such as intravenous Vitamin C, Sono-Photo Dynamic Therapy, ultraviolet blood irradiation and hyperthermia, are also effective antiviral therapies.

Common botanical remedies for chronic viruses include but are not limited to: licorice root, cat's claw, oregano, thuja, St. John's wort, echinacea root, astragalus, eleuthero (or Siberian ginseng), and olive leaf, although again, the type of remedy you'll need depends on the viruses present and your individual situation. You'll want to get tested and/or consult with your doctor to find out what treatment is best for you.

Fungi

As I mentioned in Chapter 2, the Italian cancer surgeon Dr. Tullio Simoncini believes that cancer is caused principally by Candida, a fungal infection. He developed a simple therapy to treat his cancer patients using sodium bicarbonate, which he has found to be effective for killing fungal colonies. Dr. Simoncini has also devised different ways to deliver sodium bicarbonate to the body, such as by directly injecting tumors with it. He has apparently seen many people recover from cancer just by treating these infections.

Key Principle #6 | Parasites, Viruses, Fungi and Bacteria

According to one study review published in 2017, the role of fungal infections in cancer is less clear and established than it is for parasites, bacteria and viruses. However, some infections, including chronic Candida, have been implicated in certain cancers, such as squamous cell carcinomas. Candida species are also prevalent in cancers of the oral mucosa.[11]

> Sometime in the late 1990s, I was asked to see a lung cancer patient in Sacramento, California who had been admitted to the Intensive Care Unit. She had suffered a bad reaction to chemotherapy, which caused her to go into respiratory distress and kidney failure.
>
> I flew to Sacramento to see her, but when I landed, there were lots of messages on my phone and beeper (this was at a time when beepers were used to contact people!). The messages were from one of the patient's family members, who informed me that their loved one had passed away.
>
> I asked them if they wanted me to just fly back home, but to my surprise they said, "No, we want you to come look at her records."
>
> In that moment, and for some reason, my gut told me that the patient hadn't really suffered from cancer. So I asked the family to request an autopsy, which they did.
>
> A few weeks later, they phoned to tell me that they had not found a trace of cancer in her, but rather, a fungal infection in the lung!
>
> It made me wonder how often this kind of situation happens, and how often fungal infections are misdiagnosed as cancer. Some of my colleagues have treated a lot of so-called lung cancers as if they were fungal infections and their patients have actually recovered just by doing that! This illustrates the importance of looking for infections and treating them, along with the cancer.
>
> ~ Dr. Jimenez

Mold has also been linked to cancer. One study review published in 2010 in EXS confirms this, and states that mold toxins are more toxic than pesticides.[12] One cancer-causing mold is aflatoxin, which is a common mold found in some foods, and is linked to hepatocellular carcinoma, or liver cancer.[13]

Treatment for fungal infections includes both natural and pharmaceutical remedies. Yeasts such as Candida require different treatments than mold, and mold treatments are prescribed according to the species of mold and the mold toxins, or mycotoxins, that are present.

Treatments for Candida include, but are not limited to: ozone, a product made from coconut oil called monolaurin (which is also helpful for viruses), clove, oregano, lavender and myrrh oils. In addition, a low carbohydrate diet and fermented vegetables can help to restore a healthy balance of microbes to fight the infection.

Treatments for mold include, but are not limited to: ozone, botanical remedies, antifungal drugs such as nystatin and itraconazole, and nasal sprays such as ketoconazole, amphotericin B and colloidal silver. Natural remedies for mold include clove and oregano essential oils, as well as garlic. These eliminate fungus and biofilm in the sinuses and gut, where mold likes to colonize.

Mycotoxin (or mold toxin) binders are also an important component of treatment. This is because mold is a live organism that generates toxins in the body, which must be removed using different remedies than those that are used to treat the mold. Common mycotoxin binders include: bentonite clay, chlorella, zeolite, activated charcoal and medications such as cholestyramine and Welchol.

Two labs that test for mold and mycotoxins are: Real Time Laboratories, Inc. and The Great Plains Laboratory, Inc. For more information, see: RealTimeLab.com and GreatPlainsLaboratory.com, respectively. Consult with your doctor for an appropriate treatment regimen.

Bacteria

We are all reservoirs for latent or active bacterial infections. Some bacterial infections are harmless when they are kept under control by the immune system, but can become pathogenic when the immune system becomes suppressed. Like the other pathogens described in this chapter, bacteria can create conditions in your body that favor cancer, such as inflammation, DNA damage, hormonal and nutritional imbalances, and organ dysfunction. At other times, although perhaps less frequently, bacteria may directly cause cancer.

For instance, according to the American Cancer Society website, the bacterium *Helicobacter pylori*, which colonizes the stomachs of about two thirds of people worldwide, is directly linked to stomach cancer, the fifth most-common cancer in the world. However, most people that have the bacteria won't get cancer from it. And *Chlamydia trachomatis* is a sexually transmitted bacterium that has been associated with cervical cancer.[14]

Like other types of pathogenic infections, treatments for bacteria range from botanical and pharmaceutical remedies, to clinical therapies that we do at Hope4Cancer like ozone, hyperthermia, Photodynamic Therapy and ultraviolet blood irradiation.

Some common botanical remedies for bacterial infections include, but are not limited to: garlic, myrrh, thyme, oregano, anise and clove essential oils; black cumin, curcumin, phellodendron, and echinacea, among others. Again, you will want to work with your doctor to determine what you may need.

Another remedy that I really like is lapachol, which is the most active compound of Pau d'arco, a rainforest tree. It has a wide range of antimicrobial benefits. Physica Energetics also makes some wonderful antimicrobial agents, and is the product line that we most use.

On occasion, we will treat our patients' infections with antibiotics, especially when we need to be aggressive and quickly eliminate an infection. At the same time, we will also administer natural therapies to support their bodies, especially those that support the microbiome (or gut health), liver detoxification, and also the mesenchyme, or the fluid-filled network of spaces that lie between the muscles and skin, also called the extracellular matrix.

The mesenchyme is so important that scientists are now referring to it as another organ in the body! Pomegranates are one food that has been found to support the mesenchyme. In addition, we recommend other foods that support the immune system, such as sprouts and probiotic products.

A comprehensive approach using antibiotics, along with supportive therapies, is especially important for patients that arrive at our treatment center with advanced cancers.

For instance, if a woman comes to the treatment center with a cauliflower sized breast tumor, which actually happens quite often, and her breast is infected, we have to treat her systemically and topically with antibiotics. Typically, pseudomonas, *Klebsiella pneumoniae* or *Escherichia coli* bacteria are found in these tumors, and they respond well to antibiotics. We might also use intravenous silver or cold plasma ozone applied directly to the tumor area.

The Cancer Microbe
The "cancer microbe" is a generic term that has been used to describe a pleomorphic organism that has been found within cancer tumors, and which some researchers believe is a principal cause of cancer. This microbe can apparently change its shape and size based on the acidity or alkalinity of the cell. So for instance, it can appear in the tissue as a tiny round form, or as a larger form that pathologists call "Russell bodies." It can live both inside and outside of the cells.

Pathologist William Russell was perhaps the first to describe this microbe, calling it the "parasite of cancer" at the end of the nineteenth century. However, conventional medical science does not accept any research concerning the concept of a cancer microbe.

Therefore, little is yet known about the cancer microbe, but it may play an important role in cancer. In any case, many microbes have been found inside tumors, including staphylococci, streptococci, cytomegalovirus and corynebacteria—among others. For example, a study published in 2013 contends that cytomegalovirus is common in glioblastomas, a type of brain cancer.[15]

We treat microbes inside tumors with many of the same treatments that we use for cancer, and which are described throughout this chapter (including hyperthermia, ozone and our immune protocols).

Dental Infections
As we've discussed, periodontal disease (or gum infections) and root canal and cavitation infections are strongly linked to cancer. For example, 90% of all oral cancers are oral squamous cell carcinomas (OSCCs), which are often infected with bacteria[16] indicating that dental infections cause OSCCs.

As another example, a study published in *Revista ADM,* a Mexican scientific journal, reveals that there is a strong association between *Fusobacterium nucleatum*, a gram-negative anaerobic bacterium, and periodontitis. This bacterium has also been associated with colorectal cancer, but the correlation between periodontal infections and colorectal cancer is not yet clear.[17]

Many other studies indicate a correlation between dental infections and cancer. See Chapter 8 for more information on these infections, and how to treat them.

Clinical Treatments for Acute and Chronic Infections

Following are the principal antimicrobial treatments we give our patients. They are effective for treating a wide variety of pathogenic organisms and incidentally, we also use them as part of our cancer protocols. They include:

- Ozone
- Photodynamic Therapy
- Hyperthermia
- Ultraviolet blood irradiation
- Vitamin C
- Sunivera Immunotherapy
- Intravenous herbal and pharmaceutical agents

Ozone Therapy

Ozone isn't just a fantastic oxygenating or cancer-killing agent; it also kills pathogenic microbes, including bacteria, viruses, fungi and parasites, through a variety of mechanisms. For instance, it ruptures bacterial cell walls and inactivates the bacteria's enzyme control mechanisms. It kills viruses by diffusing through their protein coat into the nucleic acid core, where it damages their RNA, and oxidizes the capsid, or viral protein shell.

Many viruses, including poliovirus 1 and 2, human rotaviruses, Norwalk virus, parvoviruses, and hepatitis types A and B, as well as others, have all been shown in studies to be susceptible to ozone. Doing a rectal or vaginal treatment using an ozone level of 0.4 ppm for four minutes has been shown to kill any bacteria, virus, mold, or fungus, although the appropriate concentration of ozone and treatment time varies from person to person.

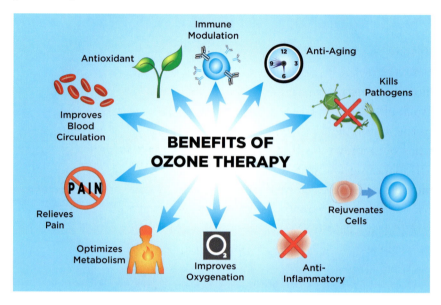

Figure 28. The many benefits of ozone therapy.

Fungal infections that have been found to be affected by ozone include: Candida, Aspergillus mold, Histoplasma, Actinomycoses, and Cryptococcus. Protozoans, or parasites that are affected by ozone include: Giardia, Cryptosporidium, and free-living amoebas, namely Acanthamoeba, Hartmonella, and Negleria, although there are likely to be many others.

Studies substantiate the effects of ozone on pathogenic microbes. For example, in one study published in 2012 in *BMC Infectious Diseases*,[18] ozone was found to inhibit the growth of six out of eight strains of bacteria, including: *Escherichia coli, Staphylococcus aureus, Enterococcus faecalis, Klebsiella pneumoniae, Acinetobacter baumannii,* and *Pseudomonas aeruginosa*.

The number of ozone treatments that are needed to treat a particular infection depends upon the infection present and each patient's individual biochemistry. Although we have found that doing treatments three-five times weekly is usually sufficient, if it's combined with the other 6 Key Principles, including a high consumption of healing foods, plenty of rest, sunshine and healthy thoughts!

Photodynamic Therapy or Antimicrobial Photodynamic Inactivation

Photodynamic Therapy is another remarkable anticancer treatment that also doubles as an antimicrobial therapy. When used against pathogens, the therapy is known as Antimicrobial Photodynamic Inactivation (PDI). It has been shown to be effective against a broad spectrum of pathogens including stronger antibiotic-resistant microbes. It selectively kills microbes without harming the body's tissues, and microbes don't adapt to it as easily as they can to other antimicrobial agents like antibiotics.

PDI principally destroys many components of pathogenic organisms, including their cell walls and membranes, protein capsids, lipid envelopes, and nucleic acids.

The benefits of PDI have been demonstrated in studies. For example, in the 1990s, three research groups discovered that Photodynamic Therapy induced fast and effective killing of gram-negative bacteria, including *Escherichia coli* and *Pseudomonas aeruginosa*, as well as fungi, and gram-positive bacteria.[19] Another bacterium that has been shown to be susceptible to it is *Staphylococcus aureus*.[20]

In addition, PDI has been found to be useful for treating periodontal pathogens, and in one study, it significantly reduced periodontal microbe counts.[21]

Hyperthermia

Hyperthermia is yet another treatment that packs a dual punch to cancer and infections. In *New Paradigms in Lyme Disease Treatment: 10 Top Doctors Reveal Healing Strategies that Work,* medical doctor Friedrich Douwes of the internationally renowned *Klinik St. Georg* in Germany shares how he inadvertently discovered that hyperthermia was incredibly effective for killing Lyme disease pathogens; two of his cancer patients found that their Lyme symptoms resolved after they received treatment for cancer![22]

Dr. Douwes has since been using hyperthermia to treat many people with chronic Lyme and other infectious diseases, in addition to cancer, and reports good outcomes. He states, "... we are able to get over 60% of our Lyme patients back to life by using hyperthermia, along with adjunct treatments... [and] another 30% improve with the treatment but require additional treatments to get better."[22]

Chronic Lyme disease is one of the most complex, disabling and yet fastest growing infectious diseases in the United States and many other developed nations, including Canada and Western Europe. More than 300,000 new cases are reported per year in the United States alone. Lyme creates conditions in the body that can lead to cancer, including inflammation, angiogenesis, high insulin levels, hormonal deregulation and connective tissue damage.

For this reason, treating Lyme is vital if you have an active infection, as indicated by a symptom evaluation and lab tests. IgeneX, Fry Labs and DNAConnexions all test for Lyme, but no test is 100% accurate. Any diagnosis should be confirmed with bioenergetic testing and/or Applied Kinesiology (muscle testing), along with a clinical evaluation. For more information on the testing labs, see: IgeneX.com, FryLabs.com, and DNAConnexions.com, respectively.

Some Lyme-literate doctors believe that most people in the United States are carriers of Lyme pathogens or have active infection. Lyme is often misdiagnosed as a variety of neurological conditions such as amyotrophic lateral sclerosis (ALS), multiple sclerosis (MS), Parkinson's, Alzheimer's, and chronic fatigue syndrome, among many others. Fortunately, with proper treatment, these conditions often reverse if and whenever caused by Lyme disease. Treating Lyme can also make recovery from cancer much easier.

Ultraviolet Blood Irradiation (UVBI)

Ultraviolet Blood Irradiation (UVBI) is a therapy in which blood is removed from the body via an arm vein, treated with ozone and ultraviolet light, and then put back into the body. The procedure is carried out in a controlled, closed system and sterile environment, so that the blood doesn't come into contact with anything outside of the body except for the ozone and ultraviolet light. UVBI has been shown to inactivate toxins and viruses, destroy harmful bacteria and fungi, and improve the blood's immune defense.

Since its discovery in the 1940s, UVBI has shown to be a remarkable and efficacious treatment for acute and moderately advanced infections. The severe oxygen deficit in cancer patients allows anaerobic pathogenic microbes to thrive, but these pathogens are highly sensitive to ultraviolet light and ozone, and respond well to this treatment.

In addition, UVBI increases oxygen absorption into the cells, and in so doing, improves circulation, decreases platelet aggregation, helps the body to eliminate toxins, and activates Vitamin D precursor molecules, all of which improve immune response.

The effects of UVBI are long lasting, and no harmful side effects have been reported. It is an exceedingly safe way to eliminate microbes naturally without the potential side effects of drugs.

Vitamin C

As mentioned in Chapter 4, most mammals make their own Vitamin C, and their bodies increase their production of it during times of illness or stress. However, we humans are one of only a few mammals that don't make our own Vitamin C. This means we need to make sure to take enough supplemental Vitamin C to be able to overcome disease.

Vitamin C plays a vital role in helping your body overcome infection, in addition to fighting cancer. It is a powerful immune support that I encourage you to take on a daily basis. To learn more about the benefits of Vitamin C and how to find your ideal daily dosage, see Chapter 4.

Sunivera Immunotherapy

Sunivera, which I described in Chapter 5, is a vital component of our antimicrobial approach because it boosts the immune system so that it can more effectively target infections. It activates macrophages, T-cells, and NK-cells. It can help to heal a number of acute and chronic infectious diseases and conditions believed to be associated with pathogenic infections such as: multiple sclerosis, rheumatoid arthritis, Lyme disease, chronic fatigue syndrome, psoriasis, warts and other autoimmune-like conditions.

Intravenous Herbal and Pharmaceutical Agents
Depending on the patient's diagnosis, we may recommend a variety of anti-infective herbal or pharmaceutical products to remove pathogens and support our other treatments.

Diagnosing Infections

Many pathogens can be difficult to detect, because they don't always show up in conventional blood, urine or stool tests. In addition, tests don't yet exist for all, or even most of the pathogenic microbes infecting us today.

In recognizing the limitations of conventional lab tests, many integrative and holistic healthcare practitioners worldwide use galvanic skin response devices or another similar type of bioenergetic testing device—to detect infections in their patients. These devices use software and a skin contact device to scan the body for the energetic frequencies of a variety of pathogenic organisms.

By itself, bio-energetic testing may be inadequate for detecting infections, but it is a valuable supportive tool in the diagnostic process.

Applied Kinesiology, or muscle testing, is also used by many practitioners to identify microbes; but again, no one single diagnostic tool can detect all infections, 100% of the time. For this reason, a combined approach using blood, urine and stool lab tests, along with bioenergetic testing and a clinical evaluation, is best. This can give you a pretty good idea what infections are affecting your health, and what to do about them.

The Role of Detoxification in Eliminating Pathogens

Dietrich Klinghardt, MD, PhD, suggests there are three major contributors to chronic disease: pathogens, toxins, and unresolved emotional conflicts. He says, **"The body always strives to achieve equilibrium between** stored unresolved emotional issues, toxins, and the presence of pathogenic microbes."[23]

According to Dr. Klinghardt, the level of pathogenic infection in the body directly correlates with its toxic burden. If this is true, then it means that simply treating the pathogens is not enough, and that the body's toxic burden and unresolved emotional conflicts must be addressed, as well.

Toxins such as heavy metals, pesticides, mycotoxins, biotoxins, glyphosate and EMFs, as well as toxic thoughts and beliefs, suppress the immune system, which creates an ideal breeding ground for pathogenic microbes. Therefore, detoxification and emotional healing also play a crucial role in helping the body to overcome pathogenic infection.

To learn more about the detoxification therapies we use and recommend, see Chapter 8. For more information about emotional healing, see Chapters 12 and 13.

Final Thoughts

Research has shown a clear association between pathogenic microbes and cancer. Some pathogens can directly cause cancer, while others create conditions in the body that favor its development.

Advanced cancer patients typically have chronic infections that deteriorate the body's ability to sustain health. This is why it's essential to find a therapeutic approach that addresses not only the pathogens and diseased cells, but also the inherent disequilibrium of the terrain, the body's toxic load, and any unresolved emotional conflicts.

SUMMARY

- Treating acute and chronic infections is crucial for reversing conditions in the body that favor cancer, and in some cases, for healing it.
- Many viruses, bacteria, parasites and fungi have been linked either directly or indirectly to cancer.
- Clinical treatments for infections include: ozone, ultraviolet blood irradiation, Vitamin C, Photodynamic Therapy, and hyperthermia.

PARASITES, VIRUSES, FUNGI AND BACTERIA:
Their Role in Cancer and How to Treat Them

Table 10.1.

Infections That Are Linked to Cancer	Treatments
Parasites	For protozoa: myrrh, clove and oregano essential oils, *Phellodendron amurense*, *Andrographis paniculata*, garlic, wormwood, *Artemisia annua* and black walnut.
	For helminths (worms): myrrh, *Artemisia annua*, wormwood, stemona, black walnut hulls, cloves, peppermints, green tea.
	For larger worms such as tapeworms: Mimosa pudica, wormseed, garlic, oregano oil, olive leaf, clove oil, grapefruit seed extract.
	Common pharmaceutical remedies for parasites include: ivermectin, albendazole, Praziquantel and metronidazole.
Viruses	Ultraviolet blood irradiation, ozone, Photodynamic Therapy, hyperthermia, immune therapy.
	Botanical remedies: licorice, cat's claw, oregano, thuja, St. John's wort, echinacea root, astragalus, eleuthero (or Siberian ginseng), and olive leaf.
Fungi (including mold, *Candida* and other yeasts)	Ultraviolet blood irradiation, ozone, Photodynamic Therapy, hyperthermia, immune therapy.
	Botanical remedies for *Candida*: coconut oil, clove, oregano, lavender and myrrh oils.
	Drug treatments for mold: antifungals such as nystatin and itraconazole, and nasal sprays such as ketoconazole, BEG spray and colloidal silver.
	Natural remedies for mold: clove, oregano essential oil and garlic, among others.
	Mycotoxin binders: bentonite clay, chlorella, zeolite, activated charcoal and medications such as Cholestyramine and Welchol.
Bacteria	Ultraviolet blood irradiation, ozone, Photodynamic Therapy, hyperthermia, immune therapy.
	Botanical remedies: garlic; myrrh, thyme oregano, anise and clove essential oils; black cumin, curcumin, *Phellodendron amurense*, echinacea and lapachol.

KEY PRINCIPLE #6 | PARASITES, VIRUSES, FUNGI AND BACTERIA

- Botanical and pharmaceutical remedies are important and useful at-home treatments.
- Because tests have not yet been developed for all pathogenic microbes that infect humans, and existing tests aren't always accurate, a diagnosis must be based upon blood, urine and stool tests, as well as a clinical and bioenergetic evaluation.
- Emotions and environmental toxins often correlate with the body's pathogenic load, so addressing these can help the body to better eliminate infections.
- Supporting the immune system with therapies such as Sunivera is an integral component of antimicrobial therapy.

QUESTIONS FOR FURTHER REFLECTION

1. Approximately what percentage of all cancer is caused by pathogenic infections?
2. How do pathogenic microbes create conditions in the body that favor cancer development?
3. Why is it important to treat infections at the same time as cancer?
4. What are some common therapies to treat viruses, bacteria and fungi?
5. What are some botanical and pharmaceutical remedies used to treat parasites?
6. How do you test for infections?
7. Name two common cancer-causing infections.

11

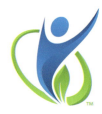

Lifestyle Tools for Healing

Overcoming cancer is as much about how you live as it is about the treatments that you do.

You can do all of the right therapies, but if your lifestyle is toxic, rushed, or stressful, or your daily habits are anything less than life-giving, it can be difficult to get well.

Yet how many people, when they get cancer or any other chronic disease, focus more upon doing the right treatments than upon improving their lifestyle and habits? **It's vital to have an effective treatment plan, but the way you live is just as important as what you do medically!**

This is actually great news, as it means that there's a lot you can do to affect your recovery, and sometimes the most powerful lifestyle tools are the simplest. For instance, you probably know by now that clean, healthy food that most closely resembles what God gave us in the Garden is foundational for healing, as are sufficient rest, sleep and exercise.

God didn't design healing to be complicated, and when you connect with Him and cultivate hobbies, habits and lifestyle practices that align with the natural laws that He has designed for your well-being, you can greatly accelerate your healing.

My maternal grandmother, Ana Teresa, who passed away at the age of 103 completely healthy, taught me three practices when I asked her about the secrets of her longevity.

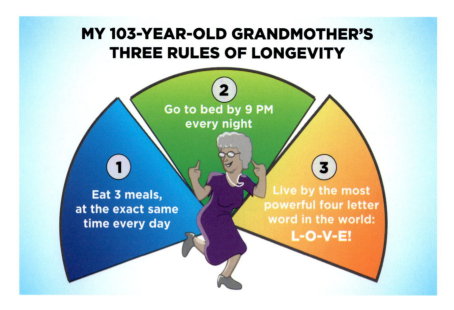

Figure 29. My grandmother's rules of longevity served her well for 103 years.

First, she always ate three meals daily, at the exact same time every day. This made sense to me because our bodies function best when we eat at set times every day. The body likes patterns and routines.

Science has even confirmed this. Two studies published in *Proceedings of the Nutrition Society* in 2016 revealed that people who ate at random times every day had higher blood pressure and a higher body mass index than people who maintained a fixed eating schedule.[1]

Gerda Pot, a professor at King's College London who worked on both studies, told *Time* magazine that appetite and digestion, as well as fat, cholesterol, and glucose metabolism all appear to be linked to circadian rhythms and follow a pattern that repeats every 24 hours.[2]

While it can be difficult in today's rushed world of ever-changing routines to maintain a fixed eating schedule, I encourage you to eat your meals at the same time every day, if you can.

In addition, in Chapter 2, I shared about the importance of thoroughly chewing your food. Studies have revealed that some of the longest-lived people on earth take one-two hours to eat a meal! This is partly

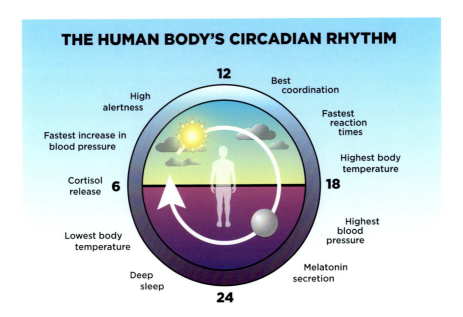

Figure 30. The science of the circadian rhythm is embedded in the fabric of life, which we ignore at our own peril. Explaining the significance of this discovery, Nobel Laureate Sir Paul Nurse said, "It's important for the basic understanding of life. Every living organism on this planet responds to the sun. All plant and also animal behavior is determined by the light-dark cycle. We on this planet are slaves to the sun. The circadian clock is embedded in our mechanisms of working, our metabolism, it's embedded everywhere, it's a real core feature for understanding life."

---

because they purposely choose to chew their food thoroughly, and in so doing, release powerful phytochemicals into their bodies.

Fruits and vegetables contain a layer of cellulose that encases and protects their life-giving phytonutrients. When you chew a lot, you more effectively break through the cellulose layer and release higher amounts of cancer-fighting phytochemicals into your body.

Nowadays, most of us don't have time to spend one-two hours chewing our food, but you can get the same amount of phytochemicals from your fruits and vegetables by blending them in a high-speed blender or Vitamix. This will release their potent nutrients in the same way as if you had chewed them for one-two hours. Drinking blended fruits and veggies also gives your digestive system a break, and gives you more energy for other activities.

The second factor my grandmother attributed to her longevity was going to bed by 9 PM every night. She was doing the right thing, because researchers now know that the body best heals, repairs and regenerates itself between 10 PM and 2 AM.

When you go to bed late, or sleep outside of those hours, your body doesn't regenerate and heal as completely as it could. In fact, studies show that people who work at night have a higher incidence of a variety of diseases, including cancer. To illustrate, a study published in February 2018 in the *European Journal of Epidemiology* found that pre-menopausal women who worked night shifts had an increased incidence of breast cancer.[3]

Like most diurnal mammals, I believe that God made us to awaken with the sun and to go to sleep shortly after nightfall. Since the invention of the light bulb, however, we have learned how to manipulate our circadian rhythms and live outside of God's original design for rest by staying up later than we were meant to. This problem has been made worse by the fact that most of us work on computers, watch TV or spend time on our cell phones at night. These activities further disrupt our body's natural sleep rhythm because the light and EMFs from electronics disrupt the function of the pineal gland, which regulates our sleep.

I know that it can be difficult to break old habits, and resist the temptation to get on your cell phone or computer at night, but I encourage you to spend less time on your electronic gadgets and go to bed a little earlier if you are accustomed to a late bedtime. This can do wonders for your healing!

The third lifestyle factor that my grandmother attributed to her longevity was that four-letter word called love! My grandmother was really connected to God; she would pray daily throughout the day, and she lived a lifestyle of loving others.

We have all been created to give and receive love. **Love is a powerful force that can heal all diseases, and loving God and intentionally seeking to love others as you love yourself is tremendously beneficial for healing.** This is simply because our highest purpose is to love and be loved. And it all starts with loving oneself!

Mark 12:30-31 says, "Love the Lord your God with all your heart, with all your soul, with all your mind, and with all your strength. The second is:

Lifestyle Tools for Healing

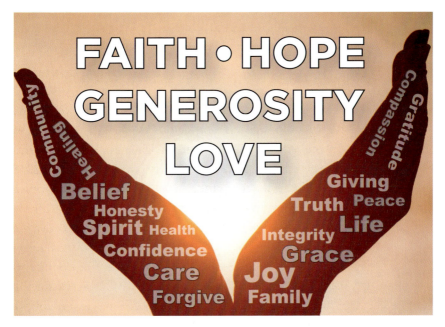

Figure 31. The Four Core Values of Hope4Cancer Treatment Centers.

Love your neighbor as yourself. There is no other command greater than these." God made us for love.

You may find that it's difficult to love others when you are suffering with cancer. Sometimes, the hardships caused by cancer can cause you to turn inward and focus only on the struggle, leaving you with little energy or time for others. Yet the more you are able to reach out to people and love them with God's love, the more you may find that love coming back to you and healing you in unexpected ways.

Finally, another thing I observed my grandmother do which I believe increased her longevity was to walk daily. She did this until the day she died. She would also get up throughout the day, saying in Spanish, "No me quiero entumir" which basically meant that she didn't want her limbs to fall asleep or to get stiff from a lack of movement.

Sometimes the simplest practices are the most difficult to cultivate, because our years-long habits become deeply entrenched in our minds and bodies. At first, you may find it difficult to change your sleep, eating and other habitual patterns. Yet with God's help, you can do all things.

His Word says, "I can do all things through him (Christ Jesus) who gives me strength" (Philippians 4:13). He can supernaturally empower you to do what you in your human weakness feel you can't do.

Proverbs 3:5-6 says, "Trust in the Lord with all your heart and lean not on your own understanding; in all your ways submit to him, and he will make your paths straight." As you do, you just may be surprised at the tremendous benefits you reap by making these few simple lifestyle changes.

Connect to God's Creation

Another powerful healing practice is to connect to God's creation and participate in nature as much as you can. There are many ways to do this.

First, if you live near a beach, park, forest or other natural setting, try to spend time there daily. For instance, if you live near the beach, take your shoes off and balance your energy by walking barefoot in the sand and grounding yourself in it. Then take in the energy of the water and waves; feel them, observe them, listen to them, breathe them in, and experience them as healing and life-giving for your body.

If you live near a park or have a garden or backyard, you can do the same. Observe the trees, flowers, and birds, or whatever surrounds you in God's creation. Spend time in that place and use all your senses to observe, smell, listen, feel and breathe in the energy of that environment.

I once had a holy man from southern Mexico come to our clinic and tell me there were two places on earth where people experienced greater healing: one was by the water, and the other was in the mountains. His observation was a testament to the power of God's creation to heal!

If you don't live near a beach, lake or the mountains, you can still reap the benefits of being in nature by going to a park or nature preserve daily, or spending as much time as you can in your backyard or garden, getting your hands in the dirt.

Another way to connect with God's creation is to hug a tree. I know! Sounds ridiculous, right? Well, far from being some hippie fad, tree hugging has actually been shown to be beneficial for balancing your body's energy!

The root system of a tree goes deep into the soil and gathers water and nutrients there, especially minerals. The energy and nutrients it receives from the ground impart energy and life to you when you make contact with the tree. Because the tree's root system goes deep, the tree also profoundly grounds you to the earth.

All parts of the tree have healing properties, including the leaves, branches, trunk and roots. Trees also absorb carbon dioxide from the environment, and release oxygen into it. So by hugging a tree, you may also improve your body's oxygenation levels.

An experience that I had overseas years ago while working in Taiwan really opened my eyes to the benefits of tree hugging. One day, I was walking to a hospital where I had been teaching and working with other doctors, and on my way there I passed a park. There was an old man, who must have been at least 90 years old, sitting on a bench next to a tree, taking his clothes off, all the way down to his underwear! He then went over to a large tree and began hugging it.

Well, I continued on my way, but when I left the clinic for a break a few hours later, I saw the old man again, sitting on the same bench, putting his clothes back on again. He had been hugging the tree for at least two or three hours! I wondered what benefit he might be getting from the tree by doing this, and it spurred me to explore tree hugging for myself. I have since become a believer in tree hugging, and my family members and I even each have our own tree to hug at home!

According to an article published on True Activist.com, author Matthew Silverstone, in his book, *Blinded by Science*, shares scientific evidence to illustrate that tree hugging can have healthful effects upon a variety of illness, including some mental illnesses, Attention Deficit Hyperactivity Disorder (ADHD), depression and headaches.

Studies cited within the book also reveal that children experience improved mental and physical health when they interact with plants. They function better cognitively and emotionally in green environments, and play more creatively in green areas.[4] We can conclude from this that tree hugging and being in a green environment is probably beneficial for people with cancer, too.

If you decide to try tree hugging, I encourage you to ask the tree for permission to hug it. I believe this connects you more deeply to the tree and honors what God has made. You might say, "Hey Mr. Tree, would you allow me to share my energy with you and receive your positive vibrations?"

When you are finished hugging the tree, say, "Thank you, Mr. Tree, for sharing your energy and vibrations."

Another way to experience nature is to bird watch. While I was in college at the University of Dallas in Irving, Texas, I took an avian ecology class, and would go bird watching twice a month. It was my favorite class! Observing and listening to the birds was such a thrilling and majestic experience, and I became so energized whenever I spent time in nature. I believe that being in nature also balances your sympathetic and parasympathetic nervous systems, which also fosters healing.

Still another activity that can connect you to nature is picking fruit or vegetables, and eating them straight off the tree or vine. I believe there's still so much we don't know about the benefits of eating fruits and veggies straight off the tree, vine or branch. But we do know that freshly picked, mature produce is likely to have more healing nutrients than produce found in the store. This is because it isn't picked prematurely, unlike supermarket produce, which is often picked off the plant or tree early so that it doesn't rot while being shipped across states or countries to your grocery store.

If you don't have a garden or fruit trees, consider attending your local farmer's market, where the fruits and veggies are likely to be fresher than what you may find in the grocery store. Ask the farm owners when they bring in their produce, and then make it a point to be there at that time. You get more nutrient-rich food this way, and attending these markets is another great way to enjoy the outdoors.

If you can't get out into nature because you live in a "concrete jungle" where there are no parks nearby, consider filling your home with plants. Then, spend some time contemplating them and their life-giving properties. Observe how they grow, from a seed into maturity, and try to see yourself in their place, growing and thriving! This will help put you in a mindset of growth and healing. Everything in creation is alive, so by focusing on what is alive, this can help you focus on living and being alive, too.

I once heard an interesting story about a classroom of fifth graders, whose teacher assigned them to go out into nature, and bring something back to her that wasn't alive.

So the kids ran out of the classroom and 30 minutes later returned with their findings. The first kid returned with a rock and, holding it out to his teacher said, "Here teacher, this rock is dead."

The teacher patiently explained to him that the rock was alive, not dead. This is interesting, because even God says in the Bible that the rocks cry out, and that all of creation, including the sun, moon and stars, praise Him (see Luke 19:40; Psalm 148:3). Could it be that all of these things are alive? I think so!

Well, the rest of the students brought back other things that they had found in nature, all of which the teacher also claimed were alive. Yet, there was one kid who didn't return to the classroom at all.

The teacher called his parents, and found out that the kid was at home. The mom put her son on the phone, and the kid said to the teacher, "I got tired of looking for something that was dead! Everything out there is really alive."

He was the only one who passed the test.

Create Art

Painting, drawing, sculpting and doing other forms of art can be very healing. You don't have to be an artist to create a painting, sculpture or drawing. You can simply draw, paint or make whatever pictures, images or forms come to mind, using colored pencils, acrylic or watercolor paint, markers, chalk, crayons and other media. Art can be very therapeutic, and in fact art therapy has become a popular way to release and process emotional trauma and troubling emotions.

If you want to use art as a way to heal trauma, you may find it valuable to work with an art therapist. These are master-level clinicians who work with people of all ages across a broad spectrum of practices. According to the American Art Therapy Association, ". . . art therapists work with people who are challenged with medical and mental health problems, as well as individuals seeking emotional, creative, and spiritual growth."

To learn more about art therapy and to find an art therapy practitioner in your area, see: ArtTherapy.org.

You may also find it fun and therapeutic to create art in a group. Taking an art class, or joining an art gathering is a great way to do this. Just remember to use non-toxic materials to create your art, as many paints, especially, can have harmful chemicals in them!

Get More Sunshine

Sunshine confers many benefits to the body. The conventional medical community has often discouraged us from getting too much sun, citing it as a cause of skin cancer. Yet the best source of Vitamin D comes from the sun, and deficiencies of Vitamin D have actually been strongly linked to a variety of cancers, as have most sunscreens, which contain cancer-causing chemicals!

God gave us the sunshine for our enjoyment and healing, and throughout most of history, humans have spent a majority of their time outdoors. Of course, too much exposure to ultraviolet light can have harmful effects upon your health, but research suggests that more disease is actually caused by a deficiency of UV rays, not an excess.

A study review published in *Environmental Health Perspectives* in 2008 confirms this.[5] According to the review, "the best-known benefit of sunlight is its ability to boost the body's Vitamin D supply, and most cases of Vitamin D deficiency are due to a lack of outdoor sun exposure. At least 1,000 different genes governing virtually every tissue in the body are now thought to be regulated by 1,25-dihydroxyvitamin D3 (1,25[OH]D), the active form of the vitamin, including several involved in calcium metabolism, and neuromuscular and immune system functioning."

The authors of the review go on to say that whereas skin cancer is associated with too much UV exposure, other cancers may be associated with too little! For instance, the researchers found that living at higher latitudes, where there is less sunlight, increases the risk of dying from Hodgkin's lymphoma, as well as from breast, ovarian, colon, pancreatic, prostate, and other cancers.

Further, a randomized clinical trial published in the *American Journal of Clinical Nutrition* in 2007 found that taking 2-to-4 times the recommended daily allowance (RDA) of 200-600 IU Vitamin D3 and calcium resulted in a 50-77% reduction in incidence rates of all types of cancers in post-menopausal women.

In addition, although excessive sun exposure has been cited as a risk factor for melanoma, continuous high sun exposure has been linked with increased survival in patients with early-stage melanoma. Interestingly, most melanomas occur on the least sun-exposed areas of the body.

These and other studies suggest that moderate exposure to sun promotes health. Anyway, would God have created such a marvelous star as the sun to shine down upon us if it were so harmful? In Scripture, God even refers to Himself as a sun, which suggests that He, as well as our earthly sun, are powerful sources of life and light. For example, Psalm 84:11 states, "For the Lord God is a sun and shield. The Lord gives grace and glory; He does not withhold the good from those who live with integrity" (HCSB).

Getting anywhere from 30-60 minutes of sunshine daily is ideal, although if you are sensitive to the sun and burn easily, you might start with just 5-10 minutes daily and increase the time slowly, if possible.

Also, don't try to get your sunshine through a window, because the glass changes the beneficial frequencies of the sun as it passes through the glass, so that your body doesn't benefit from it.

Interestingly, in Brazil there is a group of people that don't drink water or eat food on a regular basis, but instead take in the early morning sun for all of their nutritional needs. A Brazilian cardiologist even shared with me that he knew a lady who had practiced doing this for 20 years. He said that she would go out at sunrise to take in nutrients from the sun, and as a result, didn't need to eat or drink as much or as often as most people.

Discover Your Life's Purpose

You were born with what I call a God-given purpose, or reason for being. Ephesians 2:10 states, "For we are God's handiwork, created in Christ Jesus to do good works, which God prepared in advance for us to do."

Knowing your purpose, and living it out, is vital not just for health but also wholeness, because it has to do with what God created you to be and to do. Even if you don't agree with this, you would probably agree that we all need a reason to live and keep on ticking!

As I mentioned earlier in this book, you were conceived in a spark of joy that came from God, which suggests that your life has great meaning and purpose. You weren't just a random accident! As I mentioned earlier, science has even documented that when conception happens, and the sperm meets the egg, there is actually a spark of light that is emitted. I believe that light comes from God, who rejoices in your creation and the purpose for which He created you.

That purpose doesn't go away just because you get cancer, or retire from your job. Did you know that studies show that people who work and have a purpose are healthier than retired people of their same age? For instance, a study published in 2018 in *Geriatrics and Gerontology International* found that policies encouraging older people to participate in the workforce contribute to an extended healthy life expectancy.[6]

So don't retire, because having a "project purpose"—a work-based activity that God has given you to make a difference in this world—will have a profound effect on your immune system. When you tell your subconscious that it's time to retire, it sends a negative response to your immune system.

Your project purpose isn't just about you, but about helping others too (although it benefits you, too). Jesus' greatest command was "to love others as you love yourself." (Mark 12: 30-31). One way to do that is to use your gifts, talents and interests to better someone else's life or society in some way.

Again, when you are sick, it's easy to become inwardly focused, but when you use what God has given you to benefit or help others, you will be blessed as well. Jesus even said that it is more blessed to give than to receive (Acts 20:35).

That said, I've found that most cancer patients are extravagant givers who find it hard to receive from others. So perhaps the most important person that you first need to learn to give to is yourself!

In addition, giving doesn't always have to mean personal acts of service to another, although it certainly includes that. It can mean using your skills and talents to create something that will benefit humanity, as well as you.

For instance, a number of our patients write books, or become health coaches or practitioners. They make "lemonade" out of the "lemon" of cancer!

So, be cautious about retiring or even having thoughts about retirement. For example, if your doctor says you have only so much time to live, he or she may be sending a signal to your brain that it's time to retire early—in more ways than one. Refuse that idea and tell yourself that God decides when you get to come home, and because His will is for you to live out the fullness of your years, that is what you will do!

If you don't know what God has created you to do, I encourage you to quietly spend some time in His presence asking Him. Activities you enjoyed in your childhood, your personal interests, or causes that you are passionate about can provide powerful clues about what you are meant to do.

Ask yourself what your "why" is in life. Why do you do what you do, and why are you here? Embrace self-love and ask God to reveal the passions and dreams that He has put in your heart.

Sometimes, we take on jobs or projects out of fear or obligation, rather than getting in touch with our hearts, and asking God what we're really meant to do with our time. God's purpose for your life is always connected to your heart's desires, as well as to His desire to reveal Himself and impact other people's lives through you. He gave you certain interests, abilities and gifts so you would use them to better your life and the world around you.

Finally, **God didn't bring cancer upon you to teach you a lesson, although He *can* use the disease to bring about blessings into your life.** In fact, God did not cause your cancer at all. Rather, His original design for humankind, as exhibited in all its glory in the Garden of Eden, was for man and woman to live in harmony with a pure, healthy environment. As sin entered the world, and His plan became diluted and corrupted by man, disease entered the picture.

Also, disease may motivate you to pay attention to buried traumas or unhealthy habits. Or it may be a "wake up call" that helps you get in touch with whom and what God has truly called you to be.

You can trust that God's plan and purpose for your life is a good one, for He says, "For I know the plans I have for you"—this is the Lord's declaration—"plans for your welfare, not for disaster, to give you a future and a hope" (Jeremiah 29: 11, HCSB).

Cultivate Loving Relationships

Research shows that having a loving partner boosts the immune system, and that people who are in loving relationships are healthier than those who aren't. Just holding hands with someone can be so powerful!

On the other hand, toxic relationships can compromise healing. Tension, strife, dissension, abuse and other problems in relationships stress the immune system. For instance, one study published in 2016 by researchers at UCLA found that stressful friendships lead to significantly high levels of a protein that causes inflammation in the body.[7]

Another study analysis published in *Physiology and Behavior* in 2003 found that negative and hostile behaviors during marital conflict discussions were related to elevations in cardiovascular activity, alterations in stress hormones, and dysregulation of immune function.[8]

While it's normal for all of us to have problems in our relationships from time to time, it's important to seek God for help in resolving them and the toxic thoughts that go along with them.

As part of this, I encourage you to humble yourself and ask Him what you may be doing to contribute to any problems in your relationships, and what you can do to help resolve them. If you are experiencing a high level of ongoing stress in your life due to a relationship, you may also want to seek out a counselor to help you. You can never change another person's behavior, but God can, and sometimes, changing your own behavior will change theirs!

If you feel stuck due to past traumas (most of which were probably out of your control), I encourage you to research the limbic system—that part of the brain that is our "emotional center." In God's Word, when it refers to the "heart," it is talking about the limbic part of the brain—the seat of our emotions.

In recent decades, we have learned that if we are exposed to trauma when we are very young (e.g., physical or emotional abuse, neglect), we can harbor unconscious wounds and beliefs that can hold us back.

Some experts call these wounds "survival lies" because, though they are powerful, they may not be true. They are simply false constructs that were formed through limbic wounding.

For example, if you were abandoned by your father at 2 years old, you may have told yourself (subconsciously), *I cannot trust any men or father figures.* In other words, it's our heart's (i.e., our limbic system's) way of protecting us, by "mis-learning" early on that we "should never trust a man." (Put another way, just because we may believe something, does not necessarily mean it's true.)

But does this mean all men are untrustworthy? No. However, until you can name that lie and deal with it (through a qualified mental health professional), however, you may be held back in many of your relationships.

Though it's not within the scope or purpose of this book to fully explore the role of the limbic system on early cognitive and emotional formation, I encourage you to seek out caring professionals skilled in their understanding of the subject.

Comparatively, perhaps you are in a relationship where a family member, partner or friend isn't respecting you and your personal boundaries, or is causing you to feel badly in some way. If so, you may want to consider severing the relationship, or putting it on hold for a time, until you recover.

Recently, I had a patient who had to tell her best friend, who was a nurse, that she couldn't have a relationship with her anymore. The nurse had insisted that she do chemotherapy and my patient didn't want to. The nurse didn't honor or respect her friend's desire to pursue a different treatment path, and even said to her, "Why did you go to Mexico for treatment? You should be doing chemotherapy!"

My patient and the nurse had been friends for more than 20 years, but when my patient returned home after her clinic stay, she had to tell her friend in a loving way that she couldn't associate with her anymore. It was a difficult decision for her to make, but she didn't want anything to get in the way of her recovery. Sometimes self-love requires making difficult choices.

At times, it can be difficult to know whether you are in a toxic relationship that is harming you emotionally or physically. Some ways to identify whether you have serious problems in a primary relationship are: if you are unhappy at home; you don't want to speak to someone in your household or have angry thoughts toward that person; or you find excuses to be away from home and hide in your "man cave" (or "she shed").

If you are isolated or don't have many supportive friends or family members, consider cultivating some new relationships in your life. When you have cancer, it can be difficult to want to get out and socialize. I encourage you to connect with others however you can, since being in healthy relationships and community with others fosters health.

You might join a club, support group, church community, or Meetup group if you are able. Do in-person activities with others, whenever possible. There is something very healing about face-to-face interactions. If you can't do this, at least connect with someone on the phone.

Don't worry about what others might think of you because you have cancer. Meet people with the attitude and mindset that you are going to contribute something to their lives, and try not to have any expectations of them. Spend time with them simply for the sake of companionship, sharing a mutual interest or imparting the love of God to them.

People who aren't sick can't usually understand what it's like to have a long-term or challenging illness like cancer. Although they mean well, friends or family may not say the things that you need to hear, and neither will they always know how to best support you. This may cause you to feel rejected, frustrated and/or misunderstood.

If this has happened to you, **I encourage you to forgive those who have hurt you, and release any expectations that you may have of them.** We all have our flaws, and make relational mistakes. And most of the time, deep down, they mean well and just don't know the best way to help. Ephesians 4:31-32 says, "Let all bitterness and wrath and anger and clamor and slander be put away from you, along with all malice.

Be kind to one another, tender-hearted, forgiving each other, just as God in Christ also has forgiven you." This is for your sake, as much as theirs, as unforgiveness can sometimes block healing.

Instead, trust that God knows your emotional and spiritual needs, and will work to bring the right people and relationships into your life if you ask Him and trust Him to do so. He doesn't want you to be isolated or in unhealthy relationships, so seek to connect with others, and leave it up to Him to bring the right friends into your life, and to show you how to be a friend to others.

Be True to Yourself

It's important to be true to yourself in all of your decision-making. For instance, you don't want to do treatments just because your doctor or a loved one told you to. **Pursue a regimen because you believe and know they are what your body needs. So, listen to your heart when determining what treatment path to follow. As well, have faith in your body's God-given ability to heal, at the same time that you release any mentality or belief of a "quick fix."**

It took a long time for cancer to develop in your body, and you aren't going to find a fast way out of it unless you have a healing miracle (which I have seen, and which can obviously happen, too). But it is good to be patient about the process, regardless, because healing from cancer can at times be a marathon, not a sprint.

In addition, you must rely on yourself, not others, to heal you. People can be your guides or mentors, but true healing ultimately starts from within. It's not your spouse's, nor your doctor's job to get you well. They can play a tremendous role in your healing and support you, but ultimately, only God and you can heal you, not anyone else.

Identify and Resolve the Stressors in Your Life

Finally, consider any other ways in which you are exposed to stress in your daily life, and ask yourself and God what you can do to eliminate or reduce the effects of those stressors. Stress can be caused by emotional issues, but it is really anything that negatively affects your body, and can include things like: stress from harmful electromagnetic radiation; chemicals in the environment; a rushed or sedentary lifestyle; a draining job; going to bed late; maintaining poor nutritional habits; staying in unhealthy relationships; and so on.

While you can't eliminate every source of stress from your life, I encourage you to ask God what stressors most are affecting your healing, and what you can do about them. You may have 50 different causes of stress in your life, but you will likely get overwhelmed if you try to address all of them at once, which will only add to the stress in the long run!

Most long-standing positive lifestyle changes begin with baby steps, so start by working on just those factors that God may highlight to you, or what you know to be the biggest sources of stress, and go from there. Over time, you can add more and more things to your "to-do" list!

Final Thoughts

The way you live has a tremendous impact upon your healing and recovery. Cultivating simple practices such as rest, getting out in nature, taking time daily to enjoy God's creation, and creative hobbies can do wonders for your well-being. In addition, and perhaps more importantly, knowing and being able to walk out your life's purpose and having healthy relationships with others, is vital for spiritual, emotional and physical health.

You may have many things that you want to change about your life, but I encourage you to ask God what factors or issues are most important for your recovery. Start by working on those things with His help, and over time, He may show you additional things to do. By living in alignment with His will for your life, and according to the natural laws that He has created for your well-being, you will be better positioned to recover from cancer and remain well in the long run.

LIFESTYLE TOOLS FOR HEALING

Table 11.1.

Lifestyle Tools for Healing	Activity
Connect to God's creation	• Hug a tree • Bird-watch/contemplate nature • Plant a garden • Visit a farmer's market • Spend time in a park, beach, forest, or the mountains
Create art	• Paint, draw, sculpt, crochet, write, build or plant • Do art as therapy
Get sunshine	• Spend time in your backyard, your porch, a park, the beach or other recreational areas
Discover your life's purpose	• Pray/journal God's thoughts about your calling and purpose • Consider activities you enjoyed when younger and develop these • Volunteer or take the next steps toward your identified purpose • Ask yourself and God what your heart's desires are
Cultivate Loving Relationships	• Spend more time with loved ones • Make new friends: join a church, club, or support group • Disconnect from or mend unhealthy relationships

SUMMARY

- Overcoming cancer is as much about how you live as it is about the treatments you pursue.
- Cultivating hobbies, habits and lifestyle practices that align with God's will and natural laws can greatly accelerate your healing.
- Going to bed early and eating meals at the same time daily helps to balance your metabolism and align your circadian rhythm, in addition to many other benefits.

- You were created to give and receive love. Love is a powerful healing force.
- Spend time in nature as much as possible and cultivate hobbies that involve being in nature, such as hiking and gardening.
- Discovering your God-given purpose is vital not just for healing, but wholeness.
- Cultivating life-giving relationships and resolving toxic ones is foundational for wellness.

QUESTIONS FOR FURTHER REFLECTION

1. What habits do you need to eliminate or adopt to accelerate your healing journey?
2. Are there any relationships in your life that need healing or which you may need to modify?
3. Name three outdoor activities that have healing benefits.
4. Why is sunshine especially beneficial for cancer patients?
5. What is your God-given purpose, and what can you do to develop it?
6. What is the single most important lifestyle factor that you need to address in order to heal?
7. Why is giving and receiving love so important?

PAMELA'S STORY

Pamela was diagnosed with stage II-III breast cancer in 2012 at the age of 48. She lives with her two daughters and husband in Ashland, Virginia, where they farm together and live a healthy lifestyle. She credits God with restoring her marriage through cancer and the gains that she has made in her healing journey.

When I was diagnosed with stage II-III breast cancer in 2012, my two daughters were 10 and 12 years old. I was happy and healthy, and my husband and I had been doing well. So the news stunned us.

I am the youngest of six children and my uncle and mother both died of cancer, so we did not have a lot of healing success stories in our family. My mom had passed away just 21 days after her diagnosis. She was our "glue," so losing her had been devastating to me.

Because I knew what it was like to have close family members get cancer, I dreaded giving my two little girls and my husband the news about my own diagnosis. In fact, telling everyone that I had cancer was to me, worse than having it!

Fortunately, though, I had many prayer warriors, and I asked them all to pray for me. I've had so much love and support from my family, friends and several churches throughout my journey, which has really been a blessing! We all worked together, planning and preparing for the days and months ahead. I believed that God was in control and we prayed that He would give me guidance and peace.

My oncological surgeon explained that I could take one of two treatment routes. The first would be to do 14 rounds of chemotherapy to shrink the tumor, and then have a lumpectomy. The second would be to have a mastectomy, and no chemotherapy.

The only decision I was clear about in that moment was that I would never be treated with chemotherapy. I went into deep prayer about what to do, though. This was something that was so personal and I knew that only I could make the decision.

Then one day, one of my friends called and read me the Scripture, "Whether you turn to the right or to the left, your ears will hear a voice behind you saying, 'This is the way; walk in it.'" (Isaiah 30:21).

The Scripture verse came at the perfect time. After speaking to my friend and hearing the words, I made a decision to have a mastectomy.

Two and a half weeks following my surgery, my husband Doug left his job. He had worked for a large general contractor, which built schools, jails, parking decks, that sort of thing.

He came home one day and said, "I'm taking a voluntary leave of absence, to stay home to farm with you and be with you."

God had led him to do this, and little did I know then, but He was about to do something extraordinary. In fact, Doug's decision marked the beginning of a major transformation in our marriage and lives.

Now, and since November 2012, we have spent all of our days together: farming, eating three meals together daily, and raising our children. Doug takes wonderful care of all of us, and we are "side by side" in all that we do. We have raised our daughters in the Christian church and they are happy to have their father as an integral part of their lives.

The restoration of my marriage has been one of the greatest gifts God has given to me throughout this journey, because it has brought Doug and I closer together. Prior to my battle with cancer, Doug had worked 16-hour days and there was a lot of stress associated with his work. Leaving the pressure of the business allowed him to relax and focus more on his family and me, which has been good for us.

It takes a lot of work to repair a relationship. It's so wonderful for us to now be able to say we are closer than ever. We're even now able to talk to our children about our relationship; something that we could not have done before.

The journey has also brought me closer to God, and my relationship with Him has even grown stronger. So those have been some of the blessings that have happened along the way.

Shortly after my surgery, I went back to my oncologist for a checkup. I asked her if and when I would know if I was cancer-free. She said, "As of the date of your surgery, you became cancer-free. We got it all (with the surgery) so go and live your life."

At no point during my healing process did she or anyone else in the conventional medical community ever discuss with me the importance of diet or lifestyle in my recovery.

She then gave me Tamoxifen, a drug that helps to decrease estrogen in the body. She told me that I needed to take it for five years because my cancer was estrogen-driven.

Little did I know then that Tamoxifen causes liver cancer and joint pain! Within two months, I couldn't walk up a flight of steps. I'm an active person, so I told my family, "This isn't working."

So the doctor then told me to stop taking it for a while, which I did, and I ended up feeling better. Eventually, though, I had to take it again, so I lived with the joint pain the best that I could.

Everything seemed to be relatively okay for about four years, until October 7, 2016. On that day, I had some routine blood tests done, thinking that it was just going to be a normal day.

Instead, the doctor said, "We have a problem, and you need to do a scan right away."

I was totally blindsided and devastated. When I asked what was going on, they said the worst-case scenario was that the cancer had now spread to my other breast.

Unfortunately, in October 2016, I was re-diagnosed with cancer, after having been cancer-free for a number of years. But this time it had spread to my liver and under my left arm(near where the mastectomy had been performed). So, we got a second treatment opinion from another doctor, who told me that I had less than two years to live.

Now, I'm a feisty, precise, strong-willed person, and I said to him, "That is not acceptable! How long I live is not your call to make; it's God's. You're not going to tell me that I won't be here for my children in two years!" My children were now 14 and 16 years old.

Many people prayed for us again. I called a friend who had had thyroid cancer about five years earlier, and told her I needed help because the breast cancer had metastasized to my liver.

She said, "You need to see the documentary series *The Truth About Cancer*, and make sure you watch every single doctor interview in it before you make a decision about what to do next."

So my sister-in-law, husband and I sat down every morning over the next several days and watched the interviews in *The Truth About Cancer*, one right after the other.

When I saw Dr. Tony Jimenez's interview, one of the first things I noticed was that he was peaceful and calming. I knew then that I wanted to be associated with him. It was as if God had led us right to him.

The fear that had set in was now replaced by peace and God's grace and mercy, because I knew that this was the place for me. We knew we were not just going to "try" Hope4Cancer; we were going to "do" it and I was going to recover. We prayed, and then stood in agreement with God about the decision.

On November 14, 2016, my sister-in-law and I boarded a plane to the Hope4Cancer Treatment Center in Cancun, Mexico. I went for three weeks, while my husband stayed at home with the girls. I didn't ask for a reference from anyone before I went. I simply went because I felt led to go there.

Some people worry that Mexico isn't a safe place for treatment, but I found Cancun to be very safe, and the sand and sea there are beautiful. I also met many wonderful people.

When patients arrive, Dr. Tony says, "Eat the food. Enjoy the Caribbean sunshine." It's very therapeutic, and no wonder he set it up in beautiful Cancun!

I came back from the treatment center a different person, because I realized that I was supposed be healed. I was stronger and calmer, and armed with a great healing protocol. I realized, though, that my body had been compromised, and I would need to do my new protocol for life, so that I would remain healthy for life.

At Hope4Cancer, every other day, I either received intravenous Vitamin C or B-17 (Laetrile) treatments, as well as Sono-Photo Dynamic Therapy. The staff also administered many other therapies to me daily, and the doctors monitored me continually, to ensure that everything was going according to my assigned protocol.

Every other day, I received a lymphatic massage, and the staff taught me how to brush my body to stimulate the movement of lymph fluid throughout it. I also did coffee enemas, and PEMF therapy. Of all the therapies I did, Recall Healing was probably the most important. It's all about healing the emotions, which is crucial because our mind tells our body what to do.

I am headed back for my fifth visit to Hope4Cancer soon. I will be there for five days. I've visited Hope4Cancer four times since 2016. The first visit was three weeks long. I believe Dr. Tony schedules things that way, because when you do anything for three weeks, you form a habit. Treatments become a habit; eating the right food becomes a habit. Patients then take those habits home with them, to continue a healthy lifestyle there.

Most of my follow-up visits have been for four-five days at a time. The protocol is this: you arrive fasting, to do blood work and other tests, followed by a free day to enjoy Cancun while awaiting your test results.

On that day off, you can enjoy the beach and rest. The following day, you start treatments, if your doctor has ordered them. You also meet with the doctors, who will adjust your protocol if necessary, and which you will continue to follow at home. The fourth day, they pack up your prescriptions and supplements for you to take home, so you are all set to go.

When I first went to Hope4Cancer, I immediately knew it was the right place for me, and I now consider the doctors there to be my regular doctors. Every time I need something, I call their home program support line, a team that Dr. Tony has set up where people can get their questions answered. I have found that they answer my questions faster than most doctors in the US.

Also, the doctors and staff at Hope4Cancer truly love and care about you. They follow up to see how you are doing, and will also pray for you!

My daughters see strength and happiness in me now. We're living life, and I feel wonderful, so it's easy to forget that I have anything wrong with me.

We've set up an at-home clinic so I can continue to do treatments here. I also follow a very strict nutritional diet, which I switch up every several months. At first, I was on a ketogenic diet, and was consuming lots of healthy fats, such as coconut cream, in my soups and smoothies. After a while, though, I changed to a vegetarian diet.

Everyone's diet at the treatment center is individualized, so whenever other people with cancer call me for advice and ask me what they should eat, I basically just say, "Keep it clean, and make sure that your food is organic."

Juicing is probably the most important dietary practice that I follow, because the nutrients from the juice go directly to your cells. But Dr. Tony always tells patients, "Don't let food stress you out." So, for example, if you don't have time to do juicing every single day, that's okay.

Some of the treatments I continue to do at home include: hyperthermia; near infrared sauna and near infrared lamp therapies; coffee enemas; GcMAF; immune therapy; and Sonodynamic Therapy. We also have a lymph drainage machine called Vibra, which I use daily. And the most recent addition to our at-home clinic is a treadmill and rowing machine.

We're still working on fully removing the cancer, although my reports show that most of it in my liver is now gone, and any cancer at the main tumor site has been weakened (because there is no blood supply there to feed it).

I believe that by the grace of God, the cancer will soon be gone, and will be a part of my testimony to God and His goodness. I've given the battle over to Him, and received a lot of freedom from worry and doubt. Dr. Tony prayed for us while we were at Hope4Cancer, and it was exactly what I needed.

I feel like Hope4Cancer is my safe place that God sent me to, and I'm always eager to go back. I'm forever grateful for the staff there, and to God, for sending me on this path.

Another blessing of this journey is that I've been able to walk through the battle with other people, some of whom had lost hope. I've been able to give back to the world because of what I've gone through, so I don't really feel badly that this has happened to me. Indeed, God has used it all for good.

There is so much hope at Hope4Cancer. From the second you walk through their doors, you feel like you are coming home for Thanksgiving or Christmas. You feel like a family member. The staff there will hug you and tell you, "You're safe. It's okay. Now let's gets rolling!"

I remember when I first went there . . . they held my hand and said, "Listen, we don't care what you need; if you need anything at all, we are here for you. We want to do this with you."

The people who work there will even say things like, "God sent me here. I'm supposed to help people like you." The vibe there is just so positive and peaceful!

Dr. Tony and his wife, Marcy, have been assigned a major project of healing others through Jesus Christ. They are selfless, and pray for all their patients. It's a place of true comfort and hope.

If you are battling cancer, I encourage you to seek God, even if you don't already know Him—because you need Him! Then, get on your knees and ask Him to take the burden of the disease from you. Let Him have it. As soon as He takes it, freedom will come for you. The moment I gave my battle to God was when I started living again.

Anytime I feel a cancer patient giving up, I share Hebrews 12:1 with them: "Therefore, since we are surrounded by such a great cloud of witnesses, let us throw off everything that hinders and the sin that so easily entangles. And let us run with perseverance the race marked out for us."

I then tell them, "We don't give up, because that's what God commands us to do. You have to keep going. And if you stay in the center of God's will, you can be victorious!"

12

Jesus, the Resurrection, the Life and the Great Physician

KEY PRINCIPLE #7
PART 1: SPIRITUAL AND EMOTIONAL HEALING

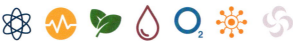

Healing your spirit and soul is foundational to cancer recovery and becoming whole, just as much as any treatment or therapy. Many of our patients and I have found that one of the best ways to do this is to cultivate a personal relationship with God and His Son, Jesus Christ. In the Bible Jesus is called "the resurrection and the life" (John 11:25), as well as the Great Physician.

The name of Jesus can elicit strong emotions in some people, either because of how religion and the world have either positively represented Him, or alternatively, misrepresented Him. Yet God doesn't support any one church as the one true way to Him.

In fact, you don't need to belong to a church or specific religion to have a relationship with God or Jesus—although I do recommend connecting with like-minded people who love God! Religion can be beneficial, but we have all been steeped so deeply in tradition that we sometimes miss that God isn't calling us to follow a set of prescribed rules; He simply wants to be in a close, personal relationship with us. This is the difference between aspects of religion (law), and an intimate relationship with a heavenly Father (love). It's the contrast between following rules and fostering relationship.

Now, I realize that you may not hold the same spiritual philosophy or beliefs as I do. That's as it should be. You are you, and I am me, and we all experience life differently. I simply want to introduce you to the God that I know, and invite you to get to know Him, too. You just may find that He's a good friend, counselor, healer and confidant who can help you—no matter where you are in your faith journey. Or, even if you've been burned or wounded by religion in the past.

This God not only wants you to know Him and His tremendous love for you, but He wants you to be healed and whole. And He can help you to get there, faster and more effectively than if you simply used medicine alone.

In this chapter, I will tell you why and how.

If you have been turned away from the idea of God or Jesus because of a negative past experience, I just want to encourage you to keep an open mind as you read. The God I know isn't a God who loves you because you do everything right or follow a certain religion or set of rules; He loves you simply because He created you! If you are a parent (or an aunt, uncle, etc.), think how much you love your child. Did you know you could multiply that feeling of love by a trillion, and it still would not equal the level of love God has for you?

That said, for most of us, our perspective of God has been influenced by how our primary caregivers treated us, or by what we've been taught by others. For instance, if you had loving parents, you may find it easy to connect with God. But if your father or mother was demanding, critical, passive or absent, you may believe that God is, as well. It's like what we talked about in Chapter 11: a limbic lie can take hold early in our development, and skew our view of what a loving Father truly looks like.

If your image of God has been distorted by your experiences with your primary caregivers or imperfect religious teachers, or you have suffered many difficult experiences in your life, you may find it difficult to want to connect with Him. If this is the case, I want to just say how sorry I am that you were treated that way. Very few things in life hurt more than to be abandoned or betrayed by the people upon whom you most relied: your parents.

The good news is, your relationship with God doesn't have to be limited by your emotional wounds or negative experiences. Otherwise, that would make Him perfectly accessible only to those who had perfectly loving parents or caregivers, right?

So I encourage you to not let your soul—or your mind and emotions—talk you out of pursuing God. He wants a relationship with you, because He simply loves you; ask Him to reveal Himself to your spirit, and then trust that He will!

Who God Is and How to Receive New Life Through Him

The God that I know and love, and whom I want to introduce to you, is made up of three persons: Father, Son and Holy Spirit. God is light and energy, as some of you may understand Him to be, but He is also a spirit with a personality and emotions, too.

God can use many tools to heal you, but I have found that nothing is more healing than knowing and experiencing His love, and I believe that we are made whole through our relationship with Him. This is because, as I mentioned in Chapter 1, our human spirit is the highest part of our being—that part of us which was designed specifically to connect to God.

John 3:16 says, "For God loved the world in this way: He gave His One and Only Son, so that everyone who believes in Him will not perish but have eternal life" (NLT).

God the Father sent Jesus Christ, His Son, to earth in the form of a man, to show the world what God was like. God also sent Jesus to become a living sacrifice for our sins (i.e., our brokenness and sicknesses), so we can be freed from their bondage and be reconciled to God the Father. Jesus died a horrible death on a cross, and was subsequently resurrected, so that we could have a relationship with the Godhead.[1]

In Hebrew, one of the original biblical languages (along with Greek and Aramaic), sin simply means "to miss the mark." We all do this daily—by having wrong or harmful beliefs, thoughts, attitudes and actions. In turn, this causes us to have trouble in our lives, and separates us from a holy and perfect God, who loves us dearly but who cannot co-abide with sin.

Because of this, and because God wants to be in a close, personal relationship with us, He made a way for us to be fully reconciled to Him. Even more, He made a way for us to be healed and empowered to live above sin, through Jesus' sacrifice. His sacrifice would make up for every harmful belief, thought or action that we would ever have, or take.

His resurrection also proved that He was who He claimed to be—the Son of God—and demonstrated that he had defeated death. Acts 1:3 states, "After He had suffered, He also presented Himself alive to them by many convincing proofs, appearing to them during 40 days and speaking about the kingdom of God" (HCSB).

So Jesus appeared to His disciples many times following His death, to prove to them and the world who He was (and is!).

Therefore, His death and subsequent resurrection into Heaven also obtained for us the privilege of being able to live forever with God in eternity after our spirit (that infinite "life spark" within us) leaves this earth!

In Revelation 1:18, Jesus says, "I am the Living One; I was dead, and now look, I am alive for ever and ever! And I hold the keys of death and Hades."

What better news could there be than to know that we can be citizens of Heaven, and that death can be just a doorway into another life?

God longs for us to accept Jesus' sacrifice, and receive Him as our Lord and Savior. When we do, we can choose to live for Jesus by giving Him reign and control over our daily lives. He then regenerates our human spirit, makes it perfect, and comes to live inside of us. Galatians 2:20 says, ". . . and I no longer live, but Christ lives in me. The life I now live in the body, I live by faith in the Son of God, who loved me and gave Himself for me."

However, while your spirit is automatically regenerated and made perfect through relationship with God, the healing of your soul and body can sometimes be a process. Yet the more you look to Him and choose to cultivate a relationship with Him, the more you can be healed, on all levels.

Jesus as the Light

Jesus also calls Himself the light. In John 8:12, Jesus says, "I am the light of the world. Whoever follows me will never walk in darkness, but will have the light of life." And 1 John 1:5 says, "This is the message we have heard from him and declare to you: God is light; and there is absolutely no darkness in Him."

One reason that we use sound and light therapy at Hope4Cancer is because we know that God is light, and He also created sound and light energy. God's light heals us. This is because, at our core, we are energetic beings, so therapies that utilize God-given energetic frequencies are powerful for healing. And when you have a relationship with God, you commune with the highest form of energy there is, and that is the light that comes from Jesus! His light can touch and heal your cells even more powerfully than any other energetic frequency.

How God Empowers You to Live Like Jesus

Just as importantly, once Jesus takes up residence inside of you, you become empowered to believe, think, and act like Him, and to overcome sin and sickness. That is God's free gift to you! In short, you are granted access to an amazing life of freedom. You may still have wounds in your soul, but you now have His Spirit inside of you to help you to overcome them, as well as the cancer.

It isn't just Jesus who lives inside of you, though. The Holy Spirit, who is the third person of the Godhead, also comes to live inside of you when you choose to be in relationship with Jesus. In John 14:16-17 Jesus speaks of the Holy Spirit, saying to His disciples, "And I will ask the Father, and He will give you another Counselor to be with you forever. He is the Spirit of truth. The world is unable to receive Him because it doesn't see Him or know Him. But you do know Him, because He remains with you and will be in you."

The Holy Spirit also empowers you to live as Jesus did, and to do the same works that Jesus did when He walked the earth, including healing the sick (including yourself!), raising the dead, and even casting out demons. Proof of this is found in Matthew 10:8, where Jesus commands his disciples, "Heal the sick, raise the dead, cleanse those with skin diseases (leprosy), drive out demons. You have received free of charge; give free of charge" (HCSB).

Another wonderful gift that you receive when you accept Jesus Christ is the right to become a son or daughter of God by spiritual adoption. Ephesians 1:5-6 says, "He predestined us to be adopted through Jesus Christ for Himself, according to His favor and will, to the praise of His glorious grace that He favored us with in the Beloved." And because we have been adopted into His Kingdom, we now have access to a higher realm, which is the heavenly realm.

In addition, Ephesians 2:6 states, "And God raised us up with Christ and seated us with him in the heavenly realms in Christ Jesus." That means right now—not at some point in your future. This means that you have access to heavenly resources, such as God's wisdom and healing power, because you are now a citizen of Heaven and a child of God.

In fact, God tells us that once we receive Jesus and the Holy Spirit, we are made a new creation. 2 Corinthians 5:17 says, "Therefore, if anyone is in Christ, he is a new creation; old things have passed away, and look, new things have come" (HCSB).

As part of becoming a new creation, God promises to give life to your physical body by His Spirit, who lives in you. Romans 8:11 says, "And if the Spirit of Him who raised Jesus from the dead lives in you, then He who raised Christ from the dead will also bring your mortal bodies to life through His Spirit who lives in you."

What is wonderful is that you will become more like God as you:

- Realize who you are as a son or daughter of God.
- Understand the spiritual riches of what you have been given as part of your inheritance in Him.
- Grow in your ability to abide (e.g., dwell, rest) and connect with Him in relationship.

I have found that people with cancer sometimes feel as if their life has been ruined, or is crumbling around them. They have thoughts of being in a coffin, or of not living long enough to see their kids grow up. They don't know that there is a better way.

This fact is another reason why Jesus' death and resurrection are so key, and why knowing what God has made available to you is so important—because it means that you can have a resurrected life, too. But the wonderful life He wants for you isn't just in the hereafter—it's here on earth, as well!

Becoming like God and surrendering fully to His Spirit and what He wants to do in your life is a process, though. Many people who have accepted Jesus Christ as their Lord and Savior don't fully realize the magnitude of the gift that has been given to them.

They may believe they've simply been given a "get out of jail free" card—a ticket to Heaven. And yes, when we receive Jesus, we now have the privilege of spending eternity with God, in a perfect place where there is no more suffering and no more tears (Revelation 21:4). This is an amazing gift—but there is more to it than that.

Because of Jesus, you can know God intimately, and have access to all the treasures of Heaven. Ephesians 1:13-14 says, "When you heard the message of truth, the gospel of your salvation, and when you believed in Him, you were also sealed with the promised Holy Spirit. He is the down payment of our inheritance, for the redemption of the possession, to the praise of His glory" (HCSB).

How to Receive Divine Healing Through God's Word and the Holy Spirit

Because the same Spirit who healed people through Jesus when He walked the earth as a man now lives in you, you can also be healed by His Spirit in you, too. In fact, God still does many healing miracles through His people today, just as He did over 2,000 years ago through Jesus. Most people believe in miracles, but what they don't know is that they are meant to be *common*, not *rare*, and are in fact so in faith communities which believe in divine healing.

When you live continually out of your spirit and in communion with God, rather than according to the history that was inscribed in your soul or your biochemistry, your soul and body start to heal, too. The limbic system needs to be renewed, and the Spirit of God wants to heal you of emotional and spiritual "cancers", just as He desires to heal you of physical cancer.

This happens for a few reasons. First, whenever you commune with God, your cells respond by vibrating at a higher resonance, or at frequencies that are healing to your body.

Secondly, when you are in relationship with God, He will begin to show you areas in your soul that need restoration. He will make you aware of any harmful beliefs, thoughts, attitudes or behaviors that you may have. What's more, by the power of the Holy Spirit He will help you—to replace those with His life-giving and loving beliefs, thoughts and behaviors!

As part of this, He will show you how to renew your mind daily. Romans 12:2 says, "Do not be conformed to this age, but be transformed by the renewing of your mind, so that you may discern what is the good, pleasing, and perfect will of God."

Thirdly, because the same Spirit that did healing miracles through Jesus lives in you, you can also speak healing to your body and expect changes to happen, especially when the words come from the Word of God (the Bible). This is because the words in the Bible are literally alive, and filled with His Spirit. In John 6:63 Jesus says, "The words I have spoken to you—they are full of the Spirit and life."

This means that the more you know, meditate upon, speak and live out the Scriptures or words that He highlights to you, the more you will live in health and wholeness because there is life in those words that will be imparted to you.

Bible Verses That Demonstrate Why Healing Is God's Will

Following are a few Bible verses that illustrate God's will to heal sickness and disease. In the Bible you will find many others.

> My soul, praise the Lord,
> and do not forget all His benefits.
> He forgives all your sin;
> He heals all your diseases.
> He redeems your life from the Pit;
> He crowns you with faithful love and compassion.
> He satisfies you with goodness;
> (so that) your youth is renewed like the eagle.
>   PSALM 103:2-5 (HCSB)
>
> Worship the LORD your God, and his blessing
> will be on your food and water. I will take away sickness
> from among you.
>   EXODUS 23:25
>
> Then they cried to the Lord in their trouble,
> and he saved them from their distress.
> He sent out his word and healed them;
> he rescued them from the grave.
> Let them give thanks to the Lord for his unfailing love
> and his wonderful deeds for mankind.
>   PSALM 107:19-21

> LORD my God, I cried to you for help, and you healed me.
> PSALM 30:2
>
> He heals the brokenhearted and binds up their wounds.
> PSALM 147:3
>
> The LORD is near the brokenhearted and saves those crushed in spirit.
> PSALM 34:18
>
> The prayer of faith will save the sick person, and the Lord will restore him to health; if he has committed sins, he will be forgiven.
> JAMES 5:15

Finally, perhaps the most important proof that Jesus gave us healing as part of His atoning work on the Cross is found in the Old Testament book of Isaiah.

Isaiah was a prophet who lived approximately 700 years before Jesus and foreknew more about His coming, life on earth, death and resurrection than any other prophet.

Isaiah 53:3-5 (HCSB) says:

> He was despised and rejected by men,
> a man of suffering who knew what sickness was.
> He was like someone people turned away from;
> He was despised, and we didn't value Him.
> Yet He Himself bore our sicknesses,
> and He carried our pains;
> but we in turn regarded Him stricken,
> struck down by God, and afflicted.
> But He was pierced because of our transgressions,

crushed because of our iniquities;
punishment for our peace was on Him,
and we are healed by His wounds.

The more that you meditate upon and speak God's Word, and have relationship with Him, the more you will have victory in every area of your life, including your health.

That said, divine healing isn't a formula, although physical healing sometimes happens once you allow God to heal your soul and restore you from any lie-based (limbic) beliefs, thoughts and behaviors.

How to Heal Your Soul Through Relationship with God

People with cancer often learn to repress negative emotions. When they do this, those emotions can get buried in their cells, where they cause disease. Healing those emotions, and uprooting the lies and toxic thoughts that caused them, with the help of God, is therefore essential.

In Chapter 13, I share how emotional conflicts and toxic emotions can cause cancer, and some additional ways to heal those using mind-body medical tools.

God will speak to you and tell you what needs to be healed in your soul, if you listen! He speaks to us through His Word, the Bible, but He can also speak to you personally in a still, small voice. In addition, He may speak to you through other people, circumstances, and dreams and visions. You know that you are hearing from God if, when you ask Him to speak to you:

1. He responds with words that line up with the Scriptures; and
2. what you hear is consistent with His attributes as a loving God.

For instance, I have found that the words God speaks to us are usually more life giving, positive and optimistic than the words that we speak to ourselves! His voice is never shaming or condemning. Let me repeat that:

God's words are never shaming or condemning.

He may point out to you something that He'd like to help you change in your life in order for you to heal—a toxic behavior or relationship, for instance—but He will never do it in a shaming or condemning way. There is a difference between guilt and shame:

1. Guilt is when you feel bad about what you have done.
2. Shame is when you feel bad about who you are.

When you feel shame, which is about your identity, that emotion is not from God.

Practice listening for the voice of God, and ask Him to speak to you. Then, journal whatever you hear that resonates with your spirit. You may want to do this in a quiet place; for example, lying face down on a yoga mat in your bedroom or a closet; while listening to some soothing instrumental music, or while you are out walking in nature.

At the same time, share your heart with Him, because He cares for you (see 1 Peter 5:7). I encourage you not just to seek Him for healing, but also to know Him. He wants to be more than a divine Santa Claus for you—He wants to be your loving Father!

This is because the highest blessing you can receive isn't your physical healing, but knowledge of His love for you. And this love is illuminated when you spend time getting to know Him.

God wants the best for you, which means seeing you prosper in all your ways. As I mentioned in Chapter 11, God says in Jeremiah 29:11, "For I know the plans I have for you"—this is the Lord's declaration—"plans for your welfare, not for disaster, to give you a future and a hope."

There is no evil in God, and it is not His will that you, or anyone you know, be sick. While He can use all circumstances for your good, He did not give you cancer to make you a better person! His death and resurrection atoned for every disease you would ever have, but you must believe Him with your whole heart and appropriate this healing by thanking Him for it, and meditating on this truth daily.

If Healing Is God's Will, Then Why Isn't Everyone Divinely Healed?

By now you may be wondering why not everyone is physically or emotionally healed through prayer or relationship with God, if healing is His will for us?

While we don't always know the answer to this question, the Bible gives us some profound insights into it. In addition, many ministers and health care practitioners who have been used greatly by God throughout history to heal have observed that certain factors play a role in whether a person receives divine healing.

For example, if you feel unworthy of healing or don't know or believe that it is God's will to heal you, then you may not receive healing through Him simply because you don't know that it's meant for you, too.

James 1:6-7 states, "But he must ask in faith without any doubting, for the one who doubts is like the surf of the sea, driven and tossed by the wind. For that man ought not to expect that he will receive anything from the Lord."

The good news is, if you have doubts about God and His will to heal you, you can still be healed through the prayers of another who has faith for healing. Proof of this is found in James 5:14-15, which says,

> Is anyone among you sick? Let them call the elders of the church to pray over them and anoint them with oil in the name of the Lord. And the prayer offered in faith will make the sick person well; the Lord will raise them up. If they have sinned, they will be forgiven.

Another hindrance to healing can be unforgiveness. At times, God may not be able to heal you if you are continually poisoning your cells with bitterness and anger toward another person, including yourself! The antidote to this is found in James 5:16, which says, "Therefore confess your sins to each other and pray for each other so that you may be healed. The prayer of a righteous person is powerful and effective."

In addition, the Bible tells us that we have a spiritual adversary in this world named Satan. He and other evil spirits can cause disease, either directly or indirectly. Most of us live according to natural laws, but there is an even higher order of spiritual laws to which we are subject, and healing sometimes depends upon knowing our adversary's spiritual tactics against us, and overcoming them.

Ephesians 6:12 says, "For our struggle is not against flesh and blood, but against the rulers, against the authorities, against the powers of this dark world and against the spiritual forces of evil in the heavenly realms."

So at times, there may be a battle in the spiritual realm for your healing. The good news is you can ask God to help you contend for the healing that Jesus made available to you through His death and resurrection, and then show you how to remove those obstacles. And then trust that He will!

For instance, evil spirits often gain access to torment or afflict us with disease through curses that have been spoken over us by others; through witchcraft rituals that a family member or ancestor has participated in, or through soul wounds that have been inflicted upon us by others.

At times, it can be enough to simply repent, or declare to God that you are turning away from the sins that opened the door for any evil spirits to afflict you, and then ask His forgiveness for entertaining those sin(s). You can also repent and ask God's forgiveness on behalf of those who harmed you or your family through a curse, ritual, or some sort of abuse, and then break that curse in the name of Jesus.

Once you do this, the evil spirit may leave, or you may need to command it to leave. In the Bible, people were sometimes healed when a demon was cast out of them. For instance, Luke 11:14 says, "Jesus was driving out a demon that was mute. When the demon left, the man who had been mute spoke, and the crowd was amazed."

The great news is that when you receive God's Spirit, you have authority over evil spirits, and can command them to leave you. This happens once you close their doors of access, such as by forgiving those who have harmed you.

This is because most spirits gain access to harass us or make us sick when we adopt harmful beliefs, thoughts and behaviors that are a result of early life wounding or traumatic events.

For example, if you put a pile of garbage in an alley, it will inevitably attract rats. If you just exterminate the rats, what will happen? That's right: the rats will come back. Similar to how cancer is a cell-level issue, and must be dealt with at its core level through a multi-pronged treatment approach, so it is with demonic harassment.

In other words, **you need to get to the root causes, and remove them (i.e., remove the garbage) through prayer, emotional and spiritual healing, and by forgiving those who have wounded you, by the power of the Holy Spirit.** And sometimes that is what it will take—divine intervention. That's particularly true if you've been badly abused or mistreated, and in your own human heart and emotions, you just can't come to forgive that other person. You need God's help.

Be aware that demonic spirits take advantage of lies that we already believe and try to reinforce those. They will encourage us to live out of our wounding, rather than through the healing that Jesus gave us access to, through His work on the Cross. Most of all, evil spirits try to get us to believe that God doesn't really love us or want us to be well, and that we have to jump through lots of hoops to receive His healing.

Nothing could be further from the truth!

Rather than try to figure out whether an evil spirit such as a demon is involved in your sickness, you may want to just ask God to show you any lie-based beliefs you may be holding onto, and help you replace those with His beliefs. As well, ask Him to heal any wounds that are allowing the enemy access to harass you. Once your emotional wounds are healed, demons often leave, although for reasons not entirely known to us. As well, you sometimes have to follow up the emotional healing by commanding them to leave, too.

In addition, you may want to work with an experienced counselor or inner healing minister to help you identify whether ancestral curses or curses that another person has spoken over you are playing a role in the disease. Such ministers are usually found in charismatic and Pentecostal churches, as well as charismatic Catholic churches.

You can also do a search online to find a trained, Bible-believing expert in the field of spiritual healing (sometimes called deliverance ministry). Like all things, make sure to work with a counselor or minister who loves God and has a reputation for being able to effectively help others. This is important, as some people have been emotionally wounded through their experiences with incompetent but well-meaning ministers.

When we aren't instantaneously healed through prayer or relationship with God, it's easy to adopt a theology (i.e., spiritual belief system) based on our personal experience, rather than upon the Word of God and what Jesus says in the Bible. Even though your experience may be telling you God doesn't heal (or heals only sometimes), it's difficult to have faith for healing if you believe that God may not want you to be well.

Wouldn't it be better to stand on the truth of His Word and what He says in the Bible, and believe that He will help you to heal, rather than assume that He may not want you to be well?

Something else to keep in mind: The Garden of Eden didn't stay so Edenic. The sins of Adam and Eve caused them to damage the intimate relationship they once had with God. As well, disease entered into the picture as a result of free will. God is a gentleman—He forces no one to believe in Him or follow His ways. And because He gave us, His children, the choice to follow Him or not, or to pursue goodness or evil, it means we live in a fallen world.

This is so relevant when it comes to cancer.

Why? Because in spite of the fact that you might do everything I've mentioned above (or in this book, for that matter), we are still just flesh and blood. We get sick, and we die. All of us. But don't confuse the sins and disease of this world with some sort of twisted desire by God to make us sick—or worse, punish us with cancer if we "don't live a good life."

God did not give you cancer. Jesus Himself says that God causes His sun to rise on the evil and the good, and sends rain on the righteous and the unrighteous (Matthew 5:45). In other words, all are susceptible to illness, even the most God-loving people in the world. And though we can improve our chances of not becoming ill by pursuing a healthy lifestyle (in spirt, mind, and body), we can't fully eliminate the chances of disease.

Anyway, whether you are physically healed or not in this lifetime, has nothing to do with His love for you; He loves you the same, whether you are healed or not!

In addition, while God may ask you to participate in your healing by repenting for unforgiveness or some other sin, I encourage you not to feel condemned or believe that you are doing something wrong if you aren't immediately healed. We are in a spiritual war here on Earth, and sometimes, people who don't even love God receive a healing miracle, while those who deeply love Him don't!

If you have observed this kind of thing, I know how painful and confounding it can be. You might think, *Why was my hateful neighbor instantaneously healed of cancer, while I remain ill?* Many of our spiritual "why" questions don't get answered on this earth, and instead only serve to separate us from God when we don't get the answers we seek.

Therefore, rather than create a philosophy about healing based on what you've experienced or observed with your five senses, I encourage you to simply get to know God and ask Him to show you His will concerning your healing. Then, meditate on those verses in the Bible that speak of who He is and His promises to you.

God didn't give you disease to teach you a lesson, so please don't listen to anyone who tells you this. Of course, God can use any situation for your benefit and to grow you through the hardships and trials that you may face (like cancer), but bringing good out of a disease isn't the same thing as believing that God is the author of it! John 10:10 says, "The thief comes only to steal and kill and destroy; I have come that they may have life, and have it to the full."

To learn more about divine healing and why it is God's will and heart to heal all those who ask Him, I recommend reading FF Bosworth's book, *Christ the Healer*, which provides a more in-depth biblical analysis of why it is God's will to heal, and how you can receive and appropriate that healing in your own life.

Abide in God, the Great Physician

In the end, sickness is destruction, not life. God is a builder and a healer, and He created you to enjoy life, be healthy, and prosper in all of your ways: relationally, financially, physically and spiritually. When you get to know Him, He will give you faith to believe Him for these things (if you don't already!). Consider 3 John 1:2, which refers to God's will for our lives and says, "Dear friend, I pray that you may enjoy good health and that all may go well with you, even as your soul is getting along well."

The more that you feed your spirit through abiding in and connecting deeply with God, living out His Word, doing the works that Jesus did—by loving other people, and healing them—the more you are likely to see His life manifest in your soul and physical body, too.

Also, **God may heal you supernaturally, but He can also anoint or bless medicine so that it becomes more effective.** For this reason, I encourage you to pray over and bless all your treatments, believing that God will cause them to work better in your body as a result.

In the end, though, I encourage you to put your hope and trust in God, not in any man or medicine, because God is ultimately the Great Physician who can lead you into all that you need to know and do for your healing. We medical doctors know a lot, but there's still much that we don't yet understand, and this is why we also need divine discernment from God. Once we can step beyond what we know in the physical realm, we can better help our patients.

I also believe that it's more important to trust and believe God for your healing than it is to do everything perfectly. God honors trust and faith, more than your ability to do everything perfectly.

It may take a while for your emotions to line up with this truth, but over time, as you determine to seek Him, you will come to progressively know Him and His will for your life. Jeremiah 29:13 states, "You will seek Me and find Me when you search for me with all your heart" (NLT).

Develop a Relationship with God Through Prayer, His Word and Community with Others

At times, you may find that your relationship with God feels empty, or like little more than a discipline or activity in which you recite a "laundry list" of requests to Him. Whenever you are at your weakest point, the enemy may try to implant lies into your mind, and tempt you to believe that your relationship with God doesn't matter. So, I encourage you to strengthen your faith as much as you can by finding time to be alone with God in prayer, spending time with prayer-minded friends, being a part of a faith community, and meditating upon His Word.

When you bring your needs to Him, be specific about what you want. 1 John 5:14-15 states, "Now this is the confidence we have before Him: Whenever we ask anything according to His will, He hears us. And if we know that He hears whatever we ask, we know that we have what we have asked Him for" (HCSB). Isn't that great news?

Another great way to know God is to meditate upon His works and attributes as described in Scripture. For example, Psalm 145:17-18 says, "The Lord is righteous in all his ways and faithful in all he does. The Lord is near to all who call on him, to all who call on him in truth."

Before you read the Bible, ask the Holy Spirit to reveal the meaning of the Scriptures to you, and to show you the verses that are meant for your life, right now. Not everything in the Bible is likely to be relevant for your life today, and you may struggle to understand certain Scriptures until the Holy Spirit highlights and illuminates their meaning to you. In any case, I encourage you to allow the beautiful, powerful words that He does give you to permeate your entire being.

You can also grow in your relationship with God by spending time with like-minded people, so I highly encourage you to consider joining a church or spiritual group that makes it their goal to love and serve God. This should be a place where you can grow, and where you feel safe and at peace. Avoid places and people that leave you with a nagging sense of condemnation or feeling like you aren't good enough.

Many people haven't learned to embrace the fact that we have been saved by God's grace—not by our works or anything we have done. This means that we can't earn God's love by anything that we do! In fact, trying to earn God's love is to essentially deny and negate what Jesus did for us on the Cross, because the Cross paid for every sin that we would ever commit.

When we receive Jesus as our Lord and Savior, however, our behavior does change, as a natural outflow of our relationship with Him. Such change is not because we are trying to please Him so that He will accept or heal us. So understand, there is nothing you can do to make Him love you more! You can't earn your healing or His favor—God already said "yes" and "amen" to your freedom, nearly 2,000 years ago when Jesus went to the Cross for you. If there is one single truth that I want to embed deeply into your mind, it is the power and perfect love that is found in Him and His living Word—the Bible.

How to Rebuild the Ruins of Your Life

When you have cancer, it is easy to feel like your life is in ruins. Yet because of Jesus Christ's death and resurrection, you now have the ability to completely rebuild those ruins! When you know Him and what He obtained for you so that you could be made whole, you can rebuild your life on a new and stronger foundation.

As part of rebuilding the "ruins" of your life, I encourage you to do the following:

1. **Believe in God, and know that something better is possible.** Jesus said, "I am the resurrection and the life. The one who believes in Me, even if he dies, will live. Everyone who lives and believes in Me will never die—ever. Do you believe this?" (John 11:25-26, HCSB). You can have life by believing in Him, here as well as in the hereafter.
2. **Be open to God rebuilding your life and restoring you.** Psalm 80:19, talks about restoration. It says, "Restore us, LORD God Almighty; make your face shine on us, that we may be saved." God's grace will meet you wherever you are. He loves you too much to let you stay where you are, and will help to rebuild and restore your life, as you seek Him daily.
3. **Grab onto faith; hold on to it, and run with it.** John 20:27-28 says, "Then [Jesus] said to Thomas, "Put your finger here; see my hands. Reach out your hand and put it into my side. Stop doubting and believe." Thomas said to him, "My Lord and my God!"

    Thomas doubted that Jesus had truly died and been resurrected back to life. That's why when Jesus appeared to him shortly following his resurrection, He told him to touch him to see that He was real. He especially had him feel his hands, scarred from the nails driven into them when he was crucified on the cross.

His message to Thomas was, "Stop doubting and believe!" Today, Thomas is often referred to as Doubting Thomas but in reality, that's not how he was. He only doubted for a little while—once when he touched Jesus' hands and saw the nail marks in His hands, he believed!

In fact, Thomas actually had a lot of faith because he ended up traveling and spreading the gospel message around the world, more than any of Jesus' other disciples!

Instead of believing in what you see, feel, or experience in the earthly realm regarding your cancer, consider how doubting Thomas believed in Jesus' resurrection. He chose to believe in the supernatural and in what didn't seem possible; and by grabbing onto faith and running with it, he spread Jesus' message far and wide. So when you are tempted to doubt, think of Thomas, and believe God for a better outcome!

4. **Get busy living.** Finally, I encourage you to see yourself as healed, and to see the greatness God has put in you. He sees wonderful things in you that perhaps you can't see in yourself. When you have cancer, it can be difficult to believe that you can heal, get over a hump or rebuild your life, but God sees and believes in much better things for you. Remember, He calls you His child! John 1:12-13 says, "Yet to all who did receive him, to those who believed in his name, he gave the right to become children of God—children born not of natural descent, nor of human decision or a husband's will, but born of God."

Final Thoughts

Mark 9:23 says, "Everything is possible for one who believes." When you come to know God and His great love for you, you can be divinely healed through relationship with Him and His miracle working power, as well as through any medicine that He leads you to take.

Above all things, though, He simply wants you to believe and trust in Him. As you do, He can and will work with you to make you whole: in body, soul and spirit. Healing can be instantaneous, or it can be a process. Regardless of the method that He uses, know that He will guide and help you, as you seek His face daily. Don't waver through difficult times, but forgive yourself if you do, and seek the strength and support of others.

Finally, be gentle with yourself and know that God loves you, whether you are healed physically on this earth or not. Don't strive to figure everything out—simply look to Him and believe and trust Him to reveal all that you need to know. Besides, in the end, the greatest healing is simply knowing that you are loved by an amazing God and that you can have eternal life through Him, in a place where there will be no more disease, suffering and tears.

> And I heard a loud voice from the throne saying, "Look! God's dwelling place is now among the people, and he will dwell with them. They will be his people, and God himself will be with them and be their God. 'He will wipe every tear from their eyes. There will be no more death' or mourning or crying or pain, for the old order of things has passed away." (Revelation 21:3-4)

Isn't this truly the best news of all?

SUMMARY

- Having a relationship with God is foundational, not only to healing your spirit and soul, but to becoming whole.
- God heals you by helping you to identify and replace any lie-based beliefs, thoughts, and behaviors with His truths.
- God can also heal you supernaturally, through His Spirit that lives in you and others.
- God's love is the most powerful healing force there is.
- God's Word has supernatural power to heal, transform and rebuild the ruins of your life.

JESUS, THE RESURRECTION, THE LIFE AND THE GREAT PHYSICIAN

God Heals:

- By revealing Himself and the Resurrection to us.
- Supernaturally, through our prayers and those of others.
- By imparting life to us when we meditate on and speak His Word.
- By helping us to replace harmful beliefs, thoughts and behaviors with His life-giving ones.
- By teaching us about who we are in Christ and the power He has given us to overcome.
- By giving life to our physical body by His Spirit in us
- By anointing and blessing medicine so that it becomes supernatural.

QUESTIONS FOR FURTHER REFLECTION

1. How can you know that it is God's will to heal you?
2. Name some Scriptures that illustrate that His will for humanity is health, not sickness?
3. What did Jesus' sacrifice on the Cross obtain for you?
4. What are some practical ways to develop a relationship with God?
5. How can you know the character and nature of God?
6. Name a few ways that God heals, both through relationship with Him as well as supernaturally.
7. Which of the four aspects of "rebuilding the ruins" resonates with you most? Which one do you need to work on cultivating more of in your life?

ERIN JESSICA'S STORY

Erin Jessica is a 35-year-old mother of four who was diagnosed with triple positive ductal carcinoma breast cancer in 2015. Her battle with cancer was triggered by multiple tragedies within her family. Despite the challenges, she is prevailing, with the help of God and her supportive family. She lives in California with her family and enjoys writing, nature and helping others to heal.

I have endured many hardships throughout my 35 years of life. By the grace of God, I have survived, but it hasn't been easy. One of the major hardships, but ironically not the worst, happened in September 2015, when I was diagnosed with a triple positive invasive ductal carcinoma in my left breast.

My daughter, Gracie, was just a year old at the time. I had been nursing her when I felt a lump in my breast. Concerned, I went to the doctor to have it checked. The doctor told me there was less than a 1% chance of getting cancer while I was nursing, so I initially dismissed the possibility.

Still, I wondered if he was wrong, and thought: *There's no way I can have any more tragedy in my life.* I was too young. Gracie's twin sister, Baylie, had passed away in my womb just a week before both she and Gracie were brought into the world. In addition, my sister had passed away from cancer when I was in my 20s, and my brother had died in a tractor accident just a year before I discovered the lump in my breast.

In some ways, though, a potential cancer diagnosis seemed like nothing when compared to everything else I had lost up until then.

Prior to the birth of my twins, everything had been going well with my pregnancy. I had had a midwife and a doctor assisting with my care, and my husband and I had already named our twins Baylie and Gracie.

But at my 33rd week of pregnancy—nearly eight months into the pregnancy—Baylie made a different kind of movement in my belly, and left the world. She woke me up during the night to say goodbye, and although I didn't know in that moment what had happened, I knew something was wrong.

The following day, my dog was sniffing me in an unusual way, and I thought, *I better check with my midwife and make sure everything is okay.*

The midwife couldn't feel Baylie's heartbeat, so I went to the hospital, and the doctors confirmed that she had passed on. I was devastated. It was a really dark time in my life, and I wanted to die right then. I knew that I couldn't, though, because I had another live baby in me, so I had to live.

The doctors kept me in the hospital for seven days, but they couldn't understand why Baylie had passed on because up until that time, the pregnancy had gone smoothly. The babies' blood pressure, ultrasounds, and other tests had always come out fine. So it was confounding.

Grace initiated labor seven days after I received the news about Baylie, so I had both of the twins at the same time. Grace came out of my body first, but initially, she didn't want to leave the womb.

When she wouldn't come out, I suspected that something was going on, and I said, "Doctor, you don't know what's going on, do you?"

She replied, "No, it's like Grace is stuck (inside your womb). She's not letting go."

When my sister passed away from brain cancer in my 20s, I remember that I wanted to die and go with her. This reminded me of that time, because it was as if Gracie didn't want to let go of her sister either. Gracie's heart rate was dropping while she was still inside the womb, and it was as if she wanted to stay there with her sister, also.

So I called my mom into the operating room and told her to "call" Grace out of my womb. She did, and to our amazement, Grace obeyed and came right out after that! She was 2 pounds 13 ounces, and able to fully breathe on her own.

Baylie came out next. She was 2 pounds 8 ounces, and absolutely perfect. It was so devastating to be so close . . . only to have to say goodbye.

But I needed to be strong, because I had a new baby to take care of, in addition to my other two children, who were 18 and 8 years old at the time.

My son, Andres, is now 22; I adopted him when he was 12 years old. And my older daughter, Leah, is now 12.

Shortly after Baylie went home to be with Jesus, my brother had the tractor accident. My body and emotions seemed to "turn off" right after that. But ironically, this was before I even *knew* what had happened to him. It was as if I had felt him die, and my body and soul were responding in the way that would best protect me from the tragedy.

I finally shut down because I just couldn't continue to grieve so many things: the loss of my baby, my sister, and now my brother. I just couldn't handle all of that and effectively continue to take care of my children, as well as breastfeed Gracie.

Fast forward to a year later. Although my doctor initially said I didn't have cancer, Jesus said, *You better go back to the doctor, because you have something going on.*

So I saw another doctor, who told me to have a mammogram; I did that, along with a very invasive biopsy. The first time I went to the clinic to do the biopsy, though, I felt such an evil presence in the place that I had to leave and reschedule the test.

I finally did the biopsy, but it ended up being a four-hour procedure and I went into shock from it. I got a hematoma on my right breast and a double breast infection, because they didn't do a proper, normal biopsy.

I decided that whatever happened, I wasn't going to go the conventional route of treatment. I had watched my sister suffer horrendous side effects from the treatments they gave her for brain cancer. They messed her up badly, and as I watched her in hospice I thought, *If something like this ever happens to me, I can't go this route.*

At that point, I still hadn't received the results of all my tests. But somehow, I knew that I had cancer. Now, I didn't yet know about alternative or integrative cancer care, but I knew there had to be a better way to treat it than with chemotherapy and radiation.

Following the biopsy, the doctors did a PET scan. Gracie was 2 years old by then, and the doctors told me I had to stop nursing: the PET scan had made me so radioactive that I could no longer breastfeed. I couldn't even sleep in the same room with my husband for a while!

While we were awaiting the biopsy results, God said to me, *It's the grief! It's the grief (that's giving you cancer), and we are going to heal it all!*

Hearing this greatly encouraged me.

After my sister had passed away from brain cancer, I bought Dr. Gerson's book *A Cancer Therapy*, and his DVD *The Gerson Miracle*, and learned about the famous Gerson cancer care treatment approach. I hadn't done any of the treatments in the book, but now, I pulled it out again and started doing some of his juicing recipes.

In the meantime, I was finally diagnosed with cancer, and a nurse gave me the names of three recommended oncologists.

As an oncology nurse explained the various treatment options, I thought: *What will all of this treatment do to me?*

I wanted to have a good quality of life, and watch my kids grow. If I did conventional treatments, I realized that I might live five years. But even so, I didn't want to die at age 38, and suffer horribly throughout those years. I wanted to enjoy life. I was depressed for obvious reasons, but I wasn't sick or bedridden, and I had children and other blessings in my life that I wanted to live for.

I then watched *The Truth About Cancer* documentary with my husband. He was completely freaked out at first by what he learned, but then he agreed that we had to go a different route with my treatment. I fell in love with Dr. Jimenez, who was featured in the documentary. I then watched some of his videos on YouTube, to learn more about his work, and I fell in love even more!

I ended up seeing the oncologists though anyway, and when I told them that I was also considering alternative cancer care, they were intimidating and unkind to me. They would say things like, "Why would you go to Mexico and choose alternative cancer care? That's like committing suicide! Why would you be so selfish and do that to your husband?"

I've discovered, though, that I'm not the only one who gets intimidated in this way. Other patients have shared how their oncologists said awful things to them when they chose alternative cancer care—even worse things that what was said to me. They use fear to control and intimidate patients into doing their treatments. It's terrible!

But shouldn't we all have the option to do the treatments that we want, without fear, intimidation and control?

I ended up applying to five alternative cancer clinics, but in the end, Dr. Tony's clinic seemed to offer the most treatments under one roof. So, I went to Hope4Cancer for the first time in May 2016.

At that time, I was only 100 pounds because I had been doing the Gerson therapy juicing protocol, which had ended up giving me pancreatitis and caused me to lose 20 pounds, so I was very thin. I was also now battling a lot of fear about what could happen to me.

I immediately fell in love with Dr. Tony and his wife, Marcy, and I felt like they loved me, too. The compassion and presence of Jesus was so evident in Dr. Tony; he just embraces and accepts people where they are at in their life's journey, which is so comforting. And the clinic just oozes the presence of Jesus; He truly walks the halls there!

So I knew that Jesus had sent me to Hope4Cancer, but after three weeks there, I returned home and fell back into my stressful lifestyle and attitude of "non-self-love." The tumor grew 30%, so I had to go back. But when I returned, it was as if I finally and truly realized I was going to be okay. I thought, *God has this!*

I pursued more therapies, and an MRI showed that the tumor was shrinking again. Some of the things I did included the AARSOTA vaccine, light therapy, IV Vitamin C, Vitamin B-17, infrared sauna and Sono-Dynamic Therapy, immune therapy injections, and Sunivera.

I continue to go back to the treatment center periodically, but I don't like to be away from my kids for long, so I also do treatments at home, as well. Some of the things I do at home include full body hyperthermia, Sono therapy, and coffee enemas. I also have a naturopath who gives me intravenous treatments, if I need them.

People ask me what is the most important treatment that I've done so far, and I tell them, self-love—falling in love with God, and discovering that Jesus loves me. Healing is also about embracing who God created me to be.

I still have a tumor, but I feel better than ever! Everyone at Hope4Cancer thinks I am a patient's daughter, not a patient, when I visit the clinic, because I'm doing so well.

A tumor isn't necessarily an indicator of how sick you are, anyway. I have met patients at Hope4Cancer who have had tumors for 15 years! Some are at the treatment center because, like me, their tumors were stable until some stressful thing in their life caused them to start growing again. Dr. Tony has told me that stress is the number one cause of cancer.

People with cancer are often terrified. I often share my experience with other patients at Hope4Cancer and tell them that fear is the enemy in this game, not the cancer. I will sometimes visit with them, and ask them straight up if they love themselves.

Some of them will just start crying, because they have so much self-hatred: from tragedies, abuse and other things that have happened to them. It's just so sad. They will say, "I hate myself. I always put myself last (in my relationships)."

I will then say to them, "Ask Jesus how to love His holy temple, which is you!" That's because He lives in those of us who believe in Him, and He loves us deeply. I tell them to ask Jesus to show them how they can love themselves as He does. He doesn't want us to suffer and torture ourselves. He wants us to enjoy this life that He died for, so we can be free.

If you are battling cancer, I encourage you to reach out and ask others for help! I tell people to do things like start a fundraiser, but they will often say things like, "I can't ask other people for help." Sadly, they are often embarrassed and ashamed that they have cancer, and don't have a lot of extra money lying around for treatments.

Well, I didn't either! I set up a fundraiser for myself, but I also have a wonderful, loving husband and family who have helped to provide for me.

Please don't feel badly about putting yourself out there, though. It's not your fault that you got sick. You have to take action, and value and love yourself enough to seek out support.

I did, and now, even though I still have a tumor, it is stable, and I feel great and optimistic about the future!

Update: On April 29, 2021, our dear friend Erin made her final journey to a wonderful place of rest. Her five-and-a-half year tryst with breast cancer ended while being surrounded by loving family and friends "singing her into Heaven." Erin left behind many friends at Hope4Cancer—doctors, nurses and staff—who, while feeling her loss, celebrate her transcendence to a place where pain and suffering do not exist anymore. Erin made her mark by living a life full of joy, laughter and energy, even during times of great challenge. We believe that it was this *joie de vivre* combined with her dedication to natural methods of healing that helped Erin defy the odds of her diagnosis for many years. We love you, Erin, and thank you for being a great example for others to follow.

13

Behavioral Emotional Spiritual Therapy (BEST)

KEY PRINCIPLE #7
PART 2: SPIRITUAL AND EMOTIONAL HEALING

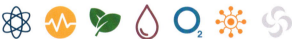

A negative thought can kill you faster than a bad germ.

ANONYMOUS

"Doctor, are you saying that emotions can cause cancer?" Patients will often ask me this question with incredulity. In my more than 25 years of serving cancer patients, I have been asked this question countless times.

My unwavering answer has always been, "Yes, they can."

Many of us have been conditioned to think that beliefs, emotions and thoughts don't play a role in disease. Yet, they are the difference between action and inaction, success and failure, health and disease, or even life and death. So, why is it a stretch to think that our thoughts couldn't cause cancer? And even if they could, how would we measure their impact and, more importantly, undo their damage?

At Hope4Cancer, we have developed a program called BEST, or Behavioral Emotional Spiritual Therapy™, to effectively address this question!

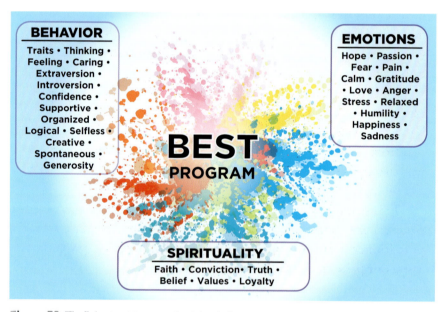

Figure 32. The Behavioral Emotional Spiritual Therapy (BEST) Program at Hope4Cancer Treatment Centers.

No two patients are alike and therefore each requires a unique healing approach. For this reason, and as part of BEST, we analyze each patient's history, personality, beliefs and behaviors, to determine how to best tailor an emotional healing program to their needs. We meet them where they are at, working in tandem with their beliefs and comfort level using different approaches, so that whichever ones we use will be most effective.

KEY PRINCIPLE #7 | BEHAVIORAL EMOTIONAL SPIRITUAL THERAPY (BEST)

In Chapter 12, I shared how you can develop a relationship with God, which is the most vital aspect of spiritual and emotional healing. Here, I share some of the tools that we use as part of the BEST program, along with a behavioral analysis, to heal emotional conflicts that are causing or contributing to our patients' cancers. These tools are based on concepts in mind-body medicine.

Interestingly, **we have found that all our cancer patients have emotional issues that are playing a role in their disease(s).** So even if you are a generally happy or peaceful person, or have had a pretty good life, I encourage you to consider the possibility that you may have an emotional issue that needs healing, too. For instance, you may have had a trauma that happened to you as a young child or when you were in your mother's womb that you don't remember, which is impacting you and your body today.

Finding the emotional conflict or the trauma that triggered the cancer is not always easy, though. Just like icebergs remain mostly hidden beneath the water, many of our emotional conflicts stay hidden from our conscious mind. Yet, they continually send strong signals to our cells via our autonomic nervous system, which then affects our biology.

In the next few pages, I will describe some techniques that practitioners use to uncover these emotional conflicts. We have several practitioners trained in the various aspects of the BEST program to assist our patients in their emotional and spiritual recovery.

How Emotions Cause Disease

Your autonomic nervous system, or that part of your brain and nervous system that is responsible for your body's automatic functions, like breathing and blood pressure, records and stores past emotional conflicts. And when you face a catastrophic emotional event or are under a lot of stress, the autonomic part of your brain sends traumatic impulses to your sympathetic nervous system.

When this happens, your body goes into what's called "sympathetic dominance" or "fight or flight" mode. In this mode, your immune and gastrointestinal systems become suppressed, and your body releases cortisol, which is a stress hormone that, when elevated for prolonged periods of time, damages your cells.

Over the long term, if the stress is prolonged, your body can get stuck in fight or flight mode, or sympathetic dominance. This results in conditions that can increase your risk of developing cancer, such as inflammation, high insulin, and high cortisol, among others. This is one way that emotions can cause cancer.

Fortunately, you can change your autonomic brain's habitual response to stress by using your conscious mind. Once you know what is causing your automatic brain to operate in sympathetic mode, you can change its programming by acknowledging and releasing the emotional trauma, and by practicing new beliefs, thoughts, and behaviors. In turn, your automatic brain will relax and begin to send healing signals to your cells.

German New Medicine

A second way emotions can cause cancer is through the shock of a sudden severe emotional conflict. The late Dr. Ryke-Geerd Hamer (1900s), a German medical doctor and Founder of German New Medicine, was one of the first physicians to discover how emotional conflicts cause cancer.

While in medical practice, Dr. Hamer's son was murdered, and shortly after this, Dr. Hamer developed testicular cancer. Dr. Hamer was suspicious of this coincidence, as he had been healthy throughout his entire life prior to this event. So he embarked on a mission to research the personal histories of thousands of cancer patients to find out whether they had suffered some type of shock, distress or trauma prior to getting cancer.

After extensively researching many thousands of patients, Dr. Hamer concluded that cancer is caused by shocking, unexpected emotional events. However, he found that if the difficult events were in any way expected, people would not become ill.

Dr. Hamer also discovered that specific emotional conflict shocks caused specific cancers. These emotional conflicts would manifest

KEY PRINCIPLE #7 | BEHAVIORAL EMOTIONAL SPIRITUAL THERAPY (BEST)

simultaneously in the psyche, brain and organ(s) where the cancer was located. These "conflict shocks" as Dr. Hamer called them, usually happened 18 months prior to the cancer diagnosis.

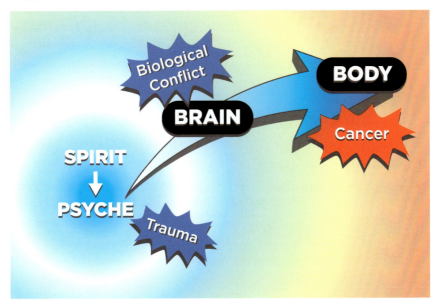

Figure 33. The trajectory of our "felt" experiences: why what we experience can manifest itself eventually as disease.

According to Dr. Hamer, the brain contains "emotional reflex centers," each of which corresponds to a specific emotion and organ in the body. He found that cancer would develop in the organ (or organs) that was related to the specific emotional center in the brain where the conflict first manifested. Once he and his patients were able to identify and resolve these emotional conflicts, the patients would often heal from their cancers.[1,2]

In my experience with thousands of cancer patients, I have found Hamer's observations and correlations to be accurate. That is why we have used his research as a reference for the development of our own healing program.

In addition, Dr. Hamer observed that people with cancer had certain psychological traits. In particular, he found that they had difficulty sharing their thoughts and emotions with others, and often hid their anger, sadness and other emotions behind a brave face. They might be described as "too nice" and would stifle emotions for the sake of avoiding conflict.

Recall Healing

Some healthcare practitioners have developed their own healing systems using principles that are based, to varying degrees, on Dr. Hamer's work. For instance, Recall Healing, created by Gilbert Renaud, PhD, is among the most well-known of these. According to Dr. Renaud's website, "In Recall Healing, as we unlock the secrets of illness, we work at identifying and solving the emotional trauma behind the condition or behavior, an important step within the healing process."

Similar to Dr. Hamer, Dr. Renaud has seen many of his clients recover from physical conditions, including cancer, once they discovered and healed from the emotional conflicts that caused them. We have incorporated aspects of Recall Healing into our BEST program and observed this to be true with our patients, as well.

We are all faced with severe and sudden life stressors from time to time, but it is how we handle them that determines whether we will get sick from them or not. For example, according to Recall Healing, as long as a conflict remains on a level that your psyche, or mind, can handle, then it won't get transferred into your body.

However, if the conflict is sudden and overwhelming, then, as a survival mechanism, your brain may "download" the effects of that conflict into your body. So where the cancer first occurs in your body can tell you a lot about what conflict you may be dealing with.

Incidentally, simply receiving a diagnosis of cancer and/or a poor prognosis can cause its own conflict shock that can stimulate the creation of a new cancer somewhere, or cause the original cancer to metastasize! This is called the "shock of the diagnosis." For this reason, it is important to resolve all conflict shocks related to the cancer you have, which you can do with the help of a BEST or Recall Healing practitioner.

Our BEST Program incorporates the concepts of Recall Healing to help our patients unravel the behavioral, emotional, and spiritual context of their disease. BEST practitioners can be reached for remote sessions from the comfort of your home via an internet telecommunication service (such as Zoom or Skype). To schedule a session, you can contact Hope4Cancer at 1-888-544-5993.

Name It, Claim It, and Dump It

At Hope4Cancer, we use a variety of techniques to help our patients resolve the conflict shock(s) that are related to their cancers. For instance, we have adopted a technique from Recall Healing that involves simply naming the conflict, claiming responsibility for it, and then "dumping" it. This means that once you know what the conflict is, you then acknowledge it as your own. It's important to do this because, even if someone else triggered or caused the conflict shock, ultimately you need to claim responsibility for what's happened to you. Once you do, you can make a conscious decision to "dump it"—or let it go.

This technique isn't just about having an "aha!" moment, though. It actually helps you to release the emotional conflict from your psyche and body. Often, the conflict causing the cancer isn't what you think it is, so it's best to work with a practitioner who can help you discover the conflict shock and release it so healing can come.

We find that once the trauma is brought to our patients' awareness, most of the work is done. They don't always need to know how to fix the problem. They simply must bring it to their awareness so their body's healing mechanisms can take over. In my experience, about 75% of all emotional conflicts can be resolved in this way.

Ho'oponopono

Hawaiian therapist Dr. Ihaleakala Hew Len developed a simple technique called *Ho'oponopono* (translated "correction" in Hawaiian), which we recommend to our patients to help them process emotional conflicts. It involves periodically thinking or speaking the following four short but powerful statements over yourself. The best part about it is that you can do it at home, on your own. The statements are broken down into four steps and are as follows:

Step 1: Repentance - "I'm sorry"
Repenting, or turning away from your sins, harmful beliefs and behaviors, or anything you believe has caused you or God sorrow or grief, is the first step to healing.

Step 2: Ask Forgiveness - "Please forgive me"
As a second step, forgive yourself and your body for the ways in which you (or your body) haven't performed in the way you expected of yourself. It is particularly important to forgive yourself (and your body) for all ways you have been mistreating yourself, as well as for anything you believe you've done (or failed to do) that has caused you unhappiness.

Step 3: Gratitude - "Thank you"
Then, thank yourself (and your body) for all that you do for yourself daily. Thank yourself for being the best you can be. Thank God for His love for you. Simply be thankful!

Step 4: Love - "I love you"
Tell yourself and your body, "I love you." Tell God and others that you love them, too! Say these things over and over and mean them!

When you put all the steps together into a full statement, it may look like this: "To whatever is going on within me that is causing me to experience this... I'm sorry, please forgive me, I love you, thank you!"

Doing this causes your body to release negative thoughts and emotions, and opens you up to complete healing.

The Power of Affirmations to Reprogram Your Brain

Speaking affirmations daily is another simple method for releasing emotional conflicts caused by trauma. Positive words help to reprogram your

KEY PRINCIPLE #7 | BEHAVIORAL EMOTIONAL SPIRITUAL THERAPY (BEST)

I CAN DO ALL THINGS

I am healthy, strong, and energetic, and I will fulfill the plans that God has for my life.

I am fully healed and restored, by the blood of Jesus Christ.

I have power over my mind, and I choose life-giving beliefs and thoughts.

I can do all things that I set my mind to accomplish daily.

All of my body's systems and organs are functioning together in perfect harmony.

I am worth loving. God loves me and I completely and fully love and accept myself.

I am safe, protected and provided for in every way.

I am thankful for the many gifts God gives me daily.

Every cell in my body is functioning according to God's original and perfect design.

I am joyful, peaceful and prosperous in every circumstance.

---

autonomic nervous system out of "fight or flight" mode and bring you into relaxation, or healing mode. They can also help you to uproot any lie-based thinking that may be encouraging disease in your body.

As I mentioned in Chapter 12, you may want to use words found in the Scriptures to do this, or if you prefer, another set of positive statements that resonate with you. Following is an example:

"I acknowledge and accept my feelings. There's nothing wrong with whatever I feel. There are no good or bad emotions. Even if I feel anger or hate, there is a reason for it. Every emotion comes directly from the integrity of my spirit."

When you have cancer, it's normal to have painful emotions, so I encourage you to feel and process those emotions. You want to do this so you can eventually release them, and so they don't stay stored in your body and harm you.

Secondly, forgiveness is an essential part of emotional healing, so consider whom you may need to forgive in your life, starting with yourself! Colossians 3:13 says, "Bear with each other and forgive one another if any of you has a grievance against someone. Forgive as the Lord forgave you." I also encourage you to forgive yourself by speaking the following statements daily:

"The supreme act of forgiveness is when I can forgive myself for all the wounds I have created in my life. Forgiveness is an act of self-love. When I begin to forgive myself, self-acceptance begins and self-love grows.

"I choose to let go of the grudge I have against (name of the person) and forgive them, and I release any judgments I have against them.

"Even though I am still very angry at (fill in the blank), I respect and love myself very much."

Following are more helpful affirmations to meditate on and/or speak. You may also want to create your own statements, using words that resonate with your spirit. (See "I Can Do All Things" on previous page.)

Fireside Chat/Guided Healing Visualization/Inner Healing Prayer

Other tools we sometimes use involve guided visualization techniques and inner healing prayer. For this, we invite our patients to close their eyes and visualize themselves as they were at the time of the traumatic event linked to the cancer, or when the conflict shock occurred.

We then ask them to visualize anyone else who was there at the time, and invite those people (person) to sit around an imaginary campfire, along with both the younger and older versions of the patient. Then, we ask them to invite a mentor or friend to sit down at the campfire with them. This should be someone they trust completely, like Jesus, or a close friend.

Next, we invite them to forgive anyone who was involved in the conflict shock or traumatic event, and then visualize their self as they are now, embracing the younger version of themselves. We then encourage them to speak words of comfort, love and reassurance over their younger self. In the meantime, their mentor is there for moral support.

KEY PRINCIPLE #7 | BEHAVIORAL EMOTIONAL SPIRITUAL THERAPY (BEST)

You can use a similar technique using prayer, and invite God or Jesus into any past situations or events that traumatized you. Once you are able to visualize yourself there, ask Him to share with you anything you need to know about the situation(s) that caused the emotional trauma. Also ask what lies you may have embraced as a result of the traumatic event, and what God wants you to know now that will heal your emotions. You might then ask Him to show you His perspective of the situation and the people involved in it.

As part of the visualization, you may see God embrace you, wipe your tears away, or even invite you to sit in His lap. While you can do this technique on your own, it is often best to invite a trusted minister who is experienced in inner healing prayer to pray and guide you through the process. Many churches have healing ministries that offer inner healing prayer, although I recommend working with someone who has been recommended by others and has a history of positive outcomes with their clients.

Testimonials of Recovery by Healing the Emotions

The effects of emotional healing in the recovery process can be profound. Many of our patients spontaneously heal, or see their recovery accelerated once they begin to deal with the emotional conflicts related to their cancers. Following are some stories of patients for whom emotional healing has made a dramatic difference in their recovery.

First, we once had a patient with cancer in her right breast. Many practitioners have found that whenever people have physical problems or symptoms on the right side of their body, it means that the emotional conflict associated with the symptom is related to a male in the person's life. When the problems are on the left side of the body, the problem is usually related to a female.

Therefore, the fact that this woman had cancer in her right breast suggested she had an issue with a male in her life. Shortly thereafter, I discovered that she was in a romantic relationship with the priest of a Catholic church. She grew up as a Catholic, so having such a relationship was "taboo" for her. It was not acceptable to the priest, either.

Well, the woman finally decided to obey her conscience and break up with him, and when she did, her breast tumor quickly disappeared!

Similarly, I had another patient with leukemia write a letter of forgiveness to his deceased father because his dad had belittled him throughout his upbringing. Shortly after he did that, and finally let go of all the trauma and hurt, the leukemia went away.

As another example, a man with prostate cancer, who was also a patient of a doctor friend of mine, was healed right while the doctor was examining him! My doctor friend had been doing a digital rectal exam and felt the man's prostate go from being enlarged to becoming normal sized, just as the patient was confessing and releasing an emotional conflict that was related to his cancer!

The doctor was amazed because the patient's prostate had shrunk back to a normal size, right as he was touching the area where the prostate was located. So he told the patient to come back in a week so he could do another ultrasound and PSA test and evaluate him again. When he did, everything was normal.

In Chapter 2, I introduced you to Donny, a former patient who had leukemia. Well, the emotional conflict behind leukemia is self-devaluation. If you'll recall, Donny's father had always told him that his brothers were better and stronger and smarter than him. He was always putting him down, and treating him as if he wasn't good enough.

Years later, while in his 20s, Donny developed leukemia. He had high white blood cell counts and did lots of chemotherapy. He finally came to Hope4Cancer after two years of chemotherapy treatment right after the doctors had told him that he would die within two weeks if he stopped the chemo. But he was dying anyway, so he stopped the treatment and decided to come see us.

I began to work with him to help him heal the emotional issues in his life, and to strengthen his spiritual life. I put him on a program involving high doses of pancreatic enzymes, and he ended up living another year, which was nothing short of miraculous.

KEY PRINCIPLE #7 | BEHAVIORAL EMOTIONAL SPIRITUAL THERAPY (BEST)

Though Donny didn't recover in the end (possibly because of the intense chemotherapy regimens that he did for so long), he was able to enjoy a good quality of life for much longer than his former doctor had anticipated, due to the healing work that we did together.

Finally, and perhaps most remarkably, a patient of mine in her 60s, who had been diagnosed with ovarian cancer, was dramatically healed after resolving a major trauma from her upbringing.

This woman had spent her younger years in France during World War II, and one day, when she was about 8 years old, some Nazi soldiers came to her house to arrest her father.

The father talked with the soldiers for a while before quietly departing the house with them, leaving the girl all alone. The girl never saw her dad again, so she became an orphan, and eventually ended up in the US with new caregivers.

Then, as an adult, she developed ovarian cancer. The main emotional conflict behind ovarian cancer has to do with loss combined with an accompanying "low blow" to the emotions. The girl had perceived her father as not loving her, rather than him negotiating his life for her freedom (which was most likely the case). So his leaving became the associated loss, and the fact that he left her without a fight was the "low blow" that devastated her. In the young girl's mind, her father had left willingly.

At the time of the event, she had thought, "My father doesn't care for me!" He didn't ask if I could go with him, and neither did he fight for me! I believe she developed cancer due to this conflict.

To help her heal, I did a guided visualization technique with her called the fireside chat. For this, I asked her to close her eyes and envision herself as that 8-year-old child again. I then invited both the adult and child versions of herself to sit around an imaginary campfire together, along with a mentor friend, who was there to support her.

I then asked her to invite her father to the campfire, as well. Then, I invited the 8-year-old girl to speak to her father from her "little girl" perspective, and forgive him. After that, I asked her to do the same thing as an adult.

Interestingly, while she was talking to her father as a child, she began to speak in French, which was her native language! Then, when I asked her to speak to her father as an adult, she began to speak to him in English. Afterward, I found out that she didn't actually remember French anymore—because when she moved to the States shortly after her father left, she no longer spoke French with anyone. So her knowledge of the language didn't come out again until she participated in the fireside chat with me.

During this process, she realized that her father hadn't left her because he didn't love her or put up a fight. Instead, he left because he actually loved her very much and wanted to save her, because he believed that if he left peacefully with the Nazis, he would spare his daughter's life.

As the woman forgave her father for apparently abandoning her in her childhood, she was able to release the trauma associated with the early life event, and was fully healed shortly thereafter.

Unfortunately, some people don't heal as quickly as she did, because they have secondary conflicts as well, which are also contributing to their cancers. Many people actually have multiple conflicts, all of which need to be resolved.

In addition, some people receive what are called "secondary gains" from being sick; meaning, they are getting some benefit out of having cancer. For instance, they may be receiving more attention from their husband or wife, or their kids or friends may be visiting them more often. This isn't usually a conscious thing, but it's important to discover so that it, too, can be resolved—if the patient is willing.

As I mentioned earlier, awareness is 75% of the healing process. So, one of the things we do is give our patients a six-page life history questionnaire to fill out. We ask them to make a chronology of their life, from the time of their birth up until the present. They write down all the conflicts and traumas they can remember from their lives; the hurts, divorces, deaths, abuses, and so on. Then we work on identifying and releasing them, especially those we believe are most strongly associated with their cancers.

Sometimes, our patients don't realize they have any emotional conflicts in their past or present that could be causing or contributing to their diseases. They may believe that they had a happy childhood, marriage, and so on, but I find that when we "dig," most often, conflicts arise.

Key Principle #7 | Behavioral Emotional Spiritual Therapy (BEST)

It's not always the severity of the conflict that matters, but what the patient felt as a result of that experience. (Remember, childhood limbic wounds don't necessarily have to be real, just perceived as real.)

To illustrate, I was once playing tag with my brother and another little boy while growing up in New Jersey. At one point, my younger brother was chasing the boy and I was running behind them both. I watched as they turned a corner and disappeared from my sight. A moment later, I heard a loud thumping noise and then a car coming to a screeching halt.

When I ran around the corner, I saw a child lying on the ground. There was blood everywhere, and people screaming. At first I thought it was my brother that had been struck by the car, but it was actually the little boy that my brother had been chasing. Tragically, the boy passed away. Of course, the event was very traumatic and devastating for both of us.

Fast forward to the present.

One day, while I was working in my clinic, I heard a car come to a screeching halt. My heart began to race, and I began to sweat as the trauma of the childhood event came rushing back to me. Nothing had happened to anyone, fortunately, but the car had come to a screeching halt, just like the one that had hit our friend when we were children. And because it was unprocessed trauma, I relived the event as if it were the first accident happening all over again.

If your "felt" experience of an event is severe, it can lead to cancer. If you are able to release the emotions behind the event, and/or the experience wasn't that impactful, it may instead lead to a cyst instead of a full-blown cancer. So it's important to process any emotions caused by events and get them healed.

Some Cancers and Their Associated Emotional Conflicts

If you'll recall, I mentioned how Dr. Hamer discovered that specific emotional conflicts lead to specific cancers. Here, I share seven of the most common cancers, and some core emotional conflicts that have been associated with each.

The correlations here were first described in Gilbert Renaud's book, *Recall Healing*, and are based largely upon Dr. Hamer's research and that of his disciple, French physician Claude Sabbah, MD, who also studied many thousands of cancer patients. However, many of the keywords included here are also a product of Dr. Renaud's work and research.

I have found these connections to correlate strongly with what I have observed in my cancer patients, as well. For more information on the emotional conflicts related to these and other types of cancer, see Dr. Renaud's book, *Recall Healing: Pyramid of Health*.

Liver Cancer

Lack and deprivation are the major themes behind liver cancer, especially being deprived of something considered vital for life, such as money, faith, food or respect. It can also be related to a fear of dying from a lack of something, such as food. Fear of financial deprivation and lack of respect are other themes. For example, you may want to research all situations in your life prior to your diagnosis in which you felt that someone disrespected you, or you disrespected yourself.

Lung Cancer

The core conflict behind lung cancer is the fear of death, fear of suffocation, or a visceral fear of something else. It can be related to fearing for loved ones that you want to "breathe for." Or, it is also related to the fear of not being able to find a way out of a bad situation, and/or feelings of insecurity and threat.

Finally, it can be caused by the conflict shock of the cancer diagnosis, which in itself is a deeply traumatic shock for many people.

Another theme, or keyword, to explore for lung cancer is "adaptation." Reflect upon situations in your life in which you may have had thoughts such as, *I can't take this anymore, I've had enough, I'm checking out*, or, *I can't adapt to this anymore*.

Breast Cancer

The conflicts surrounding breast cancer vary, depending on where the cancer is. In general, it has to do with conflicts related to the home,

KEY PRINCIPLE #7 | BEHAVIORAL EMOTIONAL SPIRITUAL THERAPY (BEST)

or the "nest," such as the relationship with one's spouse, children or other family members.

Adenocarcinomas, or cancers of the milk glands, have to do with drama in the home, such as the fear of something happening to one's children. For instance, it may have to do with fear of how a father's abusive or violent behavior is impacting the survival of the nest. Essentially, it is about conflicts involved in mothering.

Intraductal carcinomas, on the other hand, or cancers of the milk glands, have to do with a conflict of separation within the "nest," a lack of communication, or inability to convey one's love to another.

For both of these types of breast cancer, a key theme to explore is "inconceivable." For example, the drama at home may have seemed inconceivable to the wife/mother; nothing could have prepared her for it. She feels total emotional isolation deep within her soul at the moment of the drama, and feels as though she must resolve it on her own.

Lymph Node Metastases

The core conflict associated with lymph node metastases is self-devaluation and/or anxiety, and/or the fear of being attacked or not being able to defend oneself, along with the desire to seek protection.

Prostate Cancer

One core conflict behind prostate cancer is being unable to let go of something, and needing to control everything that is "vital" to the man. Other conflicts include: the man feeling as though he has violated the role of being the family guardian and protector; losing a family member; fear of his family descendants being at risk of harm; not feeling able to be the "man of the house"; lack of respect from one's partner, or violating norms of sexuality; self-reproach from sexual practices (such as extreme sexuality, conflicting sexuality, pornography, homosexuality); rape; and discomfort with one's sexuality.

Ovarian Cancer

The core conflict behind ovarian cancer is that of extreme loss, especially the loss of someone that was dearly loved by the person, such as a child or baby. The loss may have occurred through a miscarriage, abortion, stillbirth, or adoption.

Ovarian cancer is also often accompanied by a "low blow" to the emotions, and can also be about being abandoned, and then denigrated, reprimanded, or torn apart by someone of the opposite sex. Symbolically, the ovary represents the most feminine aspect of a woman, and it is therefore sensitive to being disrespected by a sexual partner.

Pancreatic Cancer

Core conflicts behind pancreatic cancer include: having a clash with a family member, struggling for "morsels" (emotional, financial or otherwise), or having a conflict related to one's inheritance. For instance, the person might think, *I was promised something, and I began to enjoy it before I even had it, but then it was given to someone else.*

Pancreatic cancer can also be about lack or a fear of lack, feeling disgraced or undeserving of material gain, and/or refusing to accept the gifts of life and abundance due to feeling unworthy of them.

Dr. Renaud has also found that it has to do with the conflict of having a double life, in some cases. For example, the person may have a wife and a lover at the same time, which creates an internal conflict in the person.

The word "pancreas" has different meanings but one of them is "by my father." Therefore, in all cases of pancreatic cancer, it is vital to explore the relationship between the client and his or her father. Dr. Renaud has found that there can be conflicts related to the client being named after the father, especially if there is a negative association between the client and his or her father, and the client wasn't recognized or acknowledged by the father.

Colon Cancer

Conflicts provoked by acts that are vile, base, ignoble, infamous, disgusting, or filthy are all associated with colon cancer. For instance, it may have to do with an inability to digest discord, or something "nasty" that can't be expelled, such as the "dirty tricks" or deceptive acts of another, or "soiling" conflicts.

The keyword or theme to explore for colon cancer is forgiveness. The person may struggle to forgive another because the conflict was so bad.

KEY PRINCIPLE #7 | BEHAVIORAL EMOTIONAL SPIRITUAL THERAPY (BEST)

Dr. Renaud notes that in many cases, the conflict is associated with the client's inability to let go of a dearly loved person who had passed away prior to his or her diagnosis. He also states that Dr. Masaru Emoto published a study in which he demonstrated that listening to the song, "Time to Say Goodbye," by Andrea Bocelli and Sarah Brightman, strongly supports the healing process of colon and rectal cancers.

Final Thoughts

Emotional and spiritual healing is vital for recovery. In my experience, nearly everyone with cancer has an emotional conflict that either caused their cancer or is contributing to it. To heal, these conflicts must be addressed and healed, through relationship with God, and by using one of the mind-body tools in this chapter, such as BEST, Recall Healing, Hoʻoponopono, affirmations and/or inner healing prayer with a trusted counselor or minister. By doing one or more of these, you will better position yourself to be more completely healed from cancer.

BEHAVIORAL EMOTIONAL SPIRITUAL THERAPY (BEST)

Tools for Emotional Healing	What It Is
Recall Healing	Identifying the "conflict shock(s)" or any sudden, severe past trauma that has led to cancer, and then "naming it, claiming it and dumping it" (the event).
Hoʻoponopono	Forgiving self through repeating the following affirmations: "I'm sorry, please forgive me, thank you."
Positive Affirmations	Speaking life-giving truths over yourself multiple times daily. Examples: "I am happy, healthy and whole," "I forgive myself and others for. . ." and "God loves me and is providing for all my needs."
Guided Healing Visualizations/Inner Healing Prayer	Visualizing past traumatic events and/or people related to past events, and then forgiving self and others through imagery and creative visualization. Inviting God into the memories to heal the memories.

SUMMARY

- The BEST program, or Behavioral Emotional Spiritual Therapy, involves analyzing patients' behaviors and personalities to tailor a healing program to their needs.
- Dr. Ryke Gerd Hamer has found that "conflict shocks" are unexpected, sudden and severe emotional conflicts that can trigger cancer. Specific emotional conflicts cause specific cancers.
- Healing the conflict shock is accomplished by identifying the specific emotional conflict that may have led to the cancer, owning it, and then releasing it. This resolves the issue more than half the time.
- Other tools for healing emotional conflicts include: counseling and ministry; reciting affirmations; forgiving those who have hurt you, including yourself; and doing inner healing prayer and/or guided imagery techniques with a qualified practitioner.

QUESTIONS FOR FURTHER REFLECTION

1. How do emotional conflicts or traumas cause cancer?
2. What is the BEST program?
3. What did Dr. Hamer discover about the relationship between emotions and cancer?
4. How can you discover what emotional conflict(s) may be causing or contributing to the cancer you battle?
5. Name three tools for healing emotional conflicts/traumas.

TRINA'S STORY

Trina is a holistic health and wellness expert who was diagnosed with ovarian cancer in 2008. She lives in Northern California with her husband, and has overcome many health battles, including Lyme disease, mold toxicity, heavy metal poisoning and cancer. Her story and teachings have been featured on The Truth About Cancer Docu-series and a number of on-line health summits. In her free time, she indulges in sweaty spin classes, five-mile beach walks with her two dogs, and dinners with the love of her life.

In 2008, my Ob-Gyn did a pelvic ultrasound on me, and without a second thought, diagnosed me with stage IV ovarian cancer—although I would later discover that it was really stage III.

When he gave me the news, I felt the room spin. I could hardly speak, and in my mind, I immediately saw a coffin. Even though this Ob-Gyn had been my doctor for years and was a really nice man, his bedside manner when he delivered the news was horrible.

He referred me to a gynecological oncologist, but I didn't go for quite some time. Intuitively, I felt like I should wait, and I'm glad that I did, because that's actually what saved my life later. (More on that in a moment.)

In the meantime, I called Dr. Tony at Hope4Cancer. I'm a holistic health practitioner and Dr. Tony and I had actually met years ago at a quantum biofeedback conference. Since then, and over the years, I had referred some of my clients with cancer to him and witnessed them having great results at his treatment centers. Because of this, I had always thought to myself, *If I ever got cancer, he'll be the first one I call.*

Dr. Tony advised me to get the tumor removed because it was the size of a melon, and to send him the pathology report. He then recommended some treatments to me.

Eventually, I also called the oncological Ob-Gyn and he recommended that I have surgery to remove my ovaries and uterus. He said that ovarian tumors don't usually get as big as mine. He also recommended chemotherapy, but I knew that there was no way I was going to do that. I had a 9-year-old son at home and I wasn't going to leave him without a mother.

I had the surgery, but the doctors kept pressing me to do chemotherapy, even though I had said "no" from the start. Three times, the oncologist called me a fool for not doing it!

I told him, "I'm working with a cancer doctor in Mexico; a doctor I have known for years and whom I really trust." I told him about Sono-Photo Dynamic Therapy and he didn't say anything.

I had surgery at a hospital in Santa Cruz, California, although I actually lived in Big Sur, California. Unfortunately, there was a wildfire near our house so we couldn't go home for five weeks following the surgery. During that time I stayed with my best friend and her husband. Eventually, I returned home and was able to check my answering machine messages. There was one from another oncologist, who informed me that I had an appointment to do chemotherapy the following day! I thought, *Wait a minute, I refused chemo!*

But they had set it up anyway! I called the doctor's office back and said, "I will not be doing chemotherapy."

Shortly thereafter, I began self-treating at home, and scheduled a visit to Hope4Cancer to consult with Dr. Tony.

He showed me how to do Sono-Photo Dynamic Therapy at home. In those days, Photodynamic Therapy consisted of rigging a bank of full-spectrum lights above the bed, which I could lower and raise via a pulley system. And Dr. Tony gave me instructions about how to make my own light bed!

So every night, I would lower the bed of lights from above, and treat myself for an hour after work. Then, I would go outside and do Sono-therapy in my outdoor tub, using an ultrasound device.

For both Sono- and Photodynamic Therapy, you first take a photosensitizing agent in the dark, and a couple of days later you expose yourself to full-spectrum lights and do an ultrasound treatment. The first time I laid down under the light bed it felt like millions of champagne bubbles were bursting through my body. It was a really pleasant feeling, and I actually enjoyed doing Photodynamic Therapy.

While my ovarian cancer was a stage III, it was a potentially highly aggressive cancer. I never researched it on purpose because I didn't want to buy into the medical community's paradigm and belief system about late-stage ovarian cancer.

Instead, I simply followed Hope4Cancer's home treatment program, and combined that with my own knowledge of holistic medical treatments. As part of that, I followed my own nutritional protocol, along with the Budwig diet. I did detoxification, quantum biofeedback and essential oil therapies, among others. I also did six injections of autologous urine therapy. Dr. Tony told me that I could expect a fever from the treatments, but I only had a short reaction after the first one, which lasted for about two minutes.

I did everything that Dr. Tony told me to do. I'm also very intuitive and I knew what support and treatments my body needed to recover.

As part of my work in helping people to recover their health, I specialize in resolving emotional conflicts that trigger cancer and other diseases. Incidentally, I discovered that my own conflict related to the ovarian cancer started when I was just 3 years old. At the time, I was abruptly taken away from my dad in the middle of the night, along with my siblings. Little did I know then, but I would not see my dad again for 43 years. This event registered on my brain, body and psyche as two conflicts: separation and loss.

In all the years that followed, I didn't know what the loss was consciously, but my brain had registered it as a trauma and it was manifesting in my ovary. And unbeknownst to me at the time, it was beginning to break down and would later develop into cancer.

Prior to being diagnosed with ovarian cancer, I also had Lyme disease. In German New Medicine, Lyme can be related to separation from one's family or clan, and ovarian cancer relates to the shock of a loss. Looking back, I realized that being taken away from my father had also triggered Lyme.

When I saw my dad for the first time, 43 years after our initial separation, he was "bleeding out" in a hospital in Florida and had asked me to come visit. So I did, and he ended up living. Shortly after I returned home, I got Lyme disease.

Ironically, in German New Medicine, when your psyche resolves the emotional conflict in your brain, that's when the disease usually manifests in your body. In other words, the presentation of the disease is actually thought to be your brain's way of recovering from the shock of the emotional conflict.

In my case, it was as if my brain had said, *The separation with your father is over, so let's go repair the body now.* That's when the Lyme-related microbes come in to do that. The doctors couldn't help me so I had to heal myself from Lyme. I used nutrition, homeopathy, detox and many other tools to get well.

Then, five years later, my family and I decided to go on a vacation to Florida, and I met with my Dad again for a few days while there. At that point, it was as if my brain said, *The conflict is over, you have your daddy back.* And then, *Let's send amino acids to that area of trauma in your brain that links to the ovary, and send the message to the ovary that it's time to heal.*

So incidentally, ovarian cancer was my body's way of telling me that it was time to heal from the loss. Conflict shocks heal in the brain first and then in the body.

I've tried to disprove that this is how the healing process works, but time and again, I've found German New Medicine to be "right on the money." I've seen many cancers mysteriously disappear with emotional healing alone, when it is combined with tools that support the body. That's one reason that I love Hope4Cancer, because the people are all about supporting, rather than killing the body through the healing process.

Fortunately, once I met my dad, my body registered the conflicts of loss and separation as being over, and I finally healed.

It's important to get to the root of traumas and the emotions that made you sick. By resolving these, you dig up the roots of the disease and you can then move on with your life.

In the end, I did natural cancer treatments for about a year. I was tested on a regular basis throughout my treatment. I did the CA 125, which is a test marker for ovarian cancer, along with PET scans. Over a short period of time, my CA 125 marker went down. I had only one scare throughout the process. The doctors found what looked like a tumor in my right pelvis where the ovary had been, but it was only a seroma, or a fluid-filled mass that had resulted from the surgery, and which was eventually reabsorbed back into my body.

I followed up with my doctors for a year or two after my surgery, but since then everything has been fine. Every scan has been clear.

I don't live in fear, because I know that the healing process is done. I also know what to do if I get sick again, so I'm at peace with things.

Now, I feel fantastic; better than ever, actually! I'm strong, healthy, and I have lots of energy. I don't ever think about cancer, whereas it once used to be the first thing that came into my mind in the morning.

At one time, I was so intensely scared, because the diagnosis was so overwhelming; it was as if my mortality was right in my face. But I never, ever researched the cancer because I didn't want to buy into what the conventional medical community had to say about it. To this day, I haven't researched the details of ovarian cancer, because I believe that fear can trigger the development of another cancer.

I listen to my intuition and that still, small voice within for guidance about all of my medical and life decisions, and I encourage anyone who is reading this to do the same. That intuition can be hard to find at first, but if you just keep reaching for it, it's there and it will tell you what to do. Sometimes, you'll have to go against the wishes of family, friends, and doctors, but if you listen to the voice within, you will find the answers that are right for you—and ultimately, the healing path that you are meant to be on.

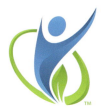

14

Putting It All Together

Healing from cancer isn't just about removing a tumor or cancer cells. It is about resolving the underlying factors that caused disease in the first place, and restoring your body, soul and spirit, using the 7 Key Principles of Cancer Therapy that I've shared with you throughout this book. When you do this, you can expect exponentially better outcomes in your recovery than if you had only taken chemotherapy drugs or underwent a surgery to remove a tumor.

Practicing the 7 Key Principles is empowering and even fun, once you integrate them into your lifestyle and they become a habit. The most important Key Principle is emotional and spiritual healing, which includes having a close relationship with God as the cornerstone and foundation.

The 7 Key Principles are also about doing the simple things: drinking pure water and breathing fresh air, as much as possible; consuming unadulterated food that resembles what our first ancestors ate; favoring vegetables and easily digestible foods; getting enough sleep; along with exercise, meditation, and prayer.

Don't cram too many activities into your days, but do those things that are essential and conducive to healing. Live according to the natural laws that God has created for your well-being. Awaken with the sun, and go to sleep earlier. Return to the simple life of our forefathers.

By following these recommendations, your immune system will become strong and balanced, and you will build up your body's foundation so it will respond more effectively to cancer treatments.

This is important, because cancer patients generally have a weakened vitality that has been highly affected by stress, financial crises, environmental toxins, vaccinations, alcohol, infections, electromagnetic fields, and nutrient-poor food, all of which have contributed to an already weakened terrain. All of these things not only lead to a greater risk and incidence of cancer, but also to a faster progression of the cancer, as well as metastatic disease.

Chemotherapy and radiation also further weaken the vitality of your body and lessen chances for long-term survival, especially when they are done as standalone therapies and your body isn't supported by the tools available through the 7 Key Principles of Cancer Therapy.

Therefore, the two most important things that you must do, before you even start any cancer treatments, is to raise your body's vitality and ability to respond to treatments using these tools. If you do that first, and then build upon that foundation, you will respond better and faster to any cancer treatments. All of the underlying causes of cancer must be removed before it can be eradicated.

Just as important, you'll want to address any "worriment" of the mind, as doctors used to call emotional conflicts in the olden days, because worry also weakens the nervous system, lowers cellular vitality and enables cancer to flourish. This involves healing any underlying emotional conflicts that are causing or contributing to the cancer.

I know it can be overwhelming to make a lot of changes at once, and to remember to do everything I've shared with you throughout this book. So, I'd like to make the process much simpler for you by creating an easy-to-follow roadmap of the tools I've presented. My hope is that this will allow you to more easily integrate them into a program—or healing "map"—that works for you.

A comprehensive healing plan incorporates all of the 7 Key Principles for wellness and includes:

1. Developing a relationship with God
2. Following the Garden Food Plan
3. Detoxifying your body of cancer-causing toxins
4. Communing with God's creation
5. Exercising
6. Oxygenating your body
7. Cultivating hobbies
8. Developing a social life
9. Discovering and living out your life's purpose
10. Doing anti-cancer treatments
11. Doing anti-microbial and immune-supportive therapies
12. Healing emotional conflicts and trauma

Many of the tools that I recommend cover multiple wellness areas. For instance, you can take a walk in the park and pray. As a result, not only will you be cultivating a relationship with God, but you'll be spending time in nature, oxygenating your body, and exercising, all at the same time.

Or, you might pray and meditate in your backyard, and find that as you are doing this, you are simultaneously receiving emotional healing from God, enjoying His creation, and getting cancer-fighting UV rays from the sun. These are just a couple of examples of how one healing tool can fulfill multiple purposes.

As you review the following tools, consider what areas of your life you need to spend more time developing. For instance, you may have a great prayer life but perhaps you haven't been diligent about exercising or spending time with friends. Or maybe you exercise, but have neglected your emotional health or relationship with God. Or maybe you need to spend a few hours every week detoxifying your body, or making healthy meals.

Don't get discouraged if you can't do everything at once, or even do it all perfectly. Perfectionism causes stress, so simply do the best you can. If you work outside of the home, you may need to do most of your therapies at night or early in the morning, before you leave for work.

If you are able, though, I encourage you to take 30 minutes during the middle of the day, perhaps during a lunch break, to get outside in nature, exercise and spend time in God's creation. We were made for the outdoors, so it's really important to do this, if you can. If you can't take a lunch break, try spending some time outdoors either before or after work.

To help you create your own roadmap, I suggest purchasing a large, laminated jumbo wall calendar or magnetic dry erase calendar, where you can post your daily activities and therapies. You may also want to purchase a separate one for your refrigerator to write down your shopping and supplement lists, and daily menus.

Finally, you'll notice that I recommend doing certain therapies or activities daily (such as following the Garden Food Plan), while others I recommend less often—anywhere from once per week to 3-5 times per week.

In addition, I recommend doing a liver-gallbladder cleanse once every few months, and a parasite cleanse once every 6-12 months. I recommend the Blessed Herbs parasite cleanses.

Other periodic therapies to consider include bodywork treatments such as acupuncture and massage.

Summary of Tools for Creating Your Own At-Home Healing Program

Following is a summary of the tools and therapies that I've shared with you throughout this book. While there are 11 categories here, all are encompassed within the 7 Key Principles of Cancer Therapy.

Choose activities or tools from each one of these category lists to do daily, multiple times per week or weekly, depending on your time, energy, degree of illness, and lifestyle commitments. Certain things, like the Garden Food Plan and spending time with God, you will want to do daily, while other things, like spending time with friends, may depend on your schedule, energy and other factors.

I recommend going through each category list and writing down those activities and tools that you know are most beneficial and feasible for you to do. Then jot those activities down on your jumbo calendar, until they become second nature to you and you no longer have to remember to do them.

Compliance is key to success and gives you the satisfaction of accomplishment and having achieved something.

In addition, if you have active cancer, I recommend that you contact a holistic-minded practitioner or Hope4Cancer to guide you in these therapies and activities.

For example, I generally recommend doing coffee enemas three times per week. You may need to do them more often if you have advanced disease; for instance, with stage III or IV cancer, or less often if you don't have much free time or are well on your way to recovery.

So you might write "coffee enema" on the Monday, Wednesday and Friday squares of your calendar, so that you remember to do it three times weekly.

Do the same with the other therapies and activities listed here.

#1 - Develop a Relationship with God

Choose one or more of the following to do daily:

1. Pray and/or do a Bible study.
2. Meditate on healing Scriptures, and then speak them aloud over yourself.
3. Listen to praise and worship music, while "soaking" in the presence of God.
4. Listen to a Bible teaching on YouTube, TV or via podcast.
5. Ask God to speak to you, and then journal His responses to you.
6. Pray about your life's purpose, and then journal whatever impressions God may give you (e.g., ideas, thoughts or revelations).
7. Pray on the phone with a friend.

#2 - Follow the Garden Food Plan

Aim to follow all of these principles daily when preparing your meals:

1. Drink fresh, clean water, preferably hydrogen-enriched water.
2. Consume ample amounts of fresh vegetables at lunch and dinner, and if possible, at breakfast, as well.

3. Enjoy fresh fruits with your meals, but make sure to eat more vegetables than fruits.
4. Have some healthy fat daily, in the form of pasture-raised butter, cold-pressed extra virgin olive oil, or avocado or coconut oil, and nuts (except for peanuts and cashews).
5. Enjoy a plant-based pea protein powder drink (GFP Nutritional) to ensure you are getting enough protein in your diet.
6. Include small to moderate amounts of healthy animal protein in your diet, such as pasture-raised chicken or wild-caught fish, if you require animal protein.
7. Make sure that all of your food is non-GMO, organic, natural, and free of artificial additives, preservatives and man-made sugars. Natural food comes directly from the ground, a tree, plant, bush or the sea!

#3 - Detoxify Your Body of Cancer-Causing Toxins

For this category, pull out your dry erase calendar and write down the specific activities that you will do each day. By the way, most of these are very relaxing, so consider them to be great "downtime" activities!

1. Coffee enema (at least 3x weekly if you are battling an advanced cancer).
2. Lymphatic drainage, using a vibrating platform, rebounder, Chi machine, or other device (at least 4-5x weekly).
3. Near-infrared sauna therapy (2-3x weekly).
4. Take toxin binders, such as zeolite, bentonite clay or activated charcoal, if applicable (daily).
5. Walk or do another form of exercise (4-5x per week, or as you are able).
6. Epsom salt baths before bedtime (using 1 pound of salt in warm water). Rub your skin vigorously to remove any grease and open up your pores)!
7. Juice vegetables, along with a little fruit, to cleanse your blood, lymphatic system and cellular matrix (5-6x weekly).
8. Clean up your home and replace all toxic chemical household products with non-toxic, natural ones (periodically).

#4 - Spend Time in God's Creation

As with #3, for this category write down the specific activities that you will pursue throughout the week.

1. Hug a tree, spend time in a garden, or pick fruit.
2. Take a walk in nature, on the beach, at a park, or in your neighborhood.
3. Go swimming in non-chemically treated water, such as in the ocean, a clean lake, or in pools treated with ozone or UV light.
4. Attend an outdoor sporting event.
5. Read a book on a park bench or in your backyard, or simply lounge in the sun in your yard.
6. Walk to the grocery store or to a local shop nearby.
7. Attend your local farmer's market.

#5 - Exercise

I encourage you to exercise outdoors, whenever possible, since you can cover several health bases this way: oxygenation, exercise, grounding and spending time in God's creation! Write down your preferred exercise(s) on your calendar, and aim to do them 4-5x weekly.

1. Take a walk.
2. Practice a mind-body exercise such as Qigong or yoga, at a park or in your backyard.
3. Go for a swim.
4. Take a Pilates or aerobics class.
5. Do some stretches or light weight lifting.
6. If you are weak, bedridden or can't tolerate much physical exercise, try moving your limbs from a seated or lying down position on your bed or a chair. Bounce your legs on a rebounder, or have your caretaker move your arms and legs.

#6 - Oxygenate Your Body

Again, you will find that there is a lot of overlap in this section with the former two categories. Whenever you exercise and spend time in God's creation while practicing proper breathing, you cover three wellness areas all at once!

However, if you are unable to exercise or go outside much, you can still oxygenate your body by practicing proper breathing and doing other activities.

1. Do some form of aerobic exercise, or mind-body exercise outdoors such as yoga or Qigong, while practicing proper breathing with your mouth closed.
2. Practice therapeutic breathing throughout the day, no matter what you are doing. Again, the key here is to keep your mouth closed, and allow your breaths to be soft and gentle.
3. Blow into balloons; try EWOT or another novel breathing activity.
4. Make sure that you are breathing properly at night by doing a sleep apnea test. If the results show you have apnea, work with your doctor to remedy it using a CPAP or other device.
5. Consume lots of live green foods, which contain high amounts of oxygen.

#7 & 8 - Cultivate a Hobby and Develop a Healthy Social Life

I recommend getting together with friends, family or other loved ones at least once a week; ideally, do a fun activity outside of the house, if you can. As well, I encourage you to spend time doing a hobby at least once a week, as your time and schedule allow. Some examples of activities that you might pursue include:

1. Going out for a meal or a movie with a friend or family member.
2. Joining a club, Bible study or other group that meets on a regular basis, anywhere from weekly to monthly.
3. Finding something that you enjoy doing at home, such as art, reading, puzzles, gardening, woodworking, volunteering for an organization, or praying for others.

4. If you are too tired to do much, consider what activities you can do from home that will uplift you, such as watching an uplifting movie or comedy show, or reconnecting via phone with old friends or acquaintances on Facebook.

#9 - Discover and Live Out Your Life's Purpose

This may be one category for which it isn't essential to do something additional daily, or even weekly. But I encourage you to periodically spend time thinking, praying about, and/or taking the next steps to further the projects, purpose, and/or calling that God has placed upon your heart. Doing this will send a message to your brain and body that you have great purpose in your life, and that you need to heal so you can fulfill that purpose.

#10 & 11 - Do Anti-Cancer, Anti-Microbial and Immune Supportive Treatments

Most likely, you will need to do some of your doctor's recommended treatments daily, and others, only three-five times weekly (such as ozone therapy). Again, you may want to pull out your calendar for this one and write down those treatments that you need to remind yourself to do, such as ozone, Sono and Photodynamic Therapy, and hyperbaric oxygen.

If you have trouble remembering to take your supplements, you may also want to create a separate calendar or agenda where you can write down the supplements you need to take daily, and when. Post the calendar or list in your kitchen or bathroom, beside your bed, or wherever you go to take your supplements.

Here's an example of what your supplement list could look like:

You may also want to purchase a pill storage box and/or some large plastic bins to store your supplements in, to better organize them and keep them all together. For example, you may find it handy to have a storage bin labeled "morning" and another labeled "evening" for those time-specific supplements. And then perhaps a third bin for those that you take at mealtimes, or on an empty stomach, between meals.

1. Take all recommended supplements (daily).
2. Do ozone therapy (3-4x per week).
3. Do Sono-Photo Dynamic Therapy (daily, in the morning or evening).
4. Do hyperbaric treatments (if possible, 3x per week).
5. Other prescribed therapies (e.g., IV Vitamin C, etc.).

#12 - Discover and Heal Emotional Conflicts/Traumas

1. Ask God to show you any harmful beliefs, thoughts or behaviors that He may want to heal in you, and then ask Him to help you replace those with His life-giving truths.
2. Work with a counselor or inner healing minister to help identify and resolve any emotional trauma.
3. Do BEST and/or Recall Healing with a trained practitioner to resolve any emotional "conflict shocks" directly related to the cancer you have.
4. Practice speaking affirmations over yourself daily, and/or meditate on Scriptures that speak about how God sees you.
5. Forgive yourself, God and others, as often as necessary!

Sample Wellness Day

Following is a short example of what your sample wellness day could look like, utilizing the 7 Key Principles. Again, this is just to give you more food for thought about how you might create your own schedule. Also, please note, the following schedule doesn't include supplements, so remember to take them throughout the day, as well!

Upon arising

- Pray, journal, meditate, spend time with God. Give Him thanks for being alive!
- Drink a glass of hydrogen water with lemon
- Do a coffee enema
- Do rectal or vaginal ozone therapy (15 minutes)

Breakfast

- Have a green smoothie. For this, mix all of the following in a blender:
  - 1 scoop of plant (pea) protein powder (GFP Nutrition)
  - 1 scoop of Vita LF Powder
  - 1 apple (or other fruit)
  - 1 carrot
  - 1 celery stalk
  - ½ avocado
  - ½-1 cup of kale and/or spinach
  - Add 8-12 ounces of water, and stevia or another natural sweetener like monk fruit for taste, if desired.
- Drink some decaffeinated green or turmeric tea, or lemon water
- Have two pasture-raised eggs and sautéed spinach, if you need some animal protein

Mid-morning

- Take a 30-60 minute walk in the park, your neighborhood or on the beach; garden, or read an uplifting book while sitting on your front porch. Benefits from this include exercise, oxygen, sun, grounding yourself to the Earth's healing energy, and spending time in nature. (Alternatively, you could do this in the evening, after your day's work).

Lunch

- Have a green salad. For this, combine in a medium-sized bowl:

    1 cup mixed greens
    ½ cup small, chopped artichoke hearts
    ¼ cup green or black olives
    ½ medium-sized tomato
    ½ cucumber
    ¼ cup pine nuts

- Steam ½ cup boiled or steamed Basmati rice and, if you desire, ½ cup cooked beans for additional protein
- Drink some hydrogen-enriched water and/or green or turmeric tea

Mid-afternoon or before dinner

- Rebound, use a vibrating platform or a Chi machine for lymphatic drainage (10-15 minutes)
- Do Sonodynamic Therapy

Evening

- Visit with a friend for an hour or two, on a landline or cell phone in speaker mode, or in person at a coffee shop or restaurant
- Epsom salt bath

Dr. Tony's Daily Health Habits

I like to practice what I preach, so many of the recommendations that I give to my patients for their healing, I also incorporate into my own life. The fact is, they are beneficial not just for treating cancer, but also for maintaining health. So the following is what a typical day looks like for me!

I hope that by reading this you will get an even better idea about how to formulate your own program. At the same time, realize that healing and maintaining health is a lifestyle change; it's not a one-time event that you do to overcome cancer. Once you start implementing the 7 Key Principles, however, you are likely to find that they will become a normal part of your life. I also believe they will be enjoyable as they impart life, energy, happiness and well-being to you.

Upon awakening, the first thing I do is pray and thank God for another day and the blessings that I know will happen as the day unfolds.

Then, I take my immune-boosting supplements, and have a powerful protein breakfast, which may consist of two hard-boiled or scrambled eggs and an avocado, or spinach. I like to squeeze a bit of lime, or add salt and pepper to my eggs, and I cook my eggs in raw butter or extra virgin cold-pressed olive oil, for a well-balanced meal.

Alternatively, I might make a protein smoothie using GFP Nutritional, which provides a broad range of nutrients to my body. If you have an advanced cancer, I recommend choosing a plant-based protein breakfast over animal protein from eggs, and including lots of healthy veggies and perhaps a little fruit and some coconut oil in your smoothies.

After breakfast, I will do some form of oxygen therapy. I like to either walk around my neighborhood, or do a hyperbaric oxygen treatment. Whenever I walk, I practice proper breathing as I go. In addition, I spend as much time as I can in the sun.

For lunch, I usually have an organic spinach and mixed greens salad, topped with two tablespoons of olive oil, a tablespoon of balsamic vinaigrette, and pink Himalayan salt. Along with that, I will have a baked or grilled wild-caught salmon fillet. Alternatively, I may swap my salad for some lightly steamed broccoli or asparagus, topped with butter. Add to that a glass of hydrogen-enriched water.

I try to have either a salad or cooked vegetables for both lunch and dinner. Usually, if I have a salad for lunch, I will have steamed vegetables for dinner, and vice versa.

For a tasty, power-packed snack, I make chia pudding, which involves mixing together a cup of coconut milk and four tablespoons of chia seeds, and allowing the mixture to sit for 20 minutes. I then add 30 grams of raw pecans, 28 grams of berries, and five drops of liquid stevia or a dash of monk fruit to the pudding. It is delicious!

Saturday is a "freer" day for me, and I might have a treat on that day; a bit of dark chocolate (70% or more cacao is best), or a healthy comfort food like a fruit smoothie. I encourage you to have a treat once a week, as well. Just don't go overboard and eat things like man-made sugars and processed foods, which are a no-no at all times. Instead, have a fruit smoothie, chia pudding, or coconut ice cream that has been flavored with stevia, erythritol or monk fruit—or another sugarless dessert made with all-natural ingredients.

On Sundays, I often fast and will drink only vegetable juice. Fasting has both spiritual and physical benefits. If you are physically able, you may want to consider doing this, too.

In addition, I do some of the same therapies as my patients, for health maintenance and for disease prevention, because we are all forming cancer cells in our bodies daily and are exposed to a lot of stress and environmental toxins.

For example, I do hyperbaric therapy periodically; sauna therapy twice weekly, a vibrating platform for lymphatic drainage, and occasionally, coffee enemas as I have time. I also do Photodynamic Therapy daily with the laser watch. While I don't have cancer, I like to wear the laser watch because it has many health benefits in addition to anti-cancer properties. For instance, it increases mitochondrial function and ATP production, and reduces inflammation.

I also like to use essential oils, which have powerful healing properties. My favorite is Bergamot, which is a good tranquilizer and mood stabilizer. I take lots of supplements as well, since our food supply no longer contains all of the nutrients we need to maintain optimal health.

Some of my favorite supplements include: liposomal Vitamin D, propolis and the other nutrients involved in the Sunivera protocol; basically, the same supplements that we recommend to our patients. Again, I take these for their multitude of health benefits, and to keep my immune system strong. I also take omega essential fatty acids from fish oil, which is an antioxidant.

Finally, I take time out to do enjoyable activities every week with my family, when I'm not at a medical conference. Spending time with my family is gratifying for me, as is reading. I was an athlete growing up, so I enjoy watching sports on television. On Sundays, I attend a non-denominational Christian church, which helps me to connect with God and remain centered in Him.

You need to have joy in your life and in what you do. Sadly, all too often, people don't enjoy their jobs and day-to-day lives. If this describes you, ask God what He may want to change in your life, and to help you do it, so that you can do and be all that He, and you, want you to be!

When you are walking in His perfect will, you will experience fulfillment and joy in all that you do.

Be Encouraged!

There is much hope for your recovery when you follow the 7 Key Principles of Cancer Therapy that are outlined in this book, especially when you stay connected to God and simply believe!

We have seen many healing miracles and full recoveries at our treatment centers, as well as cancers that have remained stable over many years. For even those patients that aren't healed, our non-toxic treatment approach has often allowed them to live fuller and more active lives, for much longer than what they otherwise would have.

At Hope4Cancer, we believe that with God, all things are possible (Matthew 19:26), because we have seen and witnessed it, time and again.

May you have the courage to believe that all things are possible for you too, as you seek God's face, take His hand, and allow Him to lead you on His perfect divine path of redemption, healing and restoration.

Peace, grace and love to you, in the name of Jesus Christ.

Antonio Jimenez, MD, ND
Chief Medical Officer and Founder
Hope4Cancer Treatment Centers

S. D. G.

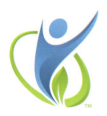

AFTERWORD

Words from a Friend and Colleague

I have had the wonderful pleasure of knowing Dr. Jimenez for more than 20 years, and I can honestly call him one of my very best friends. In fact, we refer to each other as brothers.

I've had the honor and privilege of traveling with Dr. Jimenez to several countries, participating in medical conferences with him, and co-attending many meetings. We have conducted research together and published scientific and clinical studies in medical journals.

I've also visited his cancer treatment centers dozens of times, met many of his patients, and I have a close friendship with his wife, Marcy, and all of his children.

During my visits, I've seen firsthand Dr. Jimenez's incredible bedside manner, his determination for excellent care and dedication to his patients. I've witnessed his multitude of treatment modalities and seen many positive outcomes with different types of cancer.

Dr. Jimenez described his approaches to treat cancer that emphasize natural, non-harmful therapies way back when I first met him, and he continues to improve them to this day. He also continues to travel the world to find new methods to build on his holistic arsenal.

I must sincerely tell you that the principles portrayed in this book are real. What's more, they are tried, proven, and beneficial applications, based on what I've witnessed in Dr. Jimenez's treatment centers. As mentioned in these pages, he focuses on doing what cancer cells *don't* like and administering what normal cells of the body *do* like—and that's a great recipe for recovery.

Hope for Cancer effectively elaborates the need to utilize natural and integrative means to treat cancer by incorporating the 7 Principles: using non-toxic cancer therapies; boosting the immune system; good nutrition; detoxification; oxygenation; restoration of the microbiome; spiritual and emotional healing. As well, these pages reveal a myriad of key diagnostic tests which provide clues and evidence on where and to what extent cancers occur.

Dr. Jimenez gives a marvelous exposé on the importance of a strong belief in God in the healing process. He masterfully unfolds Bible passages that give many examples, analogies and representations in relation to his cancer treatments and recovery. Dr. Jimenez's belief in the Lord's Word reveals his conviction in one of the most important treatment modalities Hope4Cancer Treatment Centers can offer its patients: Faith.

The book's premise is much like the conductor of a magnificent symphony leading musicians to orchestrate harmony and balance that results in a masterpiece of beautiful music. As the experienced practitioner ("the conductor"), Hope4Cancer Treatment Centers masterfully assembles special therapies along with their impeccable staff (the "orchestra"), which results in healing and harmony that improves one's quality of life ("the masterpiece").

Bob Settineri, MS
Founder and President, Sierra Productions
Biomedical Communications and Research

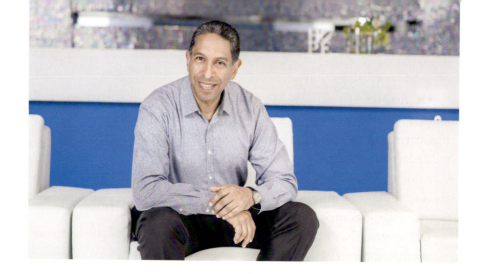

ABOUT THE AUTHOR

DR. ANTONIO JIMENEZ, MD, ND, is the Founder and Chief Medical Officer of the Hope4Cancer Treatment Centers—a world leader at the frontier of integrative oncology—with locations in Tijuana and Cancun, Mexico. Established in 2000, the Tijuana center is a certified inpatient Hospital and the Cancun center, founded in 2015, serves outpatients at one of the premier medical tourism destinations in the world. For more than 25 years, Dr. Jimenez has dedicated his life to the study, clinical research, and implementation of non-toxic and integrative strategies to treat cancer, chronic infections, and immune disorders. Today, he is one of the most trusted voices in the world of integrative cancer therapy.

Dr. Jimenez received his MD at the Autonomous University of Guadalajara Faculty of Medicine in Mexico, and ND from the Trinity School of Natural Health, Indiana, USA. In addition to Mexico, he also has a medical license in Spain. His 7 Key Principles of Cancer Therapy™ has formed the basis for his comprehensive, integrative protocols that include tumor-selective treatments such as Sono-Photo Dynamic Therapy and several biological immunotherapies. With his diverse toolbox of non-toxic therapies, he targets both the cancer and the biological terrain that causes it and feeds its growth. These clinically applied principles are consistent with scientific concepts developed in later years such as the 10 (Biological) Hallmarks of Cancer and the 4 Physical Traits of Cancer.

About the Author

Dr. Jimenez is an avid educator who has shared his wisdom with large audiences across the world. He has traveled to more than 70 countries learning, training and researching new approaches to treat cancer. In 2020, Dr. Jimenez launched a free webinar series through which he educates global audiences on wide-ranging topics on healing at all three levels—the body, the mind, and the spirit. He actively educates his medical staff that includes over 25 MD physicians.

Dr. Jimenez has been featured in numerous online symposiums, docuseries, interviews, and online featured documentaries. He was honored by the Truth About Cancer organization with a Lifetime Achievement Award in 2016 and featured in their 2016 and 2017 Live Symposiums. He was a featured participant/traveling medical expert in their docuseries *Quest for the Cures: Final Chapter* (2021), *Eastern Medicine – Journey Through Asia* (2019), *The Truth About Cancer: A Global Quest* (2015) and *The Quest for the Cures ... Continues* (2014). He was honored as an invited speaker for the last several years at celebrity Fran Drescher's Cancer Schmancer Health Summit events, and also featured on the Ask Dr. Nandi show. His work has been published in several peer-reviewed articles.

Dr. Jimenez is a Diplomat of the Canadian Society for Bioregulatory Medicine, a Founding Member of the North American Academy of Neural Therapy, and the International Scientific Advisor for Burg Apotheke (Germany). Dr. Jimenez is a member of numerous associations including the American Academy of Anti-Aging Medicine (A4M), the International Photodynamic Association (IPA), the Society of Immunotherapy for Cancer (SITC), the American College for the Advancement of Medicine (ACAM), the International Organization of Integrative Cancer Physicians (IOICP), The Androgen Society, The International Society of Medical Laser Applications (ISLA), the California Naturopathic Association (CNA), the International Iridology Practitioners Association (IIPA), and the Society of Progressive Medical Education (SOPMed). He is also an Honorary Member of the Portuguese Society of Integrative Medicine.

To learn more about Dr. Antonio Jimenez or the Hope4Cancer Treatment Centers, go to http://www.hope4cancer.com.

ENDNOTES

Preface
1. James JA. New, evidence-based estimate of patient harms associated with hospital care. *J. Patient Saf.* 2013;9(3): 122–128. doi: 10.1097/PTS.0b013e3182948a69.

Chapter 1
1. Morgan G, Ward R, Barton M. The contribution of cytotoxic chemotherapy to five year survival in adult malignancies. *J Clin Oncol.* 2004;16:549–560.
2. Byrd RC. Positive therapeutic effects of intercessory prayer in a coronary care unit population. *South Med J.* 1988;81(7):826–829. doi:10.1097/00007611-198807000-00005.
3. 1) Dantzer R, Kelley KW. Stress and immunity: an integrated view of relationships between the brain and the immune system. *Life Sci* 1989;44:1995-2008.
2) Kiecolt-Glaser JK, McGuire L, Robles TF, Glaser R. Emotions, morbidity, and mortality: new perspectives from psychoneuroimmunology. *Annu Rev Psychol* 2002;53:83-107.
3) Bauer SM. Psychoneuroimmunology and cancer: an integrated review. *J Adv Nurs* 1994;19:1114-20.
4. Yang M, Brackenbury WJ. Membrane potential and cancer progression. *Front Physiol* 2013;4:185.
5. 1) Stossel R. Water and positive thoughts increase the life-giving properties of this vital resource. *NaturalNews.com.* June 4, 2011. https://www.naturalnews.com/032604_water_structure.html. Accessed January 15, 2018.
2) Adams, M. Dr. Emoto requests assistance for Japan in the form of prayer and positive intentions. *NaturalNews.com,* March 31, 2011. https://www.naturalnews.com/031908_prayer_Japan.html. Accessed January 15, 2018.

Chapter 2
1. Hanahan D, Weinberg RA. Hallmarks of cancer: the next generation. *Cell.* 2011;144(5):646–674. doi: 10.1016/j.cell.2011.02.013.
2. Ben-Jacob E, Coffey DS, Levine, H. Bacterial survival strategies suggest rethinking cancer cooperativity. *Trends Microbiol.* 2012;20:403–410.
3. Ambrose J, Livitz M, Wessels D, Kuhl S, Lusche DF, Scherer A et al. Mediated coalescence: a possible mechanism for tumor cellular heterogeneity. *Am J Cancer Res.* 2015:5:3485–3504.
4. Melo SS, Sugimoto H, O'Connell JT, Kato N, Villanueva A Vidal A, et al. Cancer exosomes perform cell-independent microRNA biogenesis and promote tumorigenesis. *Cancer Cell.* 2014;6:707–721.
5. Nak KS, Bo YK. Psychological stress and cancer. *J Anal Sci Technol.* 2015;6(1):1. https://doi.org/10.1186/s40543-015-0070-5.
6. 232 toxic chemicals found in 10 babies. Ewg.org. July 14, 2005. https://www.ewg.org/research/body-burden-pollution-newborns#.W1J0hNhKiu4. Accessed October 3. 2018.
7. US Department of Health and Human Services. National Institutes of Health. National Cancer Institute. National Institute of Environmental Health Sciences. Cancer and the environment. what you need to know. what you can do. August 2003. https://Www.niehs.nih.gov/health/materials/cancer_and_the_environment_508.pdf. Accessed June 15, 2018.
8. Westfall S. Environmental toxins and cancer risk. *Life Extension Magazine.* February 2016.
9. Shoemaker R. *Mold Warriors.* 1st ed. Baltimore, MD: Gateway Press; 2005.

10. Wild CP, Gong YY. Mycotoxins and human disease: a largely ignored global health issue. *Carcinogenesis.* 2010;31(1):71–82.
11. Magnussen A, Parsi MA. Aflatoxins, hepatocellular carcinoma and public health. *World J Gastro.* 2013;19(10):1508–1512.
12. 1) Singh R, Gautam N, Mishra A, Gupta R. Heavy metals and living systems: an overview. *Indian J Pharmacol.* 2011;43(3):246–253.
    2) Murgueytio AM, Evans RG, Roberts D. Relationship between soil and dust lead in a lead mining area and blood lead levels. *J Expo Anal Environ Epidemiol.* 1998;8(2):173–186.
    3) Selevan SG, Landrigan PJ, Stern FB, Jones JH. Mortality of lead smelter workers. *Am J Epidemiol.* 1985;122(4):673–683.
    4) Edwards VC, Coppock RW, Zinn LL. Toxicoses related to the petroleum industry. *Vet Hum Toxicol.* 1979;21(5):328–337.
    5) Romaniuk A, Lyndin M, Sikora V, Lyndina Y, Romaniuk S, Sikora K. Heavy metals effect on breast cancer progression. *J Occup Med Toxicol.* 2017;12:32. doi: 10.1186/s12995-017-0178-1. eCollection 2017.
13. Aktar MW, Sengupta D, Chowdhury A. Impact of pesticides use in agriculture: their benefits and hazards. *Interdiscip Toxicol.* 2009;2(1):1–12.
14. 1) Belpomme D, Irigaray P, Hardell L, Clapp R, Montagnier L, Epstein S et al. The multitude and diversity of environmental carcinogens. *Environ Res.* 2007;105(3):414–429.
    2) Hung LJ, Chan TF, Wu CH, Chiu HF, Yang CY. Traffic air pollution and risk of death from ovarian cancer in Taiwan: fine particulate matter (PM2.5) as a proxy marker. *J Toxicol Environ Health A.* 2012;75(3):174–182.
15. 1) Schecter A, Startin J, Wright C, Kelly M, Päpke O, Lis A et al. Dioxins in U.S. food and estimated daily intake. *Chemosphere.* 1994;29(9–11):2261–2265.
    2) Rauscher-Gabernig E, Mischek D, Moche W, Prean M. Dietary intake of dioxins, furans and dioxin-like PCBs in Austria. *Food Addit Contam Part A Chem Anal Control Expo Risk Assess.* 2013;30(10):1770-9.
16. Dingley KH, Ubick EA, Chiarappa-Zucca ML, Nowell S, Abel S, Ebeler SE et al. Effect of dietary constituents with chemopreventive potential on adduct formation of a low dose of the heterocyclic amines PhIP and IQ and phase II hepatic enzymes. *Nutr Cancer.* 2003;46(2):212–221.
17. Ananthaswamy HN, Pierceall, WE. Molecular mechanisms of ultraviolet radiation carcinogenesis. *Photochem Photobiol.* 1990;52(6):1119–1136
18. 1) Gandhi G, Kaur G, Nisar U. A cross-sectional case control study on genetic damage in individuals residing in the vicinity of a mobile phone base station. *Electromagn Biol Med.* 2014;9:1–11.
    2) Hou Q, Wang M, Wu S, Ma X, An G, Liu H et al. Oxidative changes and apoptosis induced by 1800-MHz electromagnetic radiation in NIH/3T3 cells. *Electromagn Biol Med.* 2015;34(1):85–92.
    3) Liu C, Duan W, Xu S, Chen C, He M, Zhang L et al. Exposure to 1800 MHz radiofrequency electromagnetic radiation induces oxidative DNA base damage in a mouse spermatocyte-derived cell line. *Toxicol Lett.* 2013;218(1):2–9.
    4) Liu C, Gao P, Xu SC, Wang Y, Chen CH, He MD et al. Mobile phone radiation induces mode-dependent DNA damage in a mouse spermatocyte-derived cell line: a protective role of melatonin. *Int J Radiat Biol.* 2013;89(11):993–1001.
    5) Volkow ND, Tomasi D, Wang GJ, Vaska P, Fowler JS, Telang F et al. Effects of cell phone radiofrequency signal exposure on brain glucose metabolism. *JAMA.* 2011;305(8):808–813.
    6) Hardell L, Carlberg M, Hansson Mild K. Pooled analysis of two case-control studies on the use of cellular and cordless telephones and the risk of benign brain tumours diagnosed during 1997–2003. *Int J Oncol.* 2006;28(2):509–518. doi: 10.1186/2052-336X-12-15.

19. Mihai CT, Rotinberg P, Brinza F, Vochita G. Extremely low-frequency electromagnetic fields cause DNA strand breaks in normal cells. *J Environ Health Sci Eng*. 2014;12:15. doi: 10.1186/2052-336X-12-15.
20. Yakymenko I, Sidorik E. Risks of carcinogenesis from electromagnetic radiation of mobile telephony devices. *Exp Oncol*. 2010;32(2):54–60.
21. Environmental Toxins and Cancer Risk. *Life Extension Magazine*. February 2016. Accessed on December 20, 2017 from: http://www.lifeextension.com/magazine/2016/2/environmental-toxins-and-cancer-risk/page-01.
22. Ames BN, Shigenaga MK, Hagen TM. Oxidants, antioxidants, and the degenerative diseases of aging. *Proc Natl Acad Sci U S A*. 1993;90(17):7915–7922.
23. Helbock HJ, Beckman KB, Shigenaga MK, Walter PB, Woodall AA, Yeo HC et al. DNA oxidation matters: the HPLC-electrochemical detection assay of 8-oxo-deoxyguanosine and 8-oxo-guanine. *Proc Natl Acad Sci U S A*. 1998;95(1):288–293.
24. 1) Liu S, Li S, Du Y. Polychlorinated biphenyls (PCBs) enhance metastatic properties of breast cancer cells by activating Rho-associated kinase (ROCK). *PLoS One*. 2010;5(6):e11272.
    2) Larsen JC. Risk assessments of polychlorinated dibenzo- p-dioxins, polychlorinated dibenzofurans, and dioxin-like polychlorinated biphenyls in food. *Mol Nutr Food Res*. 2006;50(10):885–896.
    3) Hosnijeh FS, Heederik D, Vermeulen R. A review of the role of lymphoma markers and occupational and environmental exposures. *Vet Q*. 2012;32(2):61–73.
25. American Cancer Society. Can infections cause cancer? https://www.cancer.org/cancer/cancer-causes/infectious-agents/infections-that-can-lead-to-cancer/intro.html. Accessed December 27, 2017.
26. IARC Working Group on the Evaluation of Carcinogenic Risks to Humans. Biological agents. Volume 100 B: a review of human carcinogens. *IARC Monogr Eval Carcinog Risks Hum*. 2012;100(Pt B):1–441.
27. Mager, DL. Bacteria and cancer: cause, coincidence or cure? a review. *J Transl Med*. 2006;4:14.
28. Lipton, B. 2005. *The Biology of Belief: Unleashing The Power of Consciousness, Matter and Miracles*. 1st ed. Authors Pub Corp.; 2005.

Chapter 3

1. Draper G, Vincent T, Kroll ME, Swanson J. Childhood cancer in relation to distance from high voltage power lines in England and Wales: a case-control study. *BMJ*. 2005;330(7503):1290.
2. American Cancer Society. Understanding radiation risk from imaging tests. https://www.cancer.org/treatment/understanding-your-diagnosis/tests/understanding-radiation-risk-from-imaging-tests.html. Accessed January 15, 2018.
3. Brenner D, Hall E. Computed tomography — an increasing source of radiation exposure. *N Engl J Med*. 2007;357:2277–2284. doi: 10.1056/NEJMra072149.
4. Shyamala K, Girish HC, Murgod S. Risk of tumor cell seeding through biopsy and aspiration *cytology. J Int Soc Prev Community Dent*. 2014;4(1): 5–11.
5. Krawczyk N, Meier-Stiegen F., Banys M., Neubauer H., Ruckaeberle E., Fehm T. Expression of stem cell and epithelial-mesenchymal transition markers in circulating tumor cells of breast cancer patients. *Biomed Res Int*. 2014; Article ID 415721.
6. Rawal S, Yang Y-P, Cote R, Agarwal A. Identification and quantitation of circulating tumor cells. *Annu Rev Anal Chem*. 2017; 10(1):321-343.
7. Zhou L, Dicker DT, Matthew E, El-Deiry WS, Alpaugh RK. Circulating tumor cells: silent predictors of metastasis. *F1000 Res*. 2017 Aug 14;6. pii: F1000 Faculty Rev-1445.
8. Miller AB, Wall C, Baines CJ, Sun P, To T, Narod SA. Twenty-five year follow-up for breast cancer incidence and mortality of the Canadian National Breast Screening Study: randomised screening trial. *BMJ*. 2014;348 doi: https://doi.org/10.1136/bmj.g366.

9. Morgan G, Ward R, Barton, M. The contribution of cytotoxic chemotherapy to five year survival in adult malignancies. *Clin Oncol (R Coll Radiol).* 2004;16(8):549–560.
10. Karagiannis GS, Pastoriza JM, Wang Y, Harney AS, Entenberg D, Pignatelli J et al. Neoadjuvant chemotherapy induces breast cancer metastasis through a TMEM-mediated mechanism. *Sci Transl Med.* 2017; 9: 397.

Chapter 4

1. Ojima I, Chakravarty S, Inoue T, Lin S, He L., Horwitz et al. A common pharmacophore for cytotoxic natural products that stabilize microtubules. *Proc Natl Acad Sci. USA* 1999;96:4256-61.
2. Jimenez A, Chakravarty S. Seven Key Principles of Cancer Therapy: Alternative Approaches to Disease Resolution. *Forum Immun Dis Ther.* 2012;3:281-308.
3. van Straten D, Mashayekhi V, de Bruijn HS, Oliveira S, Robinson DJ. Oncologic Photodynamic Therapy: Basic Principles, Current Clinical Status and Future Directions. *Cancers* 2017; 9(2): 19; doi:10.3390/cancers9020019.
4. Wang P, Li C, Wang X, Xiong W, Feng X, Liu Q et al. Anti-metastatic and pro-apoptotic effects elicited by combination photodynamic therapy with sonodynamic therapy on breast cancer both in vitro and in vivo. *Ultrason Sonochem.* 2015;23:116–127. Epub 2014 Oct 30.
5. Sadanala KC, Chaturvedi PK, Seo YM, Kim JM, Jo YS, Lee YK et al. Sono-photodynamic combination therapy: a review on sensitizers. *Anticancer Res.* 2014;34(9): 4657–4664.
6. De Francesco EM, Bonuccelli G, Maggiolini M, Sotgia F, Lisanti M. Vitamin C and antibiotics: A one-two "punch" for knocking-out cancer stem cells. University of Salford, Manchester. 12 June 2017. www.sciencedaily.com/releases/2017/06/170612094405.htm. Accessed December 13, 2018.
7. Massey, P. Research studies effect of Vitamin C on cancer cells. *Daily Herald.* April 29, 2017. http://www.dailyherald.com/entlife/20170429/research-studies-effect-of-vitamin-c-on-cancer-cells. Accessed January 1, 2018.
8. Zhou S, Wang X, Tan Y, Qiu L, Fang H, Li W. Association between Vitamin C intake and glioma risk: evidence from a meta-analysis. *Neuroepidemiology.* 2015;44(1):39–44. Epub 2015 Feb 17.
9. Fan H, Kou J, Han D, Li P, Zhang D, Wu Q et al. Association between Vitamin C intake and the risk of pancreatic cancer: a meta-analysis of observational studies. *Sci Rep.* 2015;5:13973. doi: 10.1038/srep13973.
10. Jimenez T. Dr. Tony Jimenez from Hope4Cancer on Laetrile. *CancerTutor.com.* https://cancertutor.wistia.com/medias/m82sajtcv4. Accessed January 20, 2018.
11. Song Z, Xu X. Advanced research on anti-tumor effects of amygdalin. *J Cancer Res Ther.* 2014;10 Suppl 1:3–7. doi: 10.4103/0973-1482.139743.
12. Jimenez, A. Temperature matters. Presentation for Society of Progressive Medical Education.
13. Stępień K, Ostrowski RP, Matyja E. Hyperbaric oxygen as an adjunctive therapy in treatment of malignancies, including brain tumours. *Med Oncol.* 2016;33(9):101. doi: 10.1007/s12032-016-0814-0.
14. Raa A, Stansberg C, Steen VM, Bjerkvig R, Reed RK, Stuhr LE. Hyperoxia retards growth and induces apoptosis and loss of glands and blood vessels in DMBA-induced rat mammary tumors. *BMC Cancer.* 2007;7:23.
15. Zanardi I, Borrelli E, Valacchi G, Travagli V, Bocci V. Ozone: A Multifaceted Molecule with Unexpected Therapeutic Activity. *Curr Med Chem.* 2016;23:304-14.
16. Seyfried T. *Cancer as a Metabolic Disease: On the Origin, Management, and Prevention of Cancer.* 1st ed. Hoboken, NJ: Wiley & Sons; 2012.
17. Alabaster O, Vonderhaar BK, Shafie SM. Metabolic modification by insulin enhances methotrexate cytotoxicity in MCF-7 human breast cancer cells. *Eur J Cancer Clin Oncol.* 1981;17(11):1223–1228.

18. Jiao SC, Huang J, Sun Y, Lu SX. The effect of insulin on chemotherapeutic drug sensitivity in human esophageal and lung cancer cells. [In Chinese]. *Zhonghua Yi Xue Za Zhi*. 2003;83(3):195–197.

Chapter 5
1. Vighi G, Marcucci F, Sensi L, Di Cara G, Frati F. Allergy and the gastrointestinal system. *Clin Exp Immunol*. 2008;153(Suppl 1): 3–6. doi: 10.1111/j.1365-2249.2008.03713.x.
2. Research on Sunivera/GcMAF
    1) Yamamoto N, Kumashiro R. Conversion of Vitamin D binding protein (group-specific component) to a macrophage activating factor by the stepwise action of ß-galactosidase of B cells and sialidase of T cells. *J Immunol*. 1993;151(5): 2794–2802.
    2) Noy R, Pollard JW. Tumor-associated macrophages: from mechanisms to therapy. *Immunity*. 2014;41:49–61.
    3) Sumiya YU, Inoue T, Ishikawa M, Inui T, Kuchiike D, Kubo K et al. Macrophages exhibit a large repertoire of activation states via multiple mechanisms of macrophage-activating factors. *Anticancer Res*. 2016;36(7): 3619–3623.
    4) Yamamoto N, Suyama H, Yamamoto N. Immunotherapy for prostate cancer with Gc protein-derived macrophage-activating factor, GcMAF. *Trans Oncol*. 2008;1(2):65–72.
    5) Inui T, Amitani H, Kubo K, Kuchiike D, Uto Y, Nishikata T et al. Case report: a non-small cell lung cancer patient treated with GcMAF, sonodynamic therapy and tumor treating fields. *Anticancer Res*. 2016;36(7):3767–3770.
    6) Inui T, Katsuura G, Kubo K, Kuchiike D, Chenery L, Uto Y et al. Case report: GcMAF treatment in a patient with multiple sclerosis. *Anticancer Res*. 2016;36(7):3771–3774.
    7) Inui T, Kuchiike D, Kubo K, Mette M, Uto Y, Hori H et al. Clinical experience of integrative cancer immunotherapy with GcMAF. *Anticancer Res*. 2013;33(7): 2917–2919.
    8) Inui T, Makita K, Miura H, Matsuda A, Kuchiike D, Kubo K et al. Case report: A breast cancer patient treated with GcMAF, sonodynamic therapy and hormone therapy. *Anticancer Res*. 2014;34(8):4589–4593.
    9) Amitani H, Sloan RA, Sameshima N, Yoneda K, Amitani M, Morinaga A et al. Development of colostrum MAF and its clinical application. *Neuropsychiatry* (London). 2017;7(2):640–647.
    10) Akiyama S, Inui T. Cancer immune therapy in clinic: 2016. *Clinics in Oncol*. 2016:1:1–3.
    11) Bollard CM, Gottschalk S, Leen AM, Weiss H, Straathof KC, Carrum G et al. Complete responses of relapsed lymphoma following genetic modification of tumor-antigen presenting cells and T-lymphocyte transfer. *Blood*. 2007;110(8):2838–2845.
    12) Dudley ME, Wunderlich JR, Yang JC, Sherry RM, Topalian SL, Restifo NP et al. Adoptive cell transfer therapy following non-myeloablative but lymphodepleting chemotherapy for the treatment of patients with refractory metastatic melanoma. *J Clin Oncol*. 2005;23(10):2346–2357.
    13) Brown JM, Recht L, Strober S. The promise of targeting macrophages in cancer therapy *Clin Cancer Res*. 2017;23(13):3241–3250.
3. 1) Pacini S, Punzi T, Morucci G, Gulisano M, Ruggiero M. Effects of vitamin D-binding protein-derived macrophage-activating factor on human breast cancer cells. *Anticancer Res*. 2012;32(1):45–52.
    2) Thyer L, Ward E, Smith R, Branca JJ, Morucci G, Gulisano M et al. GC protein-derived macrophage-activating factor decreases -N-acetylgalactosaminidase levels in advanced cancer patients. *Oncoimmunology*. 2013;2(8):e25769. Epub 2013 Jul 29.
4. Inui T, Makita K, Miura H, Matsuda A, Kuchiike D, Kubo K, et al. Case report: A breastcancer patient treated with GcMAF, sonodynamic therapy and hormone therapy. Anticancer Res. 2014;34(8):4589–4593.
5. Inui T, Amitani H, Kubo K, Kuchiike D, Uto Y, Nishikata T et al. Report: a non-small cell lung cancer patient treated with GcMAF, sonodynamic therapy and tumor treating fields. *Anticancer Res*. 2016:36:3767–3770.

6. Postow M, Wolchok J. Toxicities associated with checkpoint inhibitor immunotherapy. *UpToDate.com.* https://www.uptodate.com/contents/toxicities-associated-with-checkpoint-inhibitor-immunotherapy. Accessed February 3, 2018.
7. Premratanachai P, Chanchao C. Review of the anticancer activities of bee products. *Asian Pac J Trop Biomed.* 2014;4(5):337–344. doi: 10.12980/APJTB.4.2014C1262.
8. 1) Parato KA, Senger D, Forsyth PA, Bell JC. Recent progress in the battle between oncolytic viruses and tumours. *Nat Rev Cancer.* 2005;5(12):965–976.
   2) Bartlett DL, Liu Z, Sathaiah M, Ravindranathan R, Guo Z, He Y et al. Oncolytic viruses as therapeutic cancer vaccines. *Mol Cancer.* 2013;12(1):103.
   3) Melcher A, Parato K, Rooney CM, Bell JC. Thunder and lightning: immunotherapy and oncolytic viruses collide. *Mol Ther.* 2011;19(6):1008–1016.
   4) Binz E, Lauer UM. Chemovirotherapy: combining chemotherapeutics treatment with oncolytic virotherapy. *Oncolytic Virother.* 2015:4:39–48.
   5) Coffin RS. From virotherapy to oncolytic immunotherapy: where are we now? *Curr Opin Virol.* 2015;13:93–100.
9. Finck SJ, Gupta RK, Giuliano AE, Morton DL. Excretion of tumor-associated antigen(s) in the urine of patients with colon carcinoma. *J Surg Oncol.* 1982;21:81-6.

Chapter 6

1. Swanson N, Leu A, Abrahamson J Wallet B. Genetically engineered crops, glyphosate and The deterioration of health in the United States of America. *J Organic Syst.* 2014:9(2):6–37.
2. Baudry J, Assmann KE, Allès B, Seconda L, Latino-Martel P, Ezzedine K et al. Association of frequency of organic food consumption with cancer risk. Findings from the NutriNet Santé Prospective Cohort Study. *JAMA Internal Medicine.* 2018; doi: 10.1001/jamainternmed.2018.4357.
3. Drews GJ. Unfired food and tropho-therapy (food cure). Chicago, IL: Apyrtropher Publishing House; 1912.
4. Dandawate PR, Subramaniam D, Jensen RA, Ananta S. Targeting cancer stem cells and signaling pathways by phytochemicals: novel approach for breast cancer therapy. *Semin Cancer Biol.* 2016;40–41:192–208. doi: 10.1016/j.semcancer.2016.09.001. Epub 2016 Sep 5.
5. Zheng J, Zhou Y, Li Y, Xu DP, Li S, Li, HB. Spices for prevention and treatment of cancers. *Nutrients.* 2016;8(8):495. Published online 2016 Aug 12. doi: 10.3390/nu8080495.
6. Arreola R, Quintero-Fabián S, López-Roa RI, Flores-Gutiérrez EO, Reyes-Grajeda JP, Carrera-Quintanar L, Ortuño-Sahagún D. Immunomodulation and anti-inflammatory effects of garlic compounds. *J Immunol Res.* 2015;2015:401630. doi: 10.1155/2015/401630.
7. Citrus fruits shown to be antiangiogenic and reduce risk for some cancers. Eat to Beat Cancer. EattoBeat.org.www.eattobeat.org/evidence/224/citrus-fruits-shown-to-be-antiangiogenic-and-reduce-risk-for-some-cancers.html. Accessed Feb. 13, 2018.
8. Skrovankova S, Sumczynski D, Mlcek J, Jurikova T, Sochor J. Bioactive compounds and antioxidant activity in different types of berries. *Int J Mol Sci.* 2015;16(10):24673–24706. Published online 2015 Oct 16. doi: 10.3390/ijms161024673.
9. Roomi MW, Kalinovsky T, Rath M, Niedzwiecki A. A specific mixture of nutrients suppresses ovarian cancer A-2780 tumor incidence, growth, and metastasis to lungs. *Nutrients.* 2017;9(3): E303.
10. Stuart, D. Green tea found to reduce rate of some GI cancers. Research News @ Vanderbilt; October 31, 2012. https://news.vanderbilt.edu/2012/10/31/green-tea-found-to-reduce-rate-of-some-gi-cancers/. Accessed April 2, 2017.
11. Fujiki H, Watanabe T, Sueoka E, Rawangkan A, Suganuma M. Cancer prevention with green tea and its principal constituent, EGCG: from early investigations to current focus on human cancer stem cells. *Mol Cells.* 2018;41(2):73–82.

12. 1) Settineri R, Zhou J, Ji J,Ellithorpe RR, Rosenblatt S, Jimenez A, Ohta S, Ferreira, G, Nicolson GL. Hydrogenized water effects on protection of brain cells from oxidative stress and glutamate toxicity. *Am J Food Nut.*. 2018;6:9-13.
    2) Nicolson GL, de Mattos GF, Settineri R, Costa C, Ellithorpe R, Rosenblatt S, La Valle J, Jimenez A, Ohta S. Clinical effects of hydrogen administration: From animal and human diseases to exercise medicine. *Int J Clin Med.* 2016; 7:32-76.
    3) Settineri R, Jin J, Luo C, Ellithorpe RR, de Mattos GF, Rosenblatt S, La Valle J, Jimenez A, Ohta S, Nicolson GL Effects of hydrogenized water on intracellular biomarkers for antioxidants, glucose uptake, insulin signaling, and SIRT and telomerase activity. *Am J Food Nut.* 2016; 4:161-168.
13. Jayakumar R, Kanthimathi MS. Dietary spices protect against hydrogen peroxide-induced DNA damage and inhibit nicotine-induced cancer cell migration. *Food Chem.* 2012;134(3):1580-1584. doi: 10.1016/j.foodchem.2012.03.101.
14. Panda AK, Chakraborty D, Sarkar I, Khan T, Sa G. New insights into therapeutic activity and anticancer properties of curcumin. *J Exp Pharmacol.* 2017;9:31-45.
15. Amalraj A, Pius A, Gopi, S, Gopi S. Biological activities of curcuminoids, other biomolecules from turmeric and their derivatives: a review. *J Tradit Complement Med.* 2017;7(2):205-233. Published online 2016 Jun 15. doi: 10.1016/j.jtcme.2016.05.005.
16. Deng YI, Verron E, Rohanizadeh R. Molecular mechanisms of anti-metastatic activity of curcumin. *Anticancer Res.* 2016;36(11):5639-5647.
17. The benefits of curcumin in cancer treatment. Mercola.com. March 2, 2014. http://articles.mercola.com/sites/articles/archive/2014/03/02/curcumin-benefits.aspx. Accessed May 30, 2017.
18. Applegate CC, Rowles JL III, Ranard KM, Jeon S, Erdman JW Jr. Soy consumption and the risk of prostate cancer: an updated systematic review and meta-analysis. *Nutrients.* 2018;10(1):40. Published online 2018 Jan 4. doi: 10.3390/nu10010040.
19. Le Marchand L, Hankin JH, Wilkens LR, Kolonel LN, Englyst HN, Lyu LC. Dietary fiber and colorectal cancer risk. *Epidemiology.* 1997 Nov;8(6):658-65.
20. Vallejo, F. Tomas FA Barberan C Garcia V. Phenolic compound contents in edible parts of broccoli inflorescences after domestic cooking. *J Sci Food Agric.* 2003;83(14):1511-1516. doi: 10.1002/jsfa.1585.
21. Mercola, J. How Your Microwave Oven Damages Your Health In Multiple Ways. Mercola.com. May 18, 2010. https://articles.mercola.com/sites/articles/archive/2010/05/18/microwave-hazards.aspx. Accessed July 1, 2018/
22. Davis DR, Epp MD, Riordan HD. Changes in USDA food composition data for 43 garden crops, 1950 to 1999. *J Am Coll Nutr.* 2004;23(6):669-682.

Chapter 7

1. Block KI, Koch AC, Mead MN, Tothy PK, Newman RA, Gyllenhall C. Impact of antioxidant supplementation on chemotherapeutic efficacy: a systematic review of evidence from randomized controlled trials. *Cancer Treat Rev.* 2007;33(5):407-418.
2. Premratanachai P, Chanchao C. Review of the anticancer activities of bee products. *Asian Pac J Trop Biomed.* 2014;4(5):337-344. doi: 10.12980/APJTB.4.2014C1262.
3. Chen MF, Wu CT, Chen YJ, Keng PC, Chen WC. Cell killing and radiosensitization by caffeic acid phenethyl ester (CAPE) in lung cancer cells. *J Radiat Res.* 2004;45(2):253-260.
4. Xiang D, Wang D, He Y, Xie J, Zhong Z, Li Z et al. Caffeic acid phenethyl ester induces growth arrest and apoptosis of colon cancer cells via the beta-catenin/T-cell factor signaling. *Anticancer Drugs.* 2006;17(7):753-762.
5. Carr AC, Maggini S. Vitamin C and immune function. *Nutrients.* 2017;9(11):E1211. doi: 10.3390/nu9111211.
6. Ebers G. Vitamin D found to influence over 200 genes, highlighting links to disease. *Science Daily.* August 24, 2010. https://www.sciencedaily.com/releases/2010/08/100823172327.htm. Accessed June 18, 2018.

7. Pandolfi F, Franza L, Mandolini C, Conti P. Immune modulation by vitamin D: special emphasis on its role in prevention and treatment of cancer. *Clin Ther.* 2017;39(5):884–893. doi: 10.1016/j.clinthera.2017.03.012.
8. Grant WB, Holick MF. Benefits and requirements of vitamin D for optimal health: a review. *Altern Med Rev.* 2005;10(2):94–111.
9. Mills E, Wu P, Seely D, Guyatt G. Melatonin in the treatment of cancer: a systematic review of randomized controlled trials and meta-analysis. *J Pineal Res.* 2005;39(4): 360–366.
10. Amalraj A, Pius A, Gopi S, Gopia S. Biological activities of curcuminoids, other biomolecules from turmeric and their derivatives: a review. *J Tradit Complement Med.* 2017; 7(2):205–233. doi: 10.1016/j.jtcme.2016.05.005
11. McAllister SD, Soroceanu L, Desprez PY. The antitumor activity of plant-derived non-psychoactive cannabinoids. *J Neuroimmune Pharmacol.* 2015;10(2):255–267. doi: 10.1007/s11481-015-9608-y.
12. Chakravarti B, Ravi J, Ganju RK. Cannabinoids as therapeutic agents in cancer: current status and future implications. *Oncotarget.* 2014;5(15):5852–5872. doi: 10.18632/oncotarget.2233.

Chapter 8

1. Blackburn E, Eppel E. *The Telomere Effect: A Revolutionary Approach to Living Younger, Healthier, Longer*. Reprint edition. New York: Grand Central Publishing; 2018.
2. McKeown, P. *The Oxygen Advantage: the Simple, Scientifically Proven Breathing Technique*. New York: William Morrow, an imprint of Harper Collins; 2015:4–5.
3. Pelletier M, Lavalle J, Ellithorpe R, Schmidt M, Pelton R, Settineri R. MS effects of CaNa2 EDTA (Detoxamin®) suppositories on heavy metal chelation; excretion of toxic metals. Detoxamin.com. https://www.detoxamin.com/heavy-metal-chelation-study/. Accessed March 8, 2018.
4. Levy JD. *Hidden Epidemic: Silent Oral Infections Cause More Heart Attacks and Breast Cancers*. Henderson, Nevada: MedFox Publishing; 2017.
5. 1) Nolte, H. The pathogenic multi-potency of mercury. *J Nat Med.* 1988:VI(3).
2) Belyaeva EA, Dymkowska D, Wieckowski MR, Wojtczak L. Mitochondria as an important target in heavy metal toxicity in rat hepatoma AS-30D cells; *Toxicol Appl Pharmacol.* 2008;231(1):34–42.
6. Huggins, H. Root canal dangers: DNA studies confirm Dr. Weston Price's century-old findings. Weston A. Price Foundation. June 25, 2010. https://www.westonaprice.org/health-topics/dentistry/root-canal-dangers/. Accessed March 21, 2018.
7. Sofuoglu SC, Aslan G, Inal F, Sofuoglu A. An assessment of indoor air concentrations and health risks of volatile organic compounds in three primary schools. *Int J Hyg Environ Health.* 2011;214(1):36–46. doi: 10.1016/j.ijheh.2010.08.008.
8. Shoemaker R. *Mold Warriors*. 1st ed. Baltimore, MD: Gateway Press; 2005.
9. Ahmed MA, Tabana YM, Musa KB, Sandai DA. Effects of different mycotoxins on humans, cell genome and their involvement in cancer. Review. *Oncol Rep.* 2017;37(3):1321–1336. doi: 10.3892/or.2017.5424.
10. Zota AR, Aschengrau A, Rudel RA, Brody JG. Self-reported chemicals exposure, beliefs about disease causation, and risk of breast cancer in the Cape Cod Breast Cancer and Environment Study: a case-control study. *Environ Health.* 2010;9:40. doi: 10.1186/1476-069X-9-40.
11. Mannello F, Ligi D, Canale M. Aluminium, carbonyls and cytokines in human nipple aspirate fluids: possible relationship between inflammation, oxidative stress and breast cancer microenvironment. *J Inorg Biochem.* 2013;128:250–256. doi: 10.1016/j.jinorgbio.2013.07.003.
12. Kharb S, Sandhu R, Kundu ZS. Fluoride levels and osteosarcoma. *South Asian J Cancer.* 2012;1(2):76–77. doi: 10.4103/2278-330X.103717.

13. Becker R. *Cross Currents: The Perils of Electropollution*. New York: Penguin; 1990.
14. Zhang Y, Lai J, Ruan G, Chen C, Wang DW. Meta-analysis of extremely low frequency electromagnetic fields and cancer risk: a pooled analysis of epidemiologic studies. *Environ Int.* 2016;88:36–43. doi: 10.1016/j.envint.2015.12.012.

Chapter 9

1. Brand R. Biographical sketch: Otto Heinrich Warburg, PhD, MD. *Clin Orthop Relat Res.* 2010;468(11):2831–2832. doi: 10.1007/s11999-010-1533-z.
2. Warburg, O. *The prime cause and prevention of cancer.* Lecture delivered to: Nobel Laureates June 30, 1966; Lindau, Lake Constance, Germany.
3. Muz B, de la Puente P, Azab F, Azab AK. The role of hypoxia in cancer progression, angiogenesis, metastasis, and resistance to therapy. *Hypoxia* 2015; 3:83-92.
4. Litscher D, Litscher G. Laser watch: simultaneous laser acupuncture and laser blood irradiation at the wrist. *Magazine for Acupuncture and Auricular Medicine.* October 5, 2015.
5. Seyfried T. *Cancer as a Metabolic Disease: On the Origin, Management, and Prevention of Cancer.* 1st ed. New York: Wiley & Sons; 2012.
6. Clavo B, Pérez JL, López L, Suárez G, Lloret M, Rodríguez V et al. Ozone therapy for tumor oxygenation: a pilot study. *Evid Based Complement Alternat Med.* 2004;1(1):93–98.
7. Hojman P, Gehl J, Christensen JF, Pedersen BK. Molecular mechanisms linking exercise to cancer prevention and treatment. *Cell Metab.* 2018;27(1):10–21. doi: 10.1016/j.cmet.2017.09.015.
8. Lee I-M, Oguma Y. Physical activity. In: Schottenfeld D, Fraumeni JF Jr, eds. *Cancer Epidemiology and Prevention.* 3rd ed. New York: Oxford University Press; 2006:449–468.
9. Schmidt T, Jonat W, Wesch D, Oberg HH, Adam-Klages S, Keller L et al. Influence of physical activity on the immune system in breast cancer patients during chemotherapy. *J Cancer Res Clin Oncol.* 2018;144(3):579–586. doi: 10.1007/s00432-017-2573-5.
10. Fraser G. Qigong: the power to heal. CANCERactive. http://www.canceractive.com/cancer-active-page-link.aspx?n=1438. Accessed Feb. 10, 2015.
11. Wayne PM, Lee MS, Novakowski J, Osypiuk K, Ligibel J, Carlson LE, Song R. Tai chi and qigong for cancer-related symptoms and quality of life: a systematic review and meta-analysis. *J Cancer Surviv.* 2018;12(2):256–267. doi: 10.1007/s11764-017-0665-5.
12. Agarwal RP, Maroko-Afek A. Yoga into cancer care: a review of the evidence-based research. *Int J Yoga.* 2018;11(1):3–29. doi: 10.4103/ijoy.IJOY_42_17.

Chapter 10

1. American Cancer Society. Can infections cause cancer? https://www.cancer.org/cancer/cancer-causes/infectious-agents/infections-that-can-lead-to-cancer/intro.html. Accessed December 27, 2017.
2. IARC Working Group on the Evaluation of Carcinogenic Risks to Humans. Biological agents. Volume 100 B: a review of human carcinogens. *IARC Monogr Eval Carcinog Risks Hum.* 2012;100(Pt B):1–441.
3. Mager, DL. Bacteria and cancer: cause, coincidence or cure? A review. *J Transl Med.* 2006 Mar 28;4:14.
4. Sakai C, Tomitsuka E, Esumi H, Harada S, Kita K. Mitochondrial fumarate reductase as a target of chemotherapy: from parasites to cancer cells. *Biochim Biophys Acta.* 2012 May;1820(5):643-51. doi: 10.1016/j.bbagen.2011.12.013.
5. Cheeseman K, Certad G, Weitzman JB. Parasites and cancer: is there a causal link? *Med Sci* (Paris). 2016;32(10):867–873.
6. Mandong BM, Ngbea JA, Raymond V. Role of parasites in cancer. *Niger J Med.* 2013 Apr-Jun;22(2):89-92.

7. Machicado C, Marcos LA. Carcinogenesis associated with parasites other than Schistosoma, Opisthorchis and Clonorchis: a systematic review. *Int J Cancer.* 2016;138(12):2915-2921. doi: 10.1002/ijc.30028.
8. Amin, O. Interview with Dr. Omar Amin, PhD. Alternative Cancer Research Institute. https://acri.cancerdefeated.com/interview-with-dr-omar-amin-ph-d/1196/. Accessed March 21, 2018.
9. Berman TA, Schiller JT. Human papillomavirus in cervical cancer and oropharyngeal cancer: one cause, two diseases. *Cancer.* 2017;123(12):2219-2229. doi: 10.1002/cncr.30588.
10. Lawson JS, Salmons B, Glenn WK. Oncogenic viruses and breast cancer: mouse mammary tumor virus (MMTV), bovine leukemia virus (BLV), human papilloma virus (HPV), and Epstein-Barr virus (EBV). *Front Oncol.* 2018;8:1. doi: 10.3389/fonc.2018.00001.
11. Develoux M. Cancer and mycoses and literature review. [In French]. *Bull Soc Pathol Exot.* 2017;110(1):80-84. doi: 10.1007/s13149-017-0543-9.
12. Paterson RR, Lima N. Toxicology of mycotoxins. *EXS.* 2010;100:31-63.
13. Liu Y, Chung-Chou H, Chang CC, Marsh M, Wu F. Population attributable risk of aflatoxin-related liver cancer: systematic review and meta-analysis. *Eur J Cancer.* 2012;48(14):2125-2136. Published online 2012 Mar 8. doi: 10.1016/j.ejca.2012.02.009.
14. American Cancer Society. Bacteria that can lead to cancer. https://www.cancer.org/cancer/cancer-causes/infectious-agents/infections-that-can-lead-to-cancer/bacteria.html. Accessed March 21, 2018.
15. Stragliotto G, Rahbar A, Solberg NW, Lilja A, Taher C, Orrego A et al. Effects of valganciclovir as an add-on therapy in patients with cytomegalovirus-positive glioblastoma: a randomized, double-blind, hypothesis-generating study. *Int J Cancer.* 2013;133(5):1204-1213. doi: 10.1002/ijc.28111.
16. Pushalkar S, Ji X, Li Y, Estilo C, Yegnanarayana R, Singh B et al. Comparison of oral microbiota in tumor and non-tumor tissues of patients with oral squamous cell carcinoma. *BMC Microbiol.* 2012;12:144. doi: 10.1186/1471-2180-12-144.
17. de Velasco A, Porras Lira D. Fusobacterium nucleatum ¿un patógeno periodontal promotor de carcinogénesis colorrectal? *Revista ADM.* August 2016.
18. Fontes B, Cattani Heimbecker AM, de Souza Brito G, Costa SF, van der Heijden IM, Levin AS et al. Effect of low-dose gaseous ozone on pathogenic bacteria. *BMC Infect Dis.* 2012;12:358. doi: 10.1186/1471-2334-12-358.
19. Wilson B, Burns T, Pratten J, Pearson GJ. Bacteria in supragingival plaque samples can be killed by low-power laser light in the presence of a photosensitizer. *J Appl Bacteriol.* 1995;78:569-574.
20. Johnson G, Ellis E, Kim A, Muthukrishnan H, Snavely T, Pellois JP. Photoinduced membrane damage of E. coli and S. aureus by the photosensitizer-antimicrobial peptide conjugate eosin-(KLAKLAK)2. *PLoS One.* 2014;9(3):e91220. doi: 10.1371/journal.pone.0091220.
21. Akram Z, Al-Shareef SA, Daood U, Asiri FY, Shah AH, Al Qahtani MA et al. Bactericidal efficacy of photodynamic therapy against periodontal pathogens in periodontal disease: a systematic review. *Photomed Laser Surg.* 2016;34(4):137-149. doi: 10.1089/pho.2015.4076.
22. Strasheim, C. *New Paradigms in Lyme Disease Treatment: 10 Top Doctors Reveal Healing Strategies that Work.* S. Lake Tahoe CA: BioMed Publishing Group; (2016)266-271.
23. Forsgren, S. Microbes, toxins, unresolved emotional conflicts: a unifying theory. PublicHealth Alert.org. April 1, 2009. http://www.publichealthalert.org/dietrich-klinghardt---microbes-toxins-unresolved-emotional-conflicts-a-unifying-theory.html. Accessed March 27, 2018.

Chapter 11

1. 1) Pot GK, Almoosawi S, Stephen AM. Meal irregularity and cardiometabolic consequences: results from observational and intervention studies. *Proc Nutr Soc.* 2016;75(4):475-486.

2) Almoosawi S, Vingeliene S, Karagounis LG, Pot GK. Chrono-nutrition: a review of current evidence from observational studies on global trends in time-of-day of energy intake and its association with obesity. *Proc Nutr Soc.* 2016;75(4):487–500.
2. Masters, M. Why your random eating schedule is risky for your health. *Time.com.* June 30, 2016. http://time.com/4384779/random-eating-health-risk/. Accessed June 19, 2018.
3. Cordina-Duverger E, Menegaux F, Popa A, Rabstein S, Harth V, Pesch B et al. Night shift work and breast cancer: a pooled analysis of population-based case-control studies with complete work history. *Eur J Epidemiol.* 2018;33(4):369–379. doi: 10.1007/s10654-018-0368-x.
4. Froelich, A. Science proves hugging trees is good for health. TrueActivist.com. http://www.trueactivist.com/science-proves-hugging-trees-is-good-for-health/. Accessed April 4, 2018.
5. Mead MN. Benefits of sunlight: a bright spot for human health. *Environ Health Perspect.* 2008;116(4): A160–A167.
6. Tomioka K, Kurumatani N, Hosoi H. Beneficial effects of working later in life on the health of community-dwelling older adults. *Geriatr Gerontol Int.* 2018;18(2):308–314. doi: 10.1111/ggi.13184.
7. Johnson, K. Study: toxic friendships can lead to serious health problems. CBS NewYork.com. April 22, 2016. Http://newyork.cbslocal.com/2016/04/22/toxic-friendship/. Accessed April 4, 2018.
8. Robles TF, Kiecolt-Glaser JK. The physiology of marriage: pathways to health. *Physiol Behav.* 2003;79(3):409–416.

Chapters 12

1. The Godhead is often referred to as the divine essence, or divinity of God.

Chapter 13

1. Hamer RG. *Summary of the New Medicine.* Fuengirola, Malaga, Spain: Amici di Dirk; 2000.
2. Laker L. Review of the Germanic/German new medicine of the discoveries of Dr. Ryke Geerd Hamer. The German/Germanic New Medicine. http://www.newmedicine.ca/book.php. Accessed May 7, 2018.

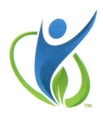

INDEX

2-butoxyethanol, toxic chemical found in household cleaning products, 244
2-Deoxyglucose (2-DG), 115
7 Key Principles of Cancer Therapy, 17, 25, 103, 113, 201, 381-382, 384, 395
Acanthamoeba, 288. *See also* fungal infections
AARSOTA, a natural, cancer-fighting vaccine-like bio-immunotherapy that uses a patient's own cancer antigens, 149-151, 156-157, 352
ablation, 161
abnormal cells, 57, 88, 102, 122
absorption, 200, 207-208, 210, 231, 291
acetogenins, natural chemicals that inhibit energy (ATP) production in the cancer cells' mitochondria, 205-206
acetyl cysteine, 131
acid-alkaline level
    acid-alkaline balance, 57, 183
    pH, 14, 183-184
acidity, 183-184, 230, 252-253, 286
Acinetobacter baumannii, 288
acrylamide, 171, 185
Actinomycoses 288. *See also* fungal infections
activated charcoal, mycotoxin binder, 284, 294, 386. *See also* mycotoxins
acupuncture, 255, 384
adaptive immune system, 107, 122, 138-139, 142-143, 151, 156-157, 206
adaptogenic herbs, 153, 204
additives, 174, 386
adenocarcinomas, 371
adenosine-5-triphosphate. *See* ATP
adrenal glands, 186, 201, 210, 414
    adrenals, 190, 414
adrenaline, 229
adversary, 338
aerobic factors
    aerobic capacity, 260, 266
    aerobic exercise, 388
    aerobic respiration, 205
aerobics, 387
Afinitor, 218
aflatoxin, 61, 243, 283. *See also* mycotoxins
Aflatoxin B. *See* mycotoxins
alarm response, 190
albendazole, 281, 294. *See also* anti-parasitic medications
albumin, 82, 94, 189, 202-203
alcohol, 15, 171, 197, 382
algae, 184, 238
alkaline, 57, 183-184
allergic reactions, 88, 90, 189
allergic responses, 191
allergies, 172, 177, 188-189, 191, 196-197, 207

allium vegetables. *See* vegetables
almonds, 49, 116, 178, 245
aloe, 187, 264
alpha-linoleic acid, 177
alpha-lipoic acid, 131
alternative, 47-48, 50, 84, 98, 115, 159, 161, 219-220, 257, 261, 281, 350-352
    cancer care, 25, 350-351
    cancer clinics, 98-99, 119, 145, 161-162, 219, 352
    medicine, 16, 19-21, 23-24, 28-30, 33, 35, 37, 39, 42-43, 47-48, 66-69, 71, 73, 75, 80, 83, 85-86, 97-98, 104, 110, 115-116, 121-122, 128, 144, 153, 155, 159, 162, 167-168, 188, 192, 195, 198, 209, 211, 215, 220, 229, 240, 254-255, 257, 280, 326, 342, 345, 347, 357-358, 377-378
    strategies, 15, 41, 54, 61, 68, 75, 142, 155, 279, 289
    therapies, 15, 21, 25-26, 34, 40, 47, 49, 51, 56, 75, 84, 86-87, 99, 101-106, 111, 115, 124-125, 129, 131, 133-135, 138, 140, 142, 145, 147-148, 150-151, 154-158, 161-162, 213, 219, 227, 229, 238, 248, 250, 252, 254, 256-257, 266-267, 275-276, 279, 282, 285, 293, 295, 297, 321-322, 329, 352, 377, 382-385, 390, 394, 396-397
    to chemotherapy, 85-86, 120, 283
    to mammography, 84
aluminum, 194, 239, 244, 272
Alzheimer's disease, 194, 290
amalgam, 57, 62, 239-240, 248, 250
AMAS test, 163
American Art Therapy Association, 305
American Cancer Society, 64, 75, 276, 285
amino acid, 131, 178, 203, 205, 378
Amin, Omar, 281
ammonia, 244
amoebas, 288
amygdalin, natural cytotoxic compound, 116-119, 135. *See also* Laetrile and Vitamin B-17
anaerobes, 253
anaerobic process, 205, 252-253, 287, 291
Andrographis paniculata, 281, 294
anemia, 82, 180, 254
angiogenesis, 54, 83, 106, 110, 120, 125, 144, 153, 177, 182, 203, 205-206, 209, 211-212, 253, 266, 280, 290
    tumor blood vessel formation, 54, 83, 120, 206, 253
anise, 187, 285, 294
antibiotics, 29, 115, 166, 180-181, 225, 272, 285-286, 289
antibodies, 138, 149, 153, 204, 282
anti-cancer effects, 66, 115, 124, 148, 175, 209, 217, 280
anti-cancer food plan, 196, 198
anti-cancer proteins, 143
antifungal drugs, 284

411

antifungal medications, 284
antigen-antibody complex, 138, 141, 149, 151, 180
antigenic proteins. *See* antigens
antigens, 77-78, 138-139, 149-151, 156-157
    antigenic proteins, 149
    cancer proteins, 77, 149
    tumor-associated antigens, 149
    tumor proteins, 78
anti-inflammatory effects, 119, 174, 176, 180, 211, 217
Antimicrobial Photodynamic Inactivation, 289. *See also* PDI
antimicrobial therapies, 111, 236, 238, 275-276, 285, 287, 289, 291, 295
antioxidants, 113-114, 116, 119, 126, 130-131, 146, 152, 172, 174, 176-177, 183-184, 199-200, 206, 212, 229, 256, 394
anti-parasitic medications
    albendazole, 281, 294
    artemisinin, 280
    ivermectin, 281, 294
    mebendazole, 280
    metronidazole, 281, 294
    praziquantel, 281, 294
antiperspirants, 244
antiviral therapies, 148, 282
anxiety, 41, 212, 260-261, 371
apoptosis, 54, 62, 64, 119-120, 125, 144, 146, 150, 153, 156, 175, 182, 187, 203, 205, 207, 211-212, 253, 276-277
appetite, 72, 120, 200, 211, 298
apples, 186, 189
appliances, 246-247
Applied Kinesiology (muscle testing), 290, 292
apricot kernels, 118
apricots, 116, 118, 135
armpits, 244
arsenic, 62, 74
Artemisia annua, 281, 294
Artemisinin, 280. *See also* anti-parasitic medications
arterial walls, 230
arthritis, 121, 292
artichoke hearts, 391
artificial
    additives, 386
    foods, 198
    fragrances, 244
    ingredients, 189, 196, 207
    products, 196
    sweeteners, 171
art therapy, 305-306
ascites, 149, 156
ascorbic acid. *See* Vitamin C
asparagus, 393
aspartame, 171
Aspergillus mold, 288. *See also* fungal infections
asthma, 237, 262
astragalus, 153, 204, 282, 294
at-home
    clinic, 322
    detoxification therapies, 229
    healing program, 384
    mold test, 243
    oxygenation therapies, 266

at-home (*continued*)
    ozone treatments, 127
    patient care program, 26
    treatment, 99
ATP, high-energy molecule and energy currency of all cells, 111, 130, 205-206, 252, 394
autoimmune diseases, 63, 168, 273, 292
Autologous Antigen Receptor Specific Oncogenic Target Acquisition. *See* AARSOTA
autologous urine therapy, 377
autonomic nervous system. *See* nervous system
avocado, 179, 386, 391, 393
avocado oil, 179
Bach flowers, 212, 217
bacteria, 294
    bacteria and cancer cells, 154
    bacteria and viruses, 132, 283
    beneficial (friendly) bacteria, 57, 202, 274
    infection-causing bacteria, 132
bacterial cell walls, 287
bacterial infection. *See* infections
bacterial overgrowth, 201
bacterium, 285, 287, 289
bananas, 172, 189, 191
barley, 189
barotrauma, 125
basil, 174
Basmati rice, 179, 392
beans, 178-179, 185, 189, 193, 392
Becker, Robert, 246
bedtime, 117, 300, 386
bee glue, 145
bee products, 146
bee propolis, 145-146, 156, 157, 203-204, 215-216, 232, 394
beef, 141, 171, 180-181
beets, 116, 186, 207
behavioral analysis, 357
Behavioral Emotional Spiritual Therapy. *See* BEST program
Bellon, Donato Perez Garcia, 129
bentonite clay, mycotoxin binder. *See* mycotoxins
benzaldehyde, 117
bergamot, 394
berries, 174, 177, 186, 393
BEST program (Behavioral Emotional Spiritual Therapy), 356-357, 360, 374, 390
beta-carotene, 176
beta-glucans, important immune modulator (found in Immune Power Plus), 153, 204
beta-glucosidase, cancer enzyme that triggers the release of cyanide from amygdalin, 117-118. *See also* Laetrile, amygdalin, Vitamin B-17
Bible, 26, 29, 33, 36, 56, 68, 96, 166, 181-182, 187, 229, 305, 325, 332-333, 335, 337-338, 340-341, 343-344, 385, 388
bile, 96-97, 234
bile duct cancer, 96
bilirubin, 234
Bio-A Curcumin Phytosome, 210
bioavailable, 178, 202, 204, 206, 216
bioenergetic testing, 290, 292
biological dentist, 239, 241-242
biomarkers, 79-80, 115

INDEX

biopsy, 71, 76-77, 83, 88, 160, 350-351
biotoxins, 293
bird watching, 304
blackberries, 174
Blackburn, Elizabeth, 226, 264
black pepper, 210
bladder cancer, 159-160, 163
bleeding, 72, 378
Blessed Herbs, parasite cleanse, 384
bloating, 192, 202, 210
blood-brain barrier, 145, 238
blood stream, 76
blood sugar, 128, 152, 172, 177, 179
blood tumor marker test, 77, 95
blood vessels, 99, 106, 109-111, 123, 187
blueberries, 174, 177, 186
body mass index, 298
Bok choy, 175
Bollinger, Ty, 48
bone marrow, 232
Bosworth, FF, 341
botanical remedies, 280-282, 284-285, 294
bouncing, 233
bowels, 72-73, 116, 201-202, 228, 231-232
brain, 33, 65-66, 84, 108, 111, 113, 116, 118, 121, 125, 131, 140, 145, 154, 169, 171, 183, 191-192, 203, 221, 230, 240, 274, 277-278, 286, 309-311, 349-351, 357-360, 362, 377-378, 389
    automatic, 358
    blood-brain barrier, 145, 238
    cancer, 65, 84, 113, 116, 118, 125, 131, 203, 278, 286, 349-351
    fog, 171, 191-192
    tumors, 33, 108, 121, 125
Brazil nuts, 178
breakfast, 193, 235, 385, 391-393
breast
    breast tumors, 124, 286, 366
    breast cancer markers, 78
    breast cancer metastases, 113
    changes in breast tissue, 84
    recurrence, 115
breathing exercises, 237, 249
broccoli, 174-175, 393
bromelain, 210
bronchitis, 73-74
Brussels sprouts, 175
Budwig diet, 377
Burdock Intrinsic. *See* drainage treatments
butter, 162, 386, 393
butternut squash, 174
Byrd, Randolph, 29
cabbage, 175
cadmium, 15, 62, 74, 238
caffeine, 229
caffeine-free, 182
calcification, 208
calcium
    absorption, 208
    metabolism, 306
Cameron, Ewan, 114
cancer cell division, 83, 205, 253, 266
cancer cells
    cloaking or shielding from immune system, 140

cancer cells (*continued*)
    communication with other cancer cells to develop drug resistance, 54
    evade the immune system, 151
    hypoxia encourages intercellular communication, 253
    innate intelligence, 55
    "lassoing", 55
    metabolism of, 66
    normal cells to cancerous ones, 56
    thrive in low oxygen environment, 252, 266
    tumor development, 55
cancer factors
    conversion of healthy cells into cancerous ones, 253
    environmental, 60-61, 69-70
    epigenetic, 37
    healing from cancer, 118
    terrain-altering, 58
    toxic, 68
    underlying, 28, 381
cancer growth
    cell growth, 54, 64, 115, 117, 125, 146, 153, 187, 253-254
    growth signals, 54
    tumor growth, 113, 120, 168, 182, 211, 259, 261
cancer-killing properties. *See* cytotoxic effects
cancer microbe, or pleomorphic organism, 286
Cancer Profile, The, 83, 95
    human chorionic gonadotropin (HCG), 83, 92
    phosphohexose isomerase enzyme (PHI), 83, 93
cancer proteins. *See* antigens
cancer recovery. *See* recovery
cancer treatments, 15, 23, 83, 101, 134, 137, 171, 201, 211, 278, 379, 382
    conventional treatments, 15, 278
    curcumin, 188
    integrative treatments, 23
    made from plants, 101
    melatonin as a cancer treatment, 209
    multifactorial approach toward, 86
Candida, 66, 177, 282-284, 288, 294. *See also* fungal infections
cannabidiol. *See* CBD
cannabinoids, 211
cannabis, 211-212, 217
carbohydrates, 172, 178-179
carbon dioxide, 228, 237, 249, 262-263, 303
carcinogens, 64, 244
carcinogenic, 64, 117, 126, 185, 194, 197, 242, 256, 266, 276
carcinomas, 120, 283, 286, 371
cardiovascular system, 179
carotenoids, 178
carpeting, 242, 244
carrots, 174, 186, 190-191, 391
cashews, 386
cassava, 116, 207
castor oil packs, 236
catalase, 114
CataZyme-7, digestive aid, 194
catechins, 182
cat's claw, 282
cauliflower, 74, 174-175, 286
cavitations, 239, 241, 250, 286

413

CBD, non-psychotropic cancer-killing treatment
  used as a sleep aid, pain reliever, and relaxant, 211-212, 216-217
    cannabidiol, 211
celery, 391
cell cycle, 64, 175, 276
cell death. *See* apoptosis
cell division, 83, 205, 253, 266
cell membrane, 55, 111, 119, 128, 179, 206
cell phones, dangers of, 247, 300
Cell Search, CTC testing laboratory, 79
cell signaling, 56
cell surface markers, 78
cellular behavior, 59, 154
cellular communication pathways, 39
cellular death. *See* apoptosis
cellular disruption
  cellular damage, 110, 126, 131, 187, 206, 209
  cellular dysfunction, 85
  cellular mutations, 277
cellular growth, 64, 276
cellular memory, 42
cellular synthesis, 150
cellulose, 299
cereals, 190
cervical cancer, 65, 282, 285
cervix, 65, 277
charcoal. *See* activated charcoal
chard, 174, 186
chelation, 49, 238-239
chemicals
  dioxin-like, 62
  endocrine-disrupting, 244
  harmful, 168, 181, 205, 245, 306
  industrial, 62
  natural, 205
  toxic, 185, 242-244, 250
chemotherapy, 14-15, 21, 27, 33, 48, 54, 59, 77-78, 84-87, 95, 97-98, 102, 120, 128-130, 140, 145, 159-160, 194, 199-200, 218, 220-222, 227, 233, 253, 261, 268-269, 283, 311, 318, 350, 366-367, 376, 381-382
  alternatives to, 85
  and radiation, 15, 33, 54, 84-87, 95, 97, 140, 200, 227, 253, 350, 382
  chemotherapy doesn't kill cancer stem cells, 87
  effect on gut health, 200
  low-dose, 86-87, 128
  with radiation and surgery, 27
chia seeds, 393
Chi machine, 233, 249-250, 386, 392
Chinese Medicine, 121
chives, 175
Chlamydia trachomatis, 65, 278, 285
chloramines, 184
chlorella, 76, 238, 264, 284, 294
chlorine, 184, 244
chlorin e6. *See* photosensitizers
chlorine, 184, 244
chlorophyll, 106, 264
chocolate. *See* dark chocolate
cholesterol, 111, 177, 179, 190, 203, 234-235, 298
cholestyramine, mycotoxin medication. *See* mycotoxin
Christ. *See* Jesus Christ

Christian, 29, 318, 394
chromosomes, 183, 226
chronic disease, 66, 126, 202, 209, 274, 279, 292, 297
chronic fatigue syndrome, 290, 292
chronic infection. *See* infections
cilantro, effective metal chelator, 238
cinnamon, 187
circadian rhythm, 298-300, 315
circulating tumor cells. *See* CTCs
circulatory system, 78-79, 232
Citrinin. *See* mycotoxins
citrus fruits, 177
Clark, Hulda, 65, 279
cleaning products, 49, 244-245, 250
cleanse, 249
  blood, 229, 386
  body of contaminants, 177
  liver and gallbladder cleanse, 234
  parasite cleanse, 384
  water cleanse, 183
Clonorchis sinenses, liver fluke, 280
clove essential oil, 281, 284-285, 294
coconut, 189, 294
  coconut ice cream, 393
  coconut milk, 49, 393
  coconut oil, 193, 284, 386, 393-4
coffee, 21, 48, 99, 118, 169, 171, 185, 229-230, 249-250, 321-322, 352, 385-386, 390, 392, 394
coffee enema, 21, 48, 99, 118, 229-230, 249-250, 321-322, 352, 385-386, 390, 394
cognitive function, 230
cold plasma ozone, 127, 257, 286
collard greens, 186
colloidal silver, antifungal nasal spray, 284, 286, 294
colon cancer, 37, 65, 84-85, 113, 117, 182, 188, 191, 201-203, 208, 212, 229, 249-250, 259, 278, 306, 372-373
colonoscopy, 84
colorectal cancer, 177, 287
Colossians, book of, 364
complementary medicine, 21, 29, 110, 209
complement cascade, 138
conflict shocks, 66, 358-360, 374, 378, 390
constipation, 73, 202
contaminants, 127, 169, 177, 184, 186, 193
conventional
  medical training, 17, 417
  medicine, 21, 28, 37, 42-43, 67, 73, 83, 85, 144, 159, 162, 220
  therapies, 21, 34, 115, 125, 417
  treatment, 24, 48, 87, 164, 269
corn-free sources, 116, 207
corn oil, 171
cortisol, 40, 190, 229, 358
corynebacteria, 286
cosmetics, 24, 244-245
cough, 73
counseling, 374
Creator (God), 29, 32, 40, 58, 66, 68, 116
cruciferous vegetables. *See* vegetables
Cryptococcus, 288. *See also* fungal infections
Cryptosporidium, parasite that causes DNA mutation, 280, 288

INDEX

CAT scan, *also known as* a CT/CAT (Computerized Tomography and Computerized Axial Tomography), 89, 160
CTCs
    circulating tumor cells, 79-80, 87, 108, 110
    silent metastatic disease, 81
CTC testing, 79
cucumber, 186, 391
cumin, 187, 285, 294
curcumin, cancer-fighting and healing compound found in turmeric. *See* photosensitizers
cyanide, cancer-killing affects when triggered by amygdalin, 116-117, 135
cyst, 369
cytokines, 64, 126, 138, 187, 256, 277
cytomegalovirus, 66, 278, 286
cytosol, 205
cytotoxic, or cancer-killing
    cytotoxic compounds, 116, 119, 217
    cytotoxic or cancer-killing properties, 104, 111, 134-135, 155, 206
    cytotoxic treatments and therapies, 105, 127-128, 138, 150, 155-156, 187, 203-204, 212, 215-216, 257, 259
dairy products, 171, 189, 196
dandelion greens, 186
dark chocolate, 174, 393
dark lettuce, 186
Davis, Donald, 195
defense system
    antioxidant defense system, 126, 256
    defense mechanisms/systems, 56, 148
dehydration, 202, 210
demons, 330, 338-339
dendritic cells, 139, 175
dental issues and cancer
    amalgams, 62, 239
    detoxification, 239
    hygiene, 242
    infections, 239, 286-287
    problems, 57
    toxins, 239, 250
deodorant, dangers of chemical-based types, 244
depression, 171, 223, 261, 303
detection, 75-76, 79, 81-84, 160, 243, 292
detoxification
    benefits, 229
    body's five means of, 228
    cellular, 260
    dental, 239
    environmental pollutants, 227
    enzymes, 182, 211
    from pathogens, 292
    heal and live long, 225, 248
    home and electromagnetic pollution, 250
    home detoxification, 249
    infrared light sauna, 131
    juicing, 229, 249
    liver, 62, 175, 285
    liver and gallbladder cleanse, 234
    negative emotions, 227
    of cells, 43
    of mold, 61, 243
    of tissue, 122

detoxification (*continued*)
    organs, 248
    pathways, 170, 205, 228
    protocol, 99
    skin as body's largest detoxification organ, 230
    sweating, 244
    therapies, 229, 250, 275, 293
diabetes, 172, 177, 179, 262
diagnostic tools/tests, 75
diaphragm, 262
diet, 37, 44-45, 48-49, 61, 67-68, 142, 155, 166, 171, 180-181, 188-189, 222, 284, 319, 322, 377, 386
    and detoxification, 142
    and exercise, 44
    and health choices, 67
    and supplements, 45
    ketogenic diet, 322
    low carbohydrate, 284
    native, 181
    non-native, 180-181
    plant-based, 166, 180
    poor nutrition, 37
    protein, 189
    vegan and non-vegan, 203
    vegetarian, 322
digestion, 171, 178, 183, 192-194, 198, 202, 216, 274, 298
digestive system, 37, 175, 182, 193, 299
digestive system cancers, 182
dioxins, 62
discomfort, 202, 371
disease
    chronic disease, 209, 292, 297
    designed to overcome disease, 69
    prevention, 45, 275, 394
    reduction, 83
    stress can lead to disease, 60
    systemic disease, 37, 121
divine healing
    divine intervention, 339
    healing and miracles, 26, 33, 36, 37, 332, 337, 345, 395
DNAConnexions, 290
Douwes, Friedrich, 289-290
Drainage Milieu. *See* drainage treatments
drainage treatments
    Burdock Intrinsic, 213
    Drainage Milieu, 213
    drainage remedies, 213, 217, 233, 249
    homeopathic drainage formulas, 213
    Lymph 1 Acute, 213
    Lymph 2 Matrix, 213
    lymphatic drainage, 106, 146, 205, 233, 249, 386, 392, 394
dreams, God-directed, 44, 309, 335
ductal carcinoma, 348
dumping, 361, 373
dysbiosis, 180, 194, 201-202
Eastern medicine, 35, 211
    cultures, 178, 236, 262
eating habits
    eating clean, 168-170
    eating rapidly, 192
    eating relaxed meals, 192
    fruits and veggies, 304

415

eating habits (*continued*)
    Garden-based, 167
    pork, 182
    red meat, 181
    schedule, 298, 413
    shellfish, 181
echinacea, 282, 285, 294
Echinococcus, parasite found in some cancers, 280
EDTA suppositories, for heavy metal removal, 135, 238
EGCG, 182, 211
Einstein, Albert, 34, 115
electrolytes, 210, 238
electromagnetic radiation, 15, 225, 249, 314
eleuthero (Siberian ginseng), antiviral botanical remedy, 282, 294
ellagic acid, 177
elliptical, 263
embryos, 35
EMF (electromagnetic field)
    EMF-protection, 247
    EMF radiation, 62
EMF-portal, 246
emotional abuse, 311
emotional and spiritual recovery, 357
emotional causes of cancer, 66
emotional conflicts, 33, 66, 292-293, 335, 357-362, 365, 368-370, 374, 377, 382-383, 390
emotional detox, 228
emotional energies, 212
emotional formation, 311
emotional healing, 373
emotional healing program, 356
emotional issues and healing, 59, 212, 293, 325, 339, 355-357, 364-365, 378, 383
emotional reflex centers, 359
emotional healing tools, 212
emotional stress, 60
emotional trauma, 57, 275, 305, 358, 360, 365, 390
emotions, 28, 32, 35, 38, 41-43, 69, 104, 154, 157, 212, 217, 223, 227, 260, 275, 295, 305, 311, 321, 326-327, 335, 339, 342, 350, 355-358, 360, 362-363, 365, 367, 369, 372, 374, 378
    and environment, 43
    catastrophic emotional event, 357
    harmful emotions, 217
    healing the, 321, 365
    mind, will and, 28, 38, 41, 104
    negative, 42, 154, 227, 260, 335
    painful, 363
    unresolved emotional conflicts, 292-293
    to heal the body, 154
    toxic, 335
    traumas and the, 378
Emoto, Masaru, 36, 373
endocrine glands, 214
endocrine system, 214
endoscopy, 44-46
endurance, 260, 263, 266
energetic frequency, 35, 65, 184, 192, 213, 248, 292, 329
energy, 25, 123, 126, 166, 171, 173, 179-180, 186, 193-194, 196-197, 230, 246-248, 252, 254-255, 257, 260, 264-265, 299, 301-304, 327, 329, 379, 384, 391-392
    currency of all cells, 205
    Earth's healing energy, 391
    energy beings, 34, 43

energy (*continued*)
    lowered energy state, 35
    meridian, 241
    metabolism, 57, 103
    of the cell, 39
    pathways, 130-131, 241
    production, 14, 111-112, 115, 131, 135, 206, 252, 255
Enhanced Permeability and Retention (EPR) Effect, 106
Enterococcus faecalis, 288
enzymatic system, 170
enzymes, 63, 182, 186, 193-194, 202, 206, 211, 216, 275, 366
    and probiotics, 202, 216, 275
    detoxification enzymes, 182, 211
    digestive, 275
    in your gut, 193
    hydrochloric acid and enzymes, 194, 216
    liver enzymes, 193
    pancreatic enzymes, 193, 366
    phase I liver enzymes, 63
    stomach acids and, 193
eosinophils, 175
Epel, Elissa, 226, 264
Ephesians, book of, 33, 307, 312, 330-331, 338
epigenetics, 37, 67
epithelial cells, 78
epithelial tumor CSCs, 78
environment, internal (having to do with the body), 205
    a cancer-disfavoring environment, 56
    acidic environment that encourages cancer growth, 252
    an environment in which abnormal cells can grow, 57
    cancer thrives in an oxygen-poor environment, 252
    create a healthier environment in your body, 252
    emotions and environmental toxins often correlate with the body's pathogenic load, 295
    environment affects our genes, 37
    environment, including our thoughts, largely affect how our genes are expressed, 67
    environment in which cancer cells can't thrive, 39
    factors that create a favorable environment in the body for the development of cancer, 57
    fear-based living fosters an environment in which cancer can occur, 60
    helpful for eliminating toxins generated by dying cancer cells and the environment, 213
    microbiome and creating an environment in which the pathogens can't flourish, 276
environment, external (having to do with factors outside the body)
    how you assimilate and utilize the nutrition in your food is affected by your environment, 192
    chemicals and toxins that you are being exposed to in your environment, 75, 314
    create a clean anti-cancer living environment that fosters health, 249
    creating a healthy living environment, 242
    today our environment and and bodies are more toxic, and we are surrounded by more negativity, 118
    environment has changed dramatically from that which God originally created, 225, 249

INDEX

environment, external (*continued*)
    God is greater than our fears, the environment, and the cancer itself, 68
    God provided us with an environment rich in anti-cancer compounds, 101
    living in harmony with our Creator and our environment, 40, 309
    microbes are ubiquitous in our environment: in the air, soil, food and water, 272
    each year new chemical and electromagnetic pollutants are introduced into the environment, 225
    none of us live entirely unaffected by the environment, 169
    observe, smell, listen, feel and breathe in the energy of that environment, 302
    our food, medicine, emotions and environment all affect our energy, 43
    reduce your exposure to EMFs in your environment, 246
    the greener your home and workplace are, the cleaner your environment, 264
    tradition of eating relaxed meals with our loved ones in a harmonious environment, 192
environmental (in the world's environment), 14-15, 37, 39, 43, 49, 57-58, 60-61, 63-64, 67, 69-70, 118, 142, 172, 174, 226-227, 234, 243-245, 252, 295, 306, 382, 394
    at least two-thirds of all cancer cases are now caused by environmental factors, 61, 69
    environmental instigators of cancer, 58
    primarily caused by environmental toxins, both chemical and electromagnetic, 37
    removing environmental toxins, toxic relationships, and undue stress, 118
    root causes of illness: spiritual, emotional, environmental and infectious, 43
    the role of environmental and lifestyle factors in gene expression, 67
    the role of environmental toxins in cancer, 60
Epsom salts, 234-235
ERMI. *Also* Environmental Moldiness Index, 243
erythritol, non-toxic sweetener, 393
escarole, 186
Escherichia coli, 278, 286, 288-289
Escobar, Jaime, 24
esophagus, 113, 129, 182
essential oils, 240, 244-245, 280-281, 284-285, 294, 377, 394
estrogen, 64, 174-176, 188, 214, 319
estrogen metabolites, 175
estrogen-receptor positive, 174
estrogen receptor sites, 174, 176
EWOT. *See* Exercise with Oxygen Therapy
exercises, 49, 154, 237, 249, 258-260, 262-263
Exercise with Oxygen Therapy, 263, 388
exhaling, 237, 262
Exodus, book of, 187, 333
exposure, 61, 75, 84, 139, 168, 226, 246, 306-307
    to a pathogen or cancer, 139
    to EMFs, 246
    to harmful radiation, 90
    to sun, 307
    to ultraviolet light, 306

expression, 15, 37, 67, 69, 170, 187, 261
    of cancer-suppressing genes, 170
    of pro-inflammatory cytokines, 187
    gene expression, 15, 67, 187
    genetic expression, 67, 261
extracellular matrix, 213, 285
extracts, 119, 156, 212
Faraday cage, 247
far infrared sauna therapy, 131
farmer's market, 304, 315, 387
fasting, 49, 128, 321, 394
fatigue, 72, 119-120, 191-192, 254, 262, 290, 292
fats, 245, 322, 386
fear, 13, 27, 42, 50, 60, 97, 169, 220, 222, 309, 320, 352-353, 370-372, 379
    fear-based living, 60
    fear is the enemy, 353
    inhibits decision-making, 50
    of dying, 370
    of financial deprivation, 370
    replacing with peace, 320
    God is greater than our fears, 68
fermentation, 201, 252-253
fermented vegetables. *See* vegetables
fever, 121-123, 135, 377
fever therapy. *See* hyperthermia
fiber, 110, 172, 177, 203, 232
fiberoptic laser technology, 109
fight or flight mode. *See* sympathetic dominance
figs, 189
filter, 184, 232
filtered water, 184, 228
filtration, 49
fireside chat, 364, 367-368
first ancestors, 166, 168, 198, 200, 258, 381
fish, non-toxic
    cold-water fish, 174
    wild-caught fish, 180, 222, 386
fish oil, 394
fitness, 260-261
flatulence, 192
flavanols, 182
flavonoids, 119, 177
flaxseed, 176-177, 179
Flora Syntropy, 146, 202
flour, 49, 171
fludeoxyglucose, 191
flukes, 280-281
fluoride, 15, 184, 244-245
folate, 177
food sensitivities, 191
forgiveness, 338, 362, 364, 366, 372
formaldehyde, 242
fragrances, 244
frankincense, 187, 221
free radicals, 15, 106, 110, 114, 152, 171, 177, 183, 187, 203, 209-210, 264
free radical scavenger, 206
free-range chicken, 181
free will, 340
fructooligosaccharide prebiotics, 202
fruits, 116, 135, 166, 172, 174, 177, 179, 186, 189, 191, 195-196, 198, 200, 222, 229, 232, 299, 304, 386
    fiber in, 232

417

fruits (*continued*)
  for your juices, 229
  organic types, 222
  straight off the tree, vine or branch, 304
Fry Labs, 290
full-body hyperthermia. *See* hyperthermia
full-dose chemotherapy, 86-87, 128
Full Spectrum Nutrition, 103, 165, 199
Fumonisins. *See* mycotoxins
fungal infections, 283-284, 288, 294
fungus, 66, 184, 284, 288
Fusobacterium nucleatum, 287
gallbladder, 65, 97, 229, 234-236, 248-250, 278
gallstones, 234
galvanic skin response devices, 292
Garcia, Donato Perez, 129
Garden-based eating and foods, 167, 170, 172
Garden Food Plan, 167, 170-172, 176-177, 179-180, 187, 196, 198, 235, 275, 383-385
Garden of Eden, 61, 165-166, 168, 178, 196, 198, 200, 271, 309, 340
  Adam and Eve, 165
  consuming food as God created it in, 166, 196, 198
  nutrition based on, 165
Garnett, Merrill, 130
gastrointestinal tract, 57, 138, 192, 201, 230, 274
  issues, problems, 180, 185
  upset, 210
GcMAF, regulatory anti-cancer, immune-supportive protein and macrophage-activating substance, 142-145, 156-157, 208, 322
  in bolstering immune system's ability to kill cancer cells, 144
  one of the most powerful anti-cancer proteins/substances, 143
  oral forms cross the blood-brain barrier, 145
  part of the Sunivera protocol, 157. *See also* Sunivera protocol
genes, 14, 37, 54, 64, 67-70, 170, 187-188, 207, 217, 276, 280, 306
  cancer-causing genes, 170
  healthy genes, 67
  tumor promoter genes, 187
  tumor suppressor genes, 187
Genesis, book of, 69, 165-166, 274
genetics, 15, 57, 67, 149, 243, 261
  genetic causes of cancer, 67
  expression, 67, 261
  factors, 57, 67
  inability to detoxify mold, 243
  pre-existing genetic factors, 57
genistein, 188
genome, 243
Genova Diagnostics, 215
German New Medicine, 66, 358, 377-378
Gerson, Max, 190-191, 351-352
GFP Nutritional, pea-based protein supplement, 194, 203, 206, 386, 391, 393
Giardia, 281, 288
gingivitis, 242
GI-supportive supplements, 202
glands, 145, 186, 201, 210, 214, 232, 241, 244, 371
glioblastoma, 212
glioma, 116, 125, 203

glucose, 76, 128, 205, 280, 298
glucose metabolism, 280, 298
gluten, 189, 198, 203
gluten-free ingredients, 179, 204
glycolysis, process by which cancer cells metabolize nutrients and create energy, 115, 252
glycolytic energy pathway, 130
glycoproteins, cancer cell-fighting mistletoe "lectins," 119
glyphosate, 168, 293
Godhead, 328, 330
gospel, 331, 345
grace, 307, 320, 322, 330, 343-344, 348-349, 395
Graham-Stetzer filters, 247
grains, 49, 169, 179, 181, 196
gram-negative bacteria, 289
gram-positive bacteria, 289
granola, 190
grapefruit, 234-235, 281, 294
grapefruit seed extract, botanical remedy for parasites/tapeworms, 281, 294
grass-fed animals, 181
gratitude, 40, 193, 198, 362
Great Plains Laboratory, 243, 284
green leafy vegetables. *See* vegetables
greens, 186, 391, 393
green tea, 182, 211, 217, 281, 294
green tea extract, 182, 211, 217
grounding, 247, 302, 391
guided healing visualizations, 364, 373-374
guided imagery, 154, 156-157, 374
guilt, 42, 336
gut-brain connection, 230
gut health, 87, 98, 140, 170, 175, 178, 189, 193-194, 200-202, 207, 216, 232, 272, 274, 277, 283-285
  beneficial bacteria in your gut, 202
  chemotherapy and radiation effects on, 200
  chronic diseases that involve a compromised gut, 202
  defense against any pathogenic organisms that enter, 274
  gluten damage to, 189
  healing and balancing gut and microbiome, 140
  healing for, 140, 170
  insufficiency of hydrochloric acid negative effects on, 193
  microbiome, gut, and the brain, 274
  rotting and fermentation in your gut, 194
  supplements that restore gut health, 201
habits, 44, 72-73, 168, 198, 231, 252, 297, 300-301, 310, 314-316, 321, 392
  lifestyle habits, 252
  old habits, 300
  unhealthy habits, 310
halting cancer cell proliferation, invasion and metastasis, 175
Hamer Herds, 66
Hamer, Ryke-Geerd, 66, 358-360, 369-370, 374
harmony, 40, 169, 309, 363
Hartmonella, 288. *See also* fungal infections
HBOT. *See* Hyperbaric Oxygen Therapy
HCL. *See* hydrochloric acid
headaches, 230, 303
healing plan, 71, 382
healthcare, 123, 229, 254, 265, 292, 360

INDEX

healthful vegetables. *See* vegetables
healthy eating, 40, 168, 222, 297, 383
hearing, 13, 20, 49, 318, 335, 351
heart, 18, 22, 29, 32, 36, 60, 72, 100, 152, 191-192, 230, 232, 262, 264, 269, 300, 302, 309, 311, 313, 315, 336, 339, 341-342, 349, 369, 389
heartbeat, 349
heart disease, 22, 230, 262, 264
heart rate, 191-192, 349
heat therapy, 122, 230
Heaven, 269, 328, 330-331
heavy metals, 39, 62, 74, 132, 180, 184, 205, 230, 237-239, 272, 279, 293
Hebrews, book of, 31, 36, 323
Helicobacter pylori, 65, 278, 285
Helixor, anti-cancer solution, 156
    See mistletoe
helminths, 280-281, 294
helper T-cells. *See* T-cells
hematocrit, 82
hematoma, 350
hemoglobin, 82, 129, 237, 252, 254-255, 262-263
hemp, 211, 217
Hepatagest, liver detoxification supplement, 146, 205
hepatic system, 229
hepatocellular carcinoma, 65, 277, 284
herbal remedies, 65-66, 280, 287, 292
herbicides, 62, 166
herbs, 35, 57, 152, 156-157, 169, 174, 187, 240, 244, 280, 384
Herceptin, 175
herpes, 65, 277, 282
herring, 181
Heterakis, parasite found in some cancers, 280
heterocyclic amines, 62
Hippocrates, 121, 192
Histoplasma, 288. *See also* fungal infections
HIV-1 virus, 65, 278
hoarseness, 73
hobbies, 297, 314-316, 383
Hodgkin's lymphoma, 65, 306
Holy Spirit, 27-29, 30-31, 36, 42, 332, 327, 330-332, 339, 343
homeopathic remedies, 35, 184, 212
homeopathy, 378
homeostasis, 112, 139, 183
homotoxicosis, 39
honey, 190, 198
Ho'oponopono, 361, 373
hormonal therapy, 144
    compounded hormone and hormone-supportive products, 215
    hormone-balancing supplement, 214
    supplemental bio-identical hormones, 215
    supplemental hormones, 214
hormone receptors, 175
hormones, 34-35, 74, 80, 166, 174, 180, 184, 203, 212, 214, 239, 311, 328, 331, 339-340, 385, 390
    and balance, 214
    and deregulation, 290
    antibiotic and hormone-free food, 180-181
    balancing the hormones, 64
    cruciferous vegetables and hormone-regulating compounds, 175

hormones (*continued*)
    hormonally influenced cancers, 174, 176
    hormonal system, 213
    hormones or antibiotics, 181
    hormone test, 215
    imbalances, 57, 64, 180, 214
    impaired hormonal and immune function, 62
    melatonin as a hormone, 209
    regulation of, 175
    serotonin, the "happiness hormone", 255
    stress hormone, 358
    synthetic hormones, 181
    toxins and hormonal imbalances, 64
Horner's Syndrome, 86
hospice, 219, 350
household cleaning products, 244-245, 250
Hoxsey, 220-221
human genome, 243
human rotaviruses, 287
human spirit. *See* spirit
hydration, 34-35, 74, 80, 166, 174, 180, 184, 203, 212, 214, 236, 239, 311, 328, 331, 339-340, 385, 390
hydrochloric acid, digestive aid supplement, 193-194, 202, 216, 275
hydrogen peroxide, 114, 135
hydrogen water
    hydrogen-enriched water, 385, 392-393
    hydrogen machine, 184
    hydrogen water, 183-184, 390
hyperbaric oxygen therapy (HBOT)
    HBOT, 124-126, 254, 256, 266
    hyperbaric chamber, 49
    hyperbaric oxygen, 124-125, 254, 256, 266, 389, 393
    hyperbaric therapy, 394
hypericin. *See* photosensitizers
hyperthermia, 105, 121-124, 135, 155, 162, 282, 285-287, 289-290, 293-294, 322, 352
    fever therapy, 121
    full-body hyperthermia, 122-123
    local hyperthermia, 123, 135
hypoxia, 266
    hypoxic, 252-253, 257
    low-oxygen environment, 57
Hypo Zymase, digestive aid, 194
iatrogenic causes of disease, 21
IgeneX, 290
illnesses, 20, 129, 303
imaging tests, 75-76, 84, 88, 95, 270
immune-boosting
    supplements, 392
    therapies, 155
immune cells, 64, 108, 114, 119, 123, 138-140, 142, 153-154, 157, 206, 232-233, 249, 256, 259, 276
    activation of macrophages, a type of immune cell, 119
    beta-glucans as immune modulators and activators of, 153
    granulocytes "engulf" cancer cells, 119
    lymphocytes, 232
    lymph fluid, 233
    recruiting immune cells, 138
    Peyer's patches, 140
    phagocytes, 138
    relaxation techniques increase the efficiency of, 154

immune cells (*continued*)
    SPDT activates immune system and recruitment of, 108
immune complement system, 54
immune function, 62, 105, 110, 114, 119, 135, 152-153, 155, 177, 204, 233, 255, 259-260, 266, 280, 310
Immune Imagery, 154, 156-158
immune markers, 154
immune modulation, 120
Immune Power Plus, recommended anti-cancer immune-boosting supplement, 152-153, 156-157, 204
immune response, 119, 130, 139, 143, 148, 150-151, 153, 156, 291
immune-supportive factors, 155-156, 383
immune surveillance, 78, 156
immune system, 15, 45, 49, 54, 56-57, 60, 64-65, 69, 82, 85, 87, 104, 108, 113-114, 120, 122-123, 126, 132, 135, 137-146, 148-157, 162, 171, 175, 180, 182, 191, 201, 203-206, 209, 211, 230, 236, 238, 240, 242, 256, 266, 272, 274-277, 279-280, 284-285, 291, 293, 295, 306, 308, 310, 354, 382, 394
    activation of, 143
    and disease prevention, 45
    boosting, 149, 291, 310
    brain and immune system, 154
    compromised immune system, 57
    deficiency, 201
    digestion, 274
    foods that support, 285
    immunomodulation, 103
    modulation, 113, 156, 120, 211
    optimization, 139
    stimulation, 132, 135, 206, 266, 230
    strengthening, 104, 142, 157
    suppression, 82, 140, 280, 293
    weakened, 65, 279
    weakened by toxins, 272
immunity, 261, 263, 266
immunoglobins, 138
immunotherapy, 142, 144-146, 148, 155, 208, 287, 291
    bio-immunotherapy, 149, 157
    conventional immunotherapies, 145
indocyanine green (ICG). *See* photosensitizers
indole-3 carbinols, hormone-regulating liver detoxification compound, 175
indoles, 176
infections, 15, 37, 57-58, 60, 64, 66, 69, 89, 91, 120, 122, 124, 138-139, 148, 239-242, 248, 272, 275-276, 278-280, 282-289, 291-295, 382
    bacterial, 284-285
    cancer-causing, 295
    cavitation, 241, 286
    chronic, 15, 37, 57-58, 272, 276, 280, 287, 293
    eliminating, 275
    first responder to gum, 286
    infection removal, 241
    parasitic infection, 281
    sub-acute, 240, 278
    susceptibility to, 120
    treating, 275, 279
    viral, 282
inflammation
    aluminum-containing antiperspirants, 244

inflammation (*continued*)
    antibiotics, hormones and systemic inflammation, 180
    antioxidants and flavonoids protect healthy cells, 177
    bacteria and inflammation, 284
    bee propolis and inflammation reduction, 216
    causes, 127, 189-190, 206
    curcumin stops angiogenesis and inflammation, 110, 187, 210
    damage to DNA, induces cancer cell proliferation, 277
    foods that lower inflammation, foster healing, 174
    free radicals and oxidative stress, 264
    fruit and reduction of, 190
    gluten inflammation and gut damage, 189
    gums and bone that surround and support the teeth, 242
    hydrogen remedy for, 184
    innate immune system response, 138
    reduction and cellular oxygen uptake, 264
    reduction of, 132, 146, 170, 177, 203, 210, 216, 255-256, 263-264, 394
    stressful friendships and, 310
    systemic inflammation, 180
infrared lamp therapy, 49, 132
infrared spectrometer, 80
injections, 19, 21, 146, 149, 151, 156, 352, 377
innate immune system, 138-139, 143, 151
innate intelligence, 53, 55, 68, 70
inner healing, 373
    inner healing minister, 339, 390
    inner healing prayer, 364-365, 373-374
insomnia, 185, 212, 217
insulin, 86-87, 127-129, 153, 190, 209, 241, 260, 290, 358
insulin potentiation therapy (IPTDL), 86, 127
integrative medicine, 16, 21, 104, 215, 294
    integrative approach, 16, 26, 95
    integrative cancer clinics, 60
    integrative cancer therapy, 101
    integrative doctor, 66, 85, 145, 191
intercellular communication, 56, 253
interferon, 114
International Academy of Biological Dentistry and Medicine, 240
International Academy of Oral Medicine and Toxicology, 240
International Agency for Research on Cancer, 64, 277
interstitial fluid, 76
intestinal flora, 140
intestines, 97, 201
intraductal carcinoma, 371
intranasal lasers, 111
invasive treatments, 14, 53, 80, 159, 161, 269, 348, 350
ionizing radiation, 15, 81
IPT (or IPTDL). *See* insulin potentiation therapy
iron, 15, 178, 195
irritability, 191-192
Isaiah, book of, 187, 318, 334
isoflavones, 188
itraconazole, antifungal medication, 284, 294
ivermectin, 281, 294. *See also* anti-parasitic medications

INDEX

Jeremiah, book of, 310, 336, 342
Jesus Christ, 236, 302, 307, 313, 323, 325, 328-331, 341, 344, 347, 363, 395
joints, 36
Jones, Robert, 240
juice, 186, 190-191, 229, 234-235, 322, 386, 394
juicing, 48, 186, 190, 229, 249-250, 322, 351-352
kale, 174-175, 186, 391
Kaposi sarcoma, 65, 277-278
kefir, 145
ketogenic diet. *See* diet
kidneys, 74, 83, 113, 186, 210, 212-213, 218, 228-229, 239, 248, 283
    flush out toxins through your kidneys, 228
    impairment of, 239
    kidney cancer, 74, 218
    kidney failure, 283
Klebsiella pneumoniae, 286, 288
Klinghardt, Dietrich, 66, 279, 292-293
Krebs cycle, 115
Kuppfer cells, 139
lactate dehydrogenase. *See* LDH
lactic acid, 205
Lactobacillus sporogenes, 202
lactose, 203
Laetrile, natural cytotoxic compound, 105, 116, 135, 219, 321. *See also* amygdalin and Vitamin B-17
Lapacho Intrinsic, lymphatic supplement, 146, 205
lapachol, botanical remedy for bacterial infections, 285, 294
laparoscopic surgery, 46
lasers, 110-111, 240, 254
laser watch, 109, 255, 394
lassoing, 55
late stage cancer, 85
laundry detergent, dangers of chemical-based types, 245
LaValley, William, 188
laxatives, 229
LDH, indirect cancer marker enzyme, 82
leafy vegetables. *See* vegetables
lectins, anti-cancer agent in mistletoe, 119
leeks, 175
left-spin molecules, 190-191
left-spin sugars, found in natural sugars, 190
legumes, 179
lemonade, 309
lemons, 177, 234
Len, Ihaleakala Hew, 361
lentils, 179
lettuce, 174, 186
leukemia, 24, 59, 65, 74, 86, 108, 212, 282, 366
Leviticus, book of, 182
licorice root, botanical remedy for viruses, 282
lie-based beliefs. *See* limbic system
life expectancy, 160, 308
lifespan, 85, 259, 266
lifestyle, 37, 43-44, 50-51, 67, 69, 74, 98, 142, 155, 222, 227, 252, 272, 297, 300, 302, 314-317, 319, 321, 340, 352, 381, 384, 392
    healthy lifestyle choices, 227
    lifestyle factors in gene expression, 67
    of loving others, 300
    practices, 297, 315
    preventative, 51

lifestyle (*continued*)
    tools for healing, 297, 315
    right attitude to foster healing, 43
    sedentary, 314
    simple changes, 302
    unhealthy, 37, 67, 74, 142, 252, 272
light-dark cycle, 299
light toxicity, 248
lignans, 176-177
limbic system
    lie-based beliefs, 59, 69, 339, 346
    lie-based thinking, 60, 363
    limbic, 310-311, 327, 332, 335, 369
limes, 177
lipid envelopes, 289
lipoic acid mineral complex, 130
lipoprotein lipase, 255
Lipton, Bruce, 67
liver, 62-63, 65, 82, 97-98, 113, 127, 131, 139, 146, 160-163, 175, 186, 201-203, 205, 213, 229-230, 234, 236, 239, 248-250, 257, 278, 280, 284-285, 319-320, 322, 370
    cleanse, 234
    detoxification, 62, 175, 285
    enzymes, 63
    flukes, 280
    liver cancer, 65, 202, 284, 319, 370
    problems, 82
    surgery, 161-163
    tumors, 127, 257
long-term immune system. *See* adaptive immune system, 139, 143, 151
low-dose chemotherapy, 86
low-level lasers, 254
low level laser therapy, or photobiomodulation, 110, 241, 254
low-oxygen environment. *See* hypoxia
lumpectomy, 318
lunch, 193, 383-385, 391, 393
lung adenocarcinoma cells, 130
lungs, 65, 83, 86, 113, 117, 129-130, 144, 146, 177, 182, 203, 212, 237, 248, 252, 256, 262-263, 278, 283, 370
    capacity, 263
    lung cancer, 65, 83, 144, 177, 203, 278, 283, 370
    metastasis, 182
    non-small cell lung cancer, 144
luteins, 176
Lymph 1 Acute. *See* drainage treatments
Lymph 3 Chronic. *See* drainage treatments
Lymph 2 Matrix. *See* drainage treatments
lymphatic drainage. *See* drainage treatments
lymphatic massage, 321
lymphatic system, 76, 138, 140, 205, 213, 218, 229, 232, 234, 236, 248-250, 386
    lymphatic fluid, 232
    lymphatic stimulants, 236
lymphatic vessels, 232
lymph fluid, 232-234, 236, 321
lymph nodes, 111, 113, 124, 127, 159, 220, 232, 257
lymphocytes, 139, 151, 175, 232
lymphoid cancers, 146
lymphoma, 65, 86, 113, 277-278, 280, 306
lysine, 182

lysis, the process of cellular breakdown, 123, 148, 156
macadamias, 178
macromolecules, 106
macronutrients, 152, 157, 204
macrophages, 119, 138-139, 142-144, 153, 157, 175, 204, 260, 291
magnesium, 152, 204, 210, 231
malaria, 280
mammogram, 83-84, 95, 350
manganese, 178
margarine, 171
marijuana, 211
markers, cancer markers, 44, 49, 77, 77-78, 82-84, 95, 149, 154, 261, 305
mass, 44, 50, 73, 87, 171, 298, 379
massage, 321, 384
Massey, Patrick B., 115
mastectomy, 318-319
Matthew, book of, 26, 68, 187, 303, 330, 340, 395
mattress, avoid chemically treated types, 242-243
McKeown, Patrick, 237, 262-263
mebendazole. *See* anti-parasitic medications
melanoma, 113, 144, 208, 212, 307
melatonin, 111, 208-209, 217
mental health, 15, 36, 45, 47, 156, 191, 258, 303, 306, 311
Merck Manual, 229
Mercola, J., 188
mercury, 15, 57, 62, 180, 238-239, 272
Meridian Valley Labs, hormone testing laboratory, 191, 215
Merkel cell polyomavirus, 65, 278
mesenchymal cells, 78
mesenchymal CTCs, 80
mesenchyme, 285
metabolism, 21, 49, 65, 98-99, 105, 113-116, 135, 155, 177, 182, 195, 200, 206-207, 216-217, 219, 238, 244, 255, 277, 282, 287, 291, 293, 321, 352, 390
    aerobic, 251
    anaerobic, 253
    balance of, 315
    cancer cells metabolize nutrients, 252
    cellular, 130
    energy, 205
    improvement of, 184
    metabolic pathway, 115
    of cancer cells, 66, 130, 280
    processes, 111, 131, 135
    waste, 108, 183
metallic-lined mesh canopy. *See* Faraday cage
metastasis, 33, 60, 78-80, 83, 97-98, 110, 146, 168, 175, 182, 203, 280
    circulating tumor cells and, 79, 89
    curcumin prevents metastases, 209
    halting of 110, 144, 175, 187, 209, 212
    into vital tissues and organs, 78
    metastases facilitated by hypoxia, 266
    tumor growth and, 113, 168, 216, 261
metastatic disease, 81, 227, 382
methotrexate, 130
metronidazole 281, 294. *See also* anti-parasitic medications
microbiome, 103, 140, 271-277, 285
    compromised microbiome, 274

microcirculation, 126, 255-256, 266
micronutrients, 130, 152
microRNA-containing exosomes, 56
microwaves, dangers of, 194
microwave towers, EMF radiation from, 62, 247
Mimosa pudica, botanical remedy for parasites (tapeworms), 281, 294
mind-body health, 154, 158, 260, 266, 335, 357, 373, 387-388
mindfulness, 260
mineral deficiencies, 57
mineral oils, 244
minerals, 57, 130, 152, 172, 177-178, 204-205, 210, 230, 238, 244, 303
mint, 174, 187
mistletoe, 105, 119-121, 133, 135, 155, 156
mitochondria, 111, 126-127, 205, 251, 257
mitochondrial dysfunction, 127, 257
mobility, 260, 266
mold toxins. *See* mycotoxins
monk fruit, natural sweetener, 391, 393
monolaurin, Candida treatment made from coconut oil, 284
mood stabilizer 394. *See also* bergamot
morning, 30, 40-41, 128, 207, 235, 237, 264, 307, 320, 379, 383, 389-390
mortality, 115, 379
motility, 83
mountains, 302, 315
mouth, 65, 237, 241, 262-263, 265, 277-278, 388
mRNA, 56
mucosa, 272, 283
mucous membranes, 138, 140
multiple sclerosis, 290, 292
muscles, 152, 159, 170-171, 183, 203, 233, 264, 285, 290, 292
muscle testing. *See* Applied Kinesiology
mushrooms, 153, 204
mycotoxin testing, 243
mycotoxins, or mold toxins
    activated charcoal, 284, 294, 386
    Aflatoxin B, 243
    bentonite clay, 284, 294, 386
    cholestyramine, 284, 294
    Citrinin, 243
    Fumonisins, 243
    mold toxin test, 243, 284
    mycotoxin, 243, 284, 294
    Patulin, 243
    Trichothecene, 243
    urine mycotoxin test, 243
    Welchol, 284, 294
    Zearalenone, 243
myeloma, 65, 277
My Green Fills, non-toxic household products, 245
myrrh essential oil, botanical remedy for parasites, 281, 284-285, 294
nagalase, cancer cell enzyme, 144
nasopharynx, 65, 277
Nathan, Neil, 244
National Cancer Institute, 61, 87, 120
natural foods, 169, 181, 386
natural laws, 56, 227, 297, 314-315, 338, 381
natural remedies, 128, 284, 294

INDEX

natural selection, 54
natural sweeteners, 174
natural therapies, 86-87, 102, 279, 285
    natural agents, 78, 240
    natural healing, 18
    natural remedies, 128, 284, 294
Nature's Carpet, 242
nature, spending time in, 51, 134, 142, 245, 302, 304, 316
naturopathic medicine, 65, 352
near infrared light, 130-131, 230
near infrared sauna therapy, 131, 230, 249
Negleria, 288. *See also* fungal infections
nephrectomy, 218
nervous system, 211, 214, 264, 357, 363, 382
    autonomic nervous system, 357, 363
    parasympathetic nervous system, 304
    sympathetic nervous system, 357
neurodegenerative diseases, 194
neurological system, 213, 277, 290
neurons, 154
neutrophils, 139, 206
New Testament, 30, 187
nickel, and heavy metal toxicity, 15
night, 18, 22, 193, 208, 237, 246-247, 262-265, 300, 349, 376-377, 383, 388
nitric oxide, immune modulator and cellular regeneration promoter, 112, 255
nitrogen, 126
nobiletin, helps stop angiogenesis, 177
nodules, 220-221
non-conventional treatments, 47
non-GMO
    fermented soy products, 188
    food, animals, 116, 180-181, 188, 204, 207, 222, 386
    pasture-raised chicken and, 181
    supplements, 207
non-food, 195
non-gluten, 179
non-gluten grains, 179
non-toxic cancer therapies, 101, 103-104, 133-134
Norwalk virus, 287
nucleic acid, 126, 287
Nurse, Paul, 72, 299, 311, 351
NutraSweet, artificial sweetener and dangers of, 171
NutrEval FMV, nutritional testing laboratory 215
nutrients, 31, 39, 54, 57, 99, 117, 146, 156, 172, 176-177, 182, 186, 188, 193-195, 200-202, 204-207, 216, 229, 237, 249, 252, 257, 260, 276, 299, 303-304, 307, 322, 393-394
    absorption and assimilation of, 202
    anti-cancer 172, 177, 182
    blocking nutrient source of tumor cells, 117
    cancer-killing, 172
    cells require ATP, or energy to absorb nutrients, 205
    depletion by frying, grilling and overcooking, 194
    effective metabolization of, 195
    finding nutrient-rich food supply, 166
    foods that contain cancer-killing types of, 172
    food supply no longer contains all of the nutrients we need, 195, 394
    freshly picked, mature produce and, 304
    from raw, fresh juice, 322
    green smoothie and, 193

nutrients (*continued*)
    green tea and, 182
    healing types of, 186, 304
    importance of receiving a broad spectrum of, 186
    in berries, 177
    in fruits, 186
    nutrient-deficient food, 195, 382
    organic soil not as nutrient-rich as years past, 195
    ozone, elimination of cancer-causing toxins and better uptake of, 257
    quick and efficient assimilation through juicing, 186
    Sunivera protocol, 142, 208, 394
    supplements and, 146, 201, 216
    targeted for reversing disease, 201
    uptake, 237, 260
    vegetables and fruits contain 30-50% less than 50 years ago, 195
nutritional approaches
    adopting good nutrition, 15
    based on the Garden of Eden, 165
    Full Spectrum Nutrition, 103, 165, 199
    individualized nutritional and immune enhancing plan, 22
    imbalances, 58, 284
    non-food factors, 195
    nutrition and exercise, 155
    primary source of, 179
    requirements, 167, 172, 200
    supplemental, 200
    targeted, 146
    unhealthy, 74
nutritional testing, 215
nuts, 49, 166, 169, 172, 178-179, 189, 196, 198, 386, 391
nystatin, antifungal medication, 284, 294
oatmeal, 179
ocular lymphoma, 65, 278
ointments, 212
Old Testament, 334
olive leaf, botanical remedy for viruses, 281-282, 294
olive oil, 174, 181, 234-235, 386, 393
olives, 391
omega-3 essential fatty acids, 177, 180-181, 394
oncogenes, 14, 187
oncolysis, cancer cell breakdown, 147
oncolytic virotherapy, viruses that selectively target cancer cells, 33, 66, 68, 87, 104, 106, 108-109, 122, 132, 134-135, 139, 141, 151, 179, 193, 346
oncotropism, 147, 156
onions, 175
Opistorchis viverrini, liver fluke, 280
oranges, 177, 189
oregano essential oil, botanical remedy for parasites and viruses, 281-282, 284-285, 294
organic vegetables. *See* vegetables
organisms
    infectious organisms, 274
    multicellular organisms, 281
    pathogenic organisms, 274, 279, 287, 289, 292
organs, 35, 37, 57, 78, 85, 97, 113, 118, 124-125, 138, 183, 201, 205, 210, 227-228, 232-234, 236-237, 239, 241, 248-249, 256, 277, 359, 363
    and oxygen therapies, 125, 256
    castor oil pack and organ toxin cleanse, 236
    detoxification, 227

organs (*continued*)
   degeneration, 233
   dysfunction, 284
   fortification of lymphatic system and, 205
   hydration, 183
   innate energy, 35
   liver and gallbladder, 234
   obstacles to healing, 201
   pathways to remove toxins, 228
   removing cellular debris from, 138
   skin, largest detoxification organ, 230
   support eliminatory pathways and, 239
   therapies that engage all detoxification organs, 248
   to cleanse the blood, organs and lymphatic system, 249
orthopedic, 246
osteosarcoma, 244
outdoors, benefits of, 44, 181, 258, 260, 304, 306, 384, 387-388
ovarian cancer, 78, 149, 182, 268-269, 367, 371-372, 375, 377-379
ovaries, 376
overweight, 265
oxygen, 101, 106, 111, 122-127, 131, 134-135, 156, 195, 205, 237, 249, 251-257, 260, 262-267, 291, 303, 388-389, 391, 393
oxygen absorption, 291
oxygenating agents, 254
oxygenation, 103, 123, 126, 131, 237, 251-253, 255, 262, 266-267, 303, 387
   cellular, 255
   improvement of, 112, 258, 288
   level, 237, 303
   of tissues, 123, 131
oxygen deprivation. *See also* hypoxia, 252-254, 262, 264
oxygen tank, 127
oxygen therapy, 67, 264
oxygen uptake, 111, 255, 260, 264, 266
ozonated water, 127
ozone, 21, 105, 124-127, 135, 144, 155, 219, 225, 240-241, 254, 256-257, 266, 284-291, 293-294, 387, 389-390
ozone generator, 127, 257
ozone therapy, 125, 127, 135, 257, 287-288, 389-390
Pacific Yew tree, compounds used for chemotherapeutic agents, 102
pain reliever, 212
painting, therapeutic benefits of, 305, 315
palladium, 131
pancoast tumor, 85
pancreas, 44-46, 49, 97, 113, 372
pancreatic cancer, 44, 96, 116, 372
pancreatitis, 352
parabens, cancer-linked preservative in some personal care/home products, 244
parasites, 15, 34-35, 74, 80, 166, 174, 180, 184, 203, 212, 214, 239, 273, 311, 328, 331, 339-340, 385, 390
   50% likelihood of parasitic infection of people in US, 281
   affected by ozone, 288
   and weakened immune system, 279
   as cause of, or linked to cancer, 65-66, 272, 279-280
   as immune system suppressors, 280
   body's first line of defense against, 138

parasites (*continued*)
   botanical remedies for, 281
   cancer causes along with viruses, fungi and bacteria, 271, 294
   cleanse, 384
   common kinds, 280
   molds and, 238
   parasitic infections, 281
   pharmaceutical remedies, 280-281, 294
   removal, 65
   testing for, 281
Parasitology, Inc., parasite testing laboratory, 281
parasympathetic nervous system. *See* nervous system
ParaWellness Research, 281
Parmenides, 121
parsley, 186
parvoviruses, 287
pasture-raised food
   butter, 386
   chicken, 181, 222, 386
   eggs, 391
pathogenic infections. *See* infections
pathogens, 19, 21-25, 28-31, 33-37, 39-41, 44-48, 50-51, 54, 56, 59, 63-70, 72-76, 78, 81-88, 96-102, 104-106, 108-111, 113-120, 122-126, 128-132, 135, 137-140, 142-146, 148-151, 154-156, 157, 160-163, 166, 168-170, 172, 175, 178, 183-184, 186-190, 192, 194-195, 200, 203-208, 212-213, 216, 218-219, 221-223, 227-232, 234, 236-237, 241-245, 248, 251-253, 256-258, 260, 262-263, 265-266, 268-270, 272, 274-275, 278-283, 287, 289-295
   anaerobic pathogenic microbes, 291
   association between pathogenic microbes and cancer, 272, 293
   cancer cells and pathogens, 138, 151
   carriers of Lyme pathogens, 290
   detection difficulties, 292
   effective treatments, 289
   emotions, environmental toxins and pathogenic load, 295
   energetic frequency of, 65
   fever to eliminate, 122
   first line of defense against, 138
   foods that feed and strengthen cancer cells and, 171
   Garden of Eden, free of disease and, 271
   how pathogens cause cancer, 64, 276
   hyperthermia treatment and, 124
   immune response specific to, 151
   infectious pathogens, 277
   initial exposure to, 139
   Lyme disease, 290
   ozone treatment of, 127
   pathogenic effect on gut-brain, 277
   pathogenic microbes, 66, 114, 153, 171, 201, 254, 271-272, 274-279, 287-288, 291-293, 295
   periodontal pathogens, 289
   those sensitive to ultraviolet light and ozone, 291
   tumor-associated types, 108
Patulin. *See* mycotoxins
Pauling, Linus, 114-115
PDI (Antimicrobial Photodynamic Activation), antimicrobial therapy used against pathogens, 289
PDIS. *See* Photodynamic Infrared Spectroscopy
PDT. *See* Photodynamic Therapy
PDT Plus. *See* Photodynamic Therapy Plus

INDEX

peaches, 116
peanuts, mold susceptibility, 178, 386
pea protein, one of most preferred sources of protein powder/supplements, 203
pears, 186, 189
pecans, 178, 393
pelvis, 84, 375, 379
pepper, natural spice
    black pepper, 210
    pepper, 169, 393
peppermint, 281, 294
peppers, 174
peptides, bee product types induce apoptosis, 146
perchloroethylene, toxic chemical found in household cleaning products, 244
periodontal disease, 242, 248, 286
periodontitis, 242, 287
personal care products, 60, 242, 244-245
perspiration. *See* sweat
pesticides, 15, 62, 166, 168, 184, 225, 283, 293
petrochemicals, 62
petrolatum, cancer-linked chemical in some personal care products, 244
PET scan, 76, 351
pH. *See* acid-alkaline level
phagocytes, immune cells that engulf cancer, 138, 154
pharmaceutical remedies, 281, 284-285, 294-295
Phellodendron amurense, botanical remedy for parasites, 281, 294
phenotype, 15
phosphatidylcholine, 210
phosphorus, 195
Photodynamic Infrared Spectroscopy (PDIS), detects both epithelial and mesenchymal CTCs within the bloodstream 80-81
Photodynamic Therapy (PDT), 82, 105-106, 108, 113, 129-130, 132, 209, 240, 254, 266 285, 287, 289, 293-294, 376-377, 389, 394
Photodynamic Therapy Plus (PDT Plus), non-toxic advanced, deep-penetrating cancer therapy, 105, 108-109, 266
photosensitizers, activators in Photodynamic Therapy, 80, 106, 109-110, 112, 129, 156, 254, 294
    chlorin e6, 80
    curcumin, 110, 174, 187-188, 209, 285, 294
    indocyanine green (ICG), 80-81, 89, 110, 112
    hypericin, 110
    riboflavin, 195
phthalates, inflammatory xenoestrogens found in plastics, 174, 183, 244
Physica Energetics, 194, 202, 207, 209-210, 213, 233, 238, 285
physical healing, 335-336
phytates, 178
phytochemicals, antioxidant and anti-inflammatory compounds found in many green leafy vegetables, 172, 176, 209, 229, 299
phytonutrients, 299
Pilates, 387
pineal gland, 300
pineapples, 186
pistachios, 178
plant-based foods, 57, 166, 198, 264
plant-based oils, 179

plaque, 230
plasma, 124, 127, 241, 257, 286
Plasmodium, parasite linked to lymphoma, 280
plastic bottles, 179, 183
platelet aggregation, 291
platelet-rich plasma, 129
Platynosomum, 280
pleomorphic organism. *See* cancer microbe
pleural fluid, 149, 156
plum seeds, 116
poliovirus 1 and 2, 287
Pollack, Gerald, 183
pollen, 145
pollutants, 61, 174, 184, 198, 225, 227, 242
pollution, 246, 250
polycyclic aromatic hydrocarbons, 62
polyester, 243
Poly-MVA nutritional supplement, 130-131, 135
polypeptides, cancer-fighting compound in mistletoe, 119
polyphenols, anti-cancer solids found in green tea leaves, 182, 211
polysaccharide-K (PSK), 153
polysaccharide-P (PSP), 153
polyunsaturated oils and fats, 171, 179
pomegranates, 285
pores, 386
pork, 182
positive affirmations, 373
post-menopause, 307
postural movements, 260
potassium, 186, 210
potatoes, 172, 174
Pot, Gerda, 298, 412-413
Pratten, J., 412
prayer, 22-23, 29, 36, 49, 317, 320, 322 29, 102, 155, 317-318, 334, 337, 339-340, 342-343, 364-365, 373-374, 381, 383
    exercise, meditation, and, 381
    improved patient outcomes, 102
    prayer of faith, 334
    prayer life, 383
    praying for others, 337, 388
    relationship with God and, 342
    therapies are potentiated and made supernatural, 102
praziquantel 281, 294. *See also* anti-parasitic medications
predators of cancer, 147
pregnancy, 83, 348-349
preventative lifestyle, 51
prevention, 51, 143, 177, 204, 208, 248, 261
Prinster, Tari, 261
probiotics, 146, 202, 216, 275, 285
processed foods, 171, 189-190, 198, 393
progesterone, 64, 214
prognosis, 26, 28, 33, 46, 59, 81-82, 161-164, 189, 360
programmed cancer cell death. *See* apoptosis
proline, 182
pro-oxidant, 113-114
prophecy, spiritual practice of, 22-23, 334
propolis. *See* bee propolis

propylene glycol, cancer-linked chemical in some personal care products, 244
prostate, 21, 33-34, 64, 78, 84, 113, 117, 124, 129, 144, 146, 159, 174-175, 188, 208, 212, 306, 366, 371
    prostate cancer 21, 33-34, 64, 78, 84, 124, 188, 366, 371
protein
    animal protein, 141, 172-174, 179-180, 198, 386, 391, 393
    plant-based protein, 172, 189, 198, 202, 393
    plant protein, 173, 193, 203
protein capsids, 289
protein powder, 189, 202, 216, 386, 391
    plant-based protein powders, 189, 202
protozoa, 281, 288, 294
Proverbs, book of, 68, 73, 202, 216, 302, 386, 391
Prozac, 72
PSA (prostate-specific antigen), 34, 77-78, 92, 366
Pseudomonas aeruginosa, 286, 288-289
psoriasis, 292
psyche, 359-361, 377-378
psychoneuroimmunology, 154
pulmonary edema, 29
pulsed LED light technology, 109
pumpkin, 174
putrefaction, 201
pyruvate, broken down glucose involved in formation of ATP, 205
qi, 35
Qigong, 260-261, 266, 387-388
quality of life, 26, 28, 45, 85, 87, 105, 113, 118-120, 152-153, 261, 351, 367
quantum biofeedback, 375, 377
quercetin, suppresses ovarian tumor incidence and growth, 182
quinoa, 49, 179
radiation, 15, 27, 33, 54, 62, 75-76, 78, 81, 83-87, 95, 97-98, 102, 140, 194, 199-200, 203, 221, 225, 227, 248-249, 253, 261, 314, 350, 382
    and surgery, 27
    chemotherapy and radiation, 33, 54, 84-87, 95, 97, 140, 200, 227, 253, 350, 382
    chemotherapy and radiation affect your gut health, 200
    do natural therapies concurrently with chemotherapy and, 87
    effects of, 76
    exposure, 84
    ionizing radiation, 15, 81
    radiation-related toxins, 74
    toxins, 76
    taking supplements during chemo or, 200
rainforest remedies, 285
Rapha Clinic, 23
raspberries, 174, 177, 186
raw vegetables. *See* vegetables
Real Time Labs, 243
reactive oxygen species, cancer-killing oxygen molecules released in light and sound cancer treatment processes 106, 126. *See also* SP-Activate
Recall Healing, 49, 321, 360-361, 370, 373, 390
receptors, 128, 148-149, 157, 174-176
recovery 17, 24, 27-29, 32, 37, 40-42, 50, 60, 64, 66, 82, 97, 114, 118, 159, 166, 189, 193, 199-200, 206, 208,

recovery (*continued*)
    210, 214, 218, 227, 248, 252, 259, 261, 278, 290, 297, 312, 314, 319, 325, 357, 365, 373, 381, 385, 395
    cancer recovery, 114, 200, 206, 325
    full recovery, 37, 42, 60
    improves recovery, 199
    recovery process, 42, 259, 365
    recovery program, 118
recovery process. *See* recovery
rectal cancer, 117, 127, 257, 288, 366, 373, 390
recurrence, 115, 163, 204, 259, 266
red blood cells, 124, 129, 251, 254-255
red meat, 141, 179, 181
regeneration, 123, 208, 263, 300, 329
regimen, 49, 166, 213, 258, 261, 284, 313, 367
ReHydrate, 210
relapse, 259
relapse rate, 259
relationships, 40, 45, 60, 118, 280, 310-316, 353
    healthy, 312, 314
    life-giving, 316
    loving, 310, 315
    new, 312
    that stress the immune system, 310
    toxic, 60, 118, 310
    unhealthy, 40, 313-315
    with God, 32, 42, 59-60, 67, 155, 212, 325-327, 329, 332, 335, 337, 340, 342-343, 346-347, 357, 373, 381, 383, 385
relax (relaxation), 131, 154, 192, 212, 217, 230, 249, 260, 266, 363, 386
relaxant, 212
remission, 37, 42, 47, 78, 114, 161, 163, 221, 269
Renaud, Gilbert, 360, 370, 372-373
renewing your mind, 332
repentance, 338, 341, 362
replenishment, electrolyte and nutrient, 130, 201, 210, 238
replicate, 147, 205
replicating, 272
replication, 203, 207, 253, 266
reprogramming, 362
resins, 62
resistance, 54, 195, 253, 262
respiration, 205, 252-253, 255
respiratory system, 73, 277, 283
restoration, 42, 318, 332, 344, 395
retirement, 309
Revelation, book of, 57, 328, 331, 346
rheumatoid arthritis, 292
rhodium, element in Poly-MVA, 131
ribcage, 195
riboflavin (Vitamin B2), 195. *See also* photosensitizers
rice-based protein supplement, 193
ricinoleic acid, medicinal compound in castor oil, 236
Rife machine, 65
Rife, Royal Raymond, 65
Romans, book of, 330, 332
ROS. *See* reactive oxygen species
rosemary, 174
roundworms, 281
rowing machine, 322
running, 200, 219, 345, 369
Russell bodies, 286. *See also* cancer microbe

INDEX

Russell, William, 286
ruthenium, 131
Sabbah, Claude, 370
sadness, 360
safflower, 179
salivary glands, 145
Salmonella typhii, 65, 278
salmon, wild-caught and cold-water preferred, 180, 393
salt, 169, 223, 230, 386, 392-393
salvation, 331
sarcoma, 65, 113, 121, 124, 277-278
sardines, low toxic load, 180-181
Satan, 338
saturated fat, 180
Savior, 329, 331, 343
scallions, 175
Schandl, Emil, 83
schistosomiasis, common cancer-associated parasite, 280
screening tools, 80-81, 110
Scripture(s), 36, 68, 333, 335, 343, 347, 363, 385, 390
sculpting, therapeutic benefits of, 305, 315
seafood, fish with scales preferred, 180
sealers, 242
secondary cancer causes, 252, 368
secretions, 145
sedentary lifestyle, 74, 233, 258-259, 314
selenium, 152, 204
self-acceptance, 364
self-devaluation, 366
self-love, 309, 312, 352, 364
self-worth, 59
senses, 169, 302, 341
sensitizer, 108
separation, 34-35, 74, 80, 166, 174, 180, 184, 203, 212, 214, 239, 311, 328, 331, 339-340, 385, 390
seroma, 379
serotonin, 255
Settineri, Robert, 398
Seventh Generation, 245
sexuality, 214, 285, 371-372
Seyfried, Thomas, 126, 257
shakes, healthful types, 49
shame, 42, 336
shampoo, dangers of chemical-based types, 244
shellfish, not recommended, 181
shock of the diagnosis, 360
Shoemaker, Ritchie, 61, 243
Siberian ginseng. *See* eleuthero
siblings, 45, 377
SIBO, small bowel bacterial overgrowth in stomach and small intestines, 201
sickness, 27-28, 61, 328-329, 333-334, 339, 341, 347
side effects, 21, 86, 95, 108, 117, 128-129, 138, 145, 150, 203, 210, 261, 291, 350
silent metastatic disease. *See* CTCs
Silverstone, Matthew, 303
Simian virus, 40, infectious agent linked to mesothelioma, brain cancers, bone cancers, lymphomas, 65, 278
Simoncini, Tullio, 66, 282
sinuses, 109, 111, 125, 138, 239, 284
sitting exercises, 259, 303, 391
skeletal system, 125
skin, 65, 108, 111, 127, 138, 182, 188, 203, 228, 230, 236, 245, 248, 257, 272, 277-278, 285, 292, 306, 330, 386
    skin cancer, 65, 278, 306
    skin conditions, 236
    skin tumors, 182
sleep
    adequate rest, 195
    aids, 212, 217
    deprivation, 209
    quality, 208
    restful, 263
    sleep apnea, 264, 267, 388
    sleeping on your side, 265
    sleep rhythm, 300
    with exercise, 297
slow cooker, 194
small intestine, 202
smoothie, 187, 193, 322, 391, 393
social intelligence (of cancer), 54
sodium, 66, 116, 210, 244, 282
sodium ascorbate. *See* Vitamin C
sodium bicarbonate, for fighting fungal infections, 66, 282
sodium hydroxide, toxic chemical found in household cleaning products, 244
SOD (superoxide dismutase), enzyme involved in the body's antioxidant defense system, 126, 256
soft drinks, 171
Solray-D Liposomal Spray, a Vitamin D supplement included in the Sunivera protocol, 146, 208
solvents, 179
Sonodynamic Therapy, non-toxic cancer therapy using sound, 49, 106-108, 113, 144, 220, 322, 392
Sono-Photo Dynamic Therapy (SPDT), non-toxic light and sound cancer therapy, 99, 105-109, 111, 113, 124, 134-135, 150, 155-156, 162, 282, 321, 376, 390
sorrow, 362
soul wounds, 58-59, 69, 338
soy, 49, 181, 188, 197
soybean oil, 179
soybeans, 180
SP-Activate, non-toxic sensitizing substance used in light and sound cancer therapies, 106, 108, 132. *See also* Sono-Photo Dynamic Therapy, Photodynamic Therapy, Photodynamic Therapy Plus
spark of joy, 32, 308
SPDT. *See* Sono-Photo Dynamic Therapy
SpectraCell, nutritional testing laboratory, 215
SpectraLyte, broad spectrum, alkalizing trace mineral formulation that replenishes electrolytes, 210, 238
spectroscopy. *See* Photodynamic Infrared Spectroscopy
spices, 174, 187, 196
spinach, 174, 186, 391, 393
spirit, human, 25, 27-32, 35-38, 40-43, 53, 58, 67, 104, 154-155, 169, 258, 325, 327-332, 334, 336, 338-339, 342-343, 346-347, 363-364, 381
Spirit. *See* Holy Spirit
Spirit of God. *See* Holy Spirit
spiritual adoption, 330
spiritual issues
    brokenness, 57-58
    healing, 103, 339-340, 373, 381

spiritual issues (*continued*)
    health, 30, 212
    spiritual therapy, 355-356, 373-374
spiritual realm, 338
spirochetes, 279
spirometer, 263, 267
spirulina, natural substances that help "mop up" the radiation toxins, 76, 264
spleen, 45, 113, 205, 213, 232
splenectomy, 47
sports, 394
sprays, 294
squash, 174
stage IV cancer, 24, 218
stamina, 260
staphylococci, 286
steamed vegetables. *See* vegetables
stemona, botanical remedy for parasites/worms, 281, 294
sternum, 124
Stevia, natural sweetener, 174, 391, 393
stimulants, 185, 236
stomach health
    acids and enzymes, 193, 201-202
    bacterial overgrowth, 201
    breakdown of food, 202
    digestive system cancers, 182
    stomach cancer, 285
stools (bowel movements), 116, 207, 231, 235
strains of bacteria, 288
Strasheim, Connie, 18, 279
streptococci, 286
Streptococcus bovis, 65, 278
stress, 13-15, 32, 40, 60, 118, 126-127, 153-154, 167, 190, 194, 204, 208, 240, 248, 252, 260-261, 264, 291, 310, 313-314, 318, 322, 353, 357-358, 382-383, 394
    alleviation of, 154
    and disease, 153, 204
    and the immune system, 310
    emotional, 60
    environmental, 15
    external, 15
    high-level, 154
    inflammatory, 15
    internal, 15
    oxidative, 126-127, 240, 252, 264
    reducing, 260-261
    systemic, 190
stressors, 15, 56, 272, 274, 313-314, 360
stress reduction, 260
stretches, 261, 387
stretching exercises, 261, 356, 387
sugarcane, alternative sweetener, 190
sugar, dangers of processed or refined, 49, 128, 152, 171-172, 177, 179, 189-191, 196, 198, 252, 386, 393
sugar oxidation, 252
suicide, 351
sulforaphane, liver-detoxifying and hormone-regulating compound found in cruciferous vegetables, 175
summer, 162
sunscreen, cancer-causing chemicals in, 306
sunshine, 40, 195, 248, 289, 306-307, 315-316, 320

super foods, 174, 198
surgery and chemotherapy, 48
surgical debridement, 240
survival mechanisms of cancer, 14, 56, 68, 70, 104-105, 138, 266, 276
sweat, 44, 249, 369
    perspiration, 132, 228
    sweating, 230, 244, 375
sweat glands, 244
sweet potatoes, 174
swimming, 387
Swiss chard, 186
sympathetic dominance, 185, 357-358
    fight or flight mode, 358
    sympathetic mode, 40, 358
    sympathetic overdrive, 277
sympathetic nervous system. *See* nervous system
sympathetic overdrive. *See* sympathetic dominance
syphilis, 129
systemic stress response, 190
Tamoxifen, 319
tapeworms, 281, 294
tapioca, 207
tap water, 184
targeted cancer response, 150
targeted cancer strategies, 85, 109, 113, 122, 128, 146-148, 150-151, 156, 201, 276
Taxol, 102
Taxotere, 102
T-cells
    T-cell, 65, 277
    T-helper cells (helper T-cells), 119
telomeres, segments of DNA located at end of chromosomes which protect them from deterioration, 183, 226-227, 255, 264
tempeh, non-GMO fermented soy product with powerful anti-cancer benefits, 188
tension, 310
terminal diagnoses, 34, 114, 144
terrain in the body
    biological, 58
    cancer and, 214
    healing and improvement, 102, 275-276
    healthy terrain, where cancer cannot survive, 69
    problems, 70
    restoration of, 66
    support for, 275
    terrain-altering factors, 58
    treat the cancer as well as the terrain, 56
    with compromised microbiome, 274
testicular cancer, 86, 358
Theileria, parasite that causes DNA mutation, 280
T-helper cells. *See* T-cells
theology, 340
thermography, non-invasive diagnostic test to assess abnormalities, 84, 88, 95, 185, 201
Think Dirty, smart device app for checking product safety, 245
three-part beings, 28
thuja, botanical remedy for viruses, 282, 294
thyroid, 57, 186, 201, 244, 320
    thyroid cancer, 320
    thyroid dysfunction, 244
tin, 239

INDEX

tinctures, 238
tinnitus, 20
tissue health, 37, 78, 85, 123-125, 138, 148, 171, 208, 227, 230, 237, 241, 255-256, 267, 277, 279, 289
    and organs, 78, 124, 227, 237
    breast, 84, 185
    connective, 114, 206, 290
    damage, 125, 290
    detoxification, 122
    healing and repair, 14, 114, 132
    oxygenation, 123, 131
    mucosal, 272
    soft, 208
tobacco, 15, 169
tofu, non-GMO fermented soy product with powerful anti-cancer benefits, 188
tolerance levels, 116, 120, 168, 263
tomatoes, 181
tonsils, 232, 239
toothpaste, dangers of chemical-based types, 244
topical cancer treatments, 109, 254
toxin binders, 75, 249, 386
toxins, 248-249, 266
    cancer-causing, 61, 98, 170, 175, 244-245, 256-257, 276, 383, 386
    chemical, 61, 132, 242, 244
    dental, 239, 250
    electromagnetic, 60
    environmental, 37, 39, 49, 57-58, 60, 63-64, 69-70, 118, 142, 172, 174, 226, 234, 252, 295, 382, 394
    indoor, 242
    mold, 61, 243, 283-284
    radiation, 76
    removal of, 108, 228-229, 236, 239-240, 248, 250, 254, 291
Toxoplasma gondii, 66, 278
training, 236
tranquilizer, 394. *See also* bergamot
trauma, 57, 59-60, 275, 305, 310, 339, 358, 360, 364-365, 368-369, 373-374, 378, 390
treadmill, 263, 322
treatment resistance, 253
tree hugging, 302-304
Trichothecene. *See* mycotoxins
Trichuris helminths, 280
triclosan, toxic chemical found in household cleaning products, 244
tripartite, 28
tumor, 13-14, 28, 33, 35, 37, 42, 44-51, 54-57, 68, 74-81, 83, 85-87, 95, 99, 106, 108-111, 113, 115, 117-121, 123-125, 127, 129, 135, 143-144, 147-149, 156, 160-162, 168, 182, 187, 206-207, 209, 211-212, 220-221, 233, 240, 245, 253, 257, 259, 261, 266, 268, 280, 282, 286, 318, 322, 352-354, 366, 376, 379, 381
    blood flow, 123-124
    cells, 35, 37, 56, 79-80, 87, 108, 110, 117, 148, 354
    external, 127, 257
    formation, 56, 187
    growth, 113, 120, 168, 182, 211, 259, 261
    metastatic, 78
    solid, 75-76, 95, 108, 113
tumor blood vessel formation. *See* angiogenesis
tumor blood vessels, 54, 83, 111, 120, 206-207, 253

tumor growth and metastasis, 168
tumor markers, 44, 49, 77, 83, 95, 149
tumor proteins. *See* antigens
turkey tail, immune-boosting mushroom, 153, 204
turmeric, powerful anti-cancer spice, 187, 209, 391-392
ultrasound, 34, 44, 76, 84, 95, 109, 111, 349, 366, 375-377
ultraviolet light, 290-291, 306
ultraviolet radiation, 62
unclean, 181-182
undigested, 201
unforgiveness, 313, 337, 341
unhealthy beliefs, 58, 275
unhealthy lifestyle, 37, 67, 74, 142, 252, 272
unhealthy nutrition, 74
unnatural foods, 166, 190
uptake, 39, 76, 106, 111, 216, 237, 255, 257, 260, 264, 266
uranium, 74, 238
urine mycotoxin test, 243. *Also see* mycotoxins
urological malignancies, 160, 163
US Wellness Meats, pasture-raised poultry, 181
uterine cancers, 214
uterus, 376
vaccines, 149-151, 352
vaginal insufflation, 257
vaginal ozone therapy, 390
vascular endothelial growth factor (VEGF), process from which tumors create blood vessels, 187
vascular system, 111, 113, 123, 187, 240
vegetables, 49, 166, 172, 174-176, 179, 186, 188-189, 195-196, 198, 200, 222, 229, 284, 299, 304, 381, 385-386, 393
    allium, 175
    cruciferous, 174-175, 188
    fermented, 284
    green leafy, 176, 186
    organic, 222, 229
    raw, 172
    steamed, 49, 393
vegetable oil, 179
vegetarian, 41, 141, 322
vessels, 54, 83, 99, 106, 109-111, 120, 123, 187, 206-207, 232-233, 253, 255
vibe, 233, 323
vibrancy, 28, 166-167
vibrating platform, 233, 249-250, 386, 392, 394
viral therapies, 147-148
virotherapy, 146-148, 155, 156-158
virus, 65-66, 132, 138, 140-141, 143, 146-149, 154, 156-157, 184, 254, 271-272, 277-279, 281-284, 287-288, 291, 293-295
visions, God-directed, 335
visualization, 154, 364-365, 367, 373
vital force, 35, 260
Vita LF Powder, nutritional supplement, 146, 204, 391
vitality, 196, 198, 382
Vitamin A, 177
Vitamin B2, 195
Vitamin B-17, natural cytotoxic compound found in the seeds of certain foods, 105, 116, 135, 352

429

Vitamin C, 21, 49, 98-99, 105, 113-116, 135, 155, 177, 182, 195, 206-207, 216-217, 219, 238, 282, 287, 291, 293, 321, 352, 390
- anti-cancer effects, 115
- ascorbic acid, 182
- benefits of, 115-116, 206, 291
- buffered forms, 116
- in large amounts, 98
- intravenous, 49, 99, 105, 114, 206, 282, 321
- IV Vitamin C, 207, 219, 352, 390
- liposomal, 206-207, 216
- non-corn, non-GMO sources, 116
- optimal dose, 207
- oral, 114-116
- pro-oxidant, 114
- sodium ascorbate, 116
- supports immune function, 135

Vitamin D, 49, 143-144, 181, 195, 207-208, 217, 255, 266, 291, 306-307, 394
- best source comes from sun, 306
- deficiencies, 306
- levels, 144, 208
- liposomal Vitamin D, 394
- metabolism, 255
- production, 255, 266
- supplementation, 144, 208
- toxicity, 208

Vitamin D3-K2 supplements, 208
Vitamin K2, 208
vitamins, 19, 21, 49, 98-99, 105, 113-116, 131, 135, 143-144, 155, 168, 172, 177-178, 181-182, 195, 205-208, 216-217, 219, 238, 255, 266, 282, 287, 291, 293, 306-307, 321, 352, 390, 394
Vitamix, 299
vomiting, 200
walnuts, 178, 281, 294
Warburg, Otto, 252
warts, 292
wastes, 54, 108, 183, 193, 230, 237, 245, 252
water, 14, 36, 49, 60, 62, 74, 76, 101, 108, 127, 134, 141, 169, 171, 181, 183-184, 193, 210, 225, 228, 230-232, 235-236, 243, 245, 249, 251, 272, 274, 302-303, 307, 333, 357, 381, 385-387, 390-393

water (continued)
- acidity in, 183
- balances your pH, 183
- before and after a sauna treatment, 230
- cell health, 183
- chlorinated and fluoridated, 171
- filtered, 184, 228
- glass-bottled, 184
- hydrogen, 183-184, 390
- in large quantities, 184
- non-chemically treated, 387
- ozonated, 127
- purified, 76
- tap water and pollutants, 184
- warm, 193, 386

water filter, 184
wavelengths, light, 106, 109-111
wavelength range, 80, 112
weakness, 156, 248-249, 266, 294, 315, 373
weight, 19, 72, 106, 170, 184, 210, 231, 265, 387
weight lifting, 387
Welchol, mycotoxin medication. *See* mycotoxins
wellness, 32, 68, 110, 181, 316, 375, 382-383, 388, 390
Western medicine, 47-48
wheatgrass, 186
whey protein powder, not recommended, 188, 202
Whipple procedure, 45
white blood cells, 129, 139, 232, 256
wholeness, 40, 308, 316, 333
windpipe, 277
wormseed, botanical remedy for parasites, 281, 294
wormwood, botanical remedy for parasites, 281, 294
worship, spiritual practice of, 333, 385
Wright, Jonathan, 191, 215
X-rays, 22, 75, 159-160, 163
yeasts, 284, 294
yogurt, 190
Zearalenone. *See* mycotoxins
zeolite, heavy metal and mycotoxin binder, 238, 284, 294, 386
zinc, immune-boosting mineral, 152-153, 178, 204

Also by Dr. Tony
Coming Soon (Q1 2022)

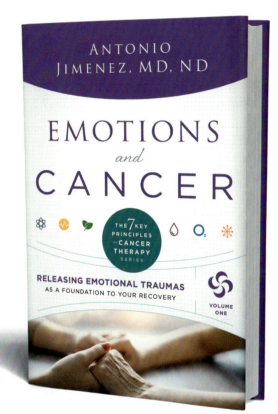

EMOTIONS AND CANCER:
RELEASING EMOTIONAL TRAUMAS AS A FOUNDATION TO YOUR RECOVERY

Discover why cancer is considered a disease of the body, mind and spirit from one of the outstanding medical icons of our generation. Get inspired by riveting stories of healing that will fill your heart with hope!

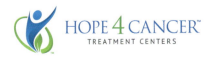 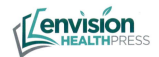

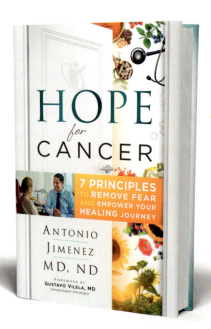
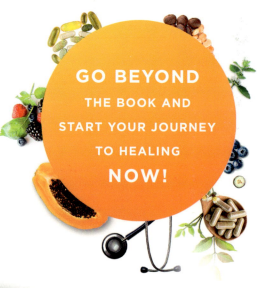

EMPOWER
YOUR HEALING TODAY!

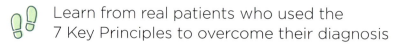
Learn from real patients who used the 7 Key Principles to overcome their diagnosis

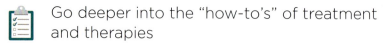
Go deeper into the "how-to's" of treatment and therapies

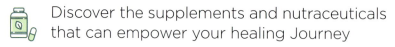
Discover the supplements and nutraceuticals that can empower your healing Journey

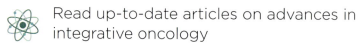
Read up-to-date articles on advances in integrative oncology

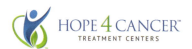

hopeforcancerbook.com